i

Error has indeed long darkened the horizon of medical science; and albeit there have been lightnings like coruscations of genius from time to time, still they have passed away, and left the atmosphere as dark as before.

— **George Macilwain**

To those who practice medicine with the sole
aspiration of easing the burden of the sufferer...
especially those who do so without acclaim.

Waters of

Bimini

By

J. Michael Jones

Table of Contents

CHAPTER ONE: ALIGNMENT

Curtis ran his fingernail across the top of the tung-oiled fir table, letting it glide to the edge, where the top dropped over the side. He was trying to feel a tiny snap from his nail catching an edge between layers of veneer. The table didn't look like it was veneered except for its size. It was massive, a full four inches thick, if not more. It was five feet wide and over fifteen feet long. It filled the center of the conference room with an awe-inspiring presence. To make such a table from what appeared to be a single piece of wood must be an illusion… so he thought.

He ran his nail over the wood again—this time with eyes closed to enhance his tactile sensitivity—as if the hard nail was the needle on an old vinyl record player and the table was the spinning LP. He felt the ridges of each salmon-colored grain, but, as he came back up over the edge to the top, he felt no juncture between thin planes of layered wood.

It can't be solid, he thought to himself, now with some uncertainty. He had been in that room many times and admired the beauty of the table but never imagined it as anything but a thick, pressboard piece encased within a thin laminate. However, he couldn't remember ever being in the room alone and never having the time to study the table or the room… until now.

These days the only place he had the privacy to think about anything except his work was sitting in the bathroom stall defecating. If he could, he would stretch out those minutes. It was unbearable to have to open the stall door and venture out into the world once more. That world was no longer his friend. Everyone wanted a piece of him, and it didn't matter to them if this constant picking would ultimately disassemble each cell of his body. They all said they "loved him"; however, he was becoming intimately acquainted with the proverbial concept of "being loved to death." Even the personal place of the company bathroom stall—his one shelter of respite—had occasionally been interrupted with intrusive voices. The stainless-steel walls left him feeling vulnerable, being so short that they exposed his ankles and pants piled around his Wallabees. He would see the toes of someone's shoes just outside the door. Then came the predictable question. "Dr. Eisner? Dr. Eisner? Sorry to bother you, but can I talk to you about my neighbor's niece? She recently had a spinal cord injury."

But now he was in physical solitude and had been for—what seemed like an endless—ninety minutes. He didn't want it to end... ever. His cellphone was off. He wasn't carrying a pager since he was not involved with clinical medicine at the time. He was alone. He closed his eyes again and fantasied that he was laying on a beach somewhere. Some deserted island where he could dwell in wonderful isolation, feeling nothing except the warmth of the equatorial sun, hearing nothing but the surf upon the sand, and thinking only about the peace of the present.

In the large room was just himself and a black, plastic, triangle speaker in the middle of the big table. On the other end of the speaker, three floors above him, was his boss, Thomas Howell. On the wall was a five-foot-by-three-foot flat-screen. It was dark but could flicker on in a second if Thomas only pushed a button to speak to him.

Curtis was about six foot even, with slightly thinning sandy-blond hair. His facial features, including his prominent nose and olive skin, made some suspect he had a Hebrew or Arab heritage, but his family—as far as he knew—was from Scotland and Sweden. The combination of features, oddly, resulted in a strikingly handsome appearance that seemed to enhance as he aged.

The doctor had been skinny his entire life, but now, sitting at a desk for eighteen hours per day and eating bites of junk food between meetings, he had developed a belly. On such a habitually thin frame, the abdominal protuberance appeared parturient. His morphing body disgusted him; nonetheless, he felt helpless to change the circumstance.

His big bright smile and green eyes was what had seduced his mother in the delivery room. They had always brought her great joy. But the whites of those eyes, now, had a network of red lines that gave them the appearance of the crimson fissures on Jupiter's ice-ball moon, Europa. The mega-doses of caffeine were giving him no gain over the want for sleep. He drank stronger and stronger cups of coffee—until one of the college students in his lab introduced him to Red Bull. It was hardly an existence anymore. It is so strange, he thought, how carefully you plan the steps of your life, but how easily you are displaced from the helm by strangers. Soon, you become just a passenger on a roller coaster, passively tossed about, while the world casts you into what they want. They all want something.

Curtis paused his thoughts and opened his eyes to look under the immense piece of furniture in front of him. He was eyeing it for some sign of fabrication, but he found none. He pushed back his chair and bent over, putting his head completely under the table. On the underside was nothing but solid wood. The bottom grains, knotholes, and quirks… matched, precisely, those on top. Either it was a very clever disguise or, indeed, the table was one monolithic piece of wood. Perhaps from one massive old-growth fir tree from the nearby North Cascades. However, his suspicion was not put completely to rest.

His mother was the first one to try and shape him. He was a shy boy. While he was still in preschool, before he had the chance to decide, his mother began to proclaim, "He wants to be a doctor. Oh, I hope so much he comes back to Jonesborough to be our doctor." Then she would smile and wink at him. He never remembered telling her he wanted to be a doctor. Maybe, when he was five, his mother had asked him, rhetorically, "You would love being a doctor wouldn't you?" To which, he gave the projected nod.

Curtis was his mom's "buddy," especially after his father suddenly left them when he was only twelve. His father seemed to have disappeared suddenly off the face of the earth, leaving Curtis with an empty room in his soul. He closed that door with the intent of never opening it again. Per his mother's explanation, his father had found, "greater satisfaction in a younger woman as many men do when they reach middle age." Curtis became the only man in his mother's new life—from that point forward. After closing the door to the room where his father's memories dwelt, he seemed to have locked out his own voice. He became a boy of few words. But time continued to march onward.

He awakened one day in a dorm bunk at the University of Tennessee studying premed. It was a track for his life that he never questioned, as if preordained by something bigger than himself. However, the studies were easy for him, and he seemed to enjoy them… but again, it could have been his mother's enjoyment being channeled into his own emotions. Maybe they were vagrant desires, which she had planted somewhere deep in his reptilian brain.

The video screen suddenly flickered on. There was Thomas Howell's high-definition face crowned by thick, coal-black hair and his trademark L-shaped hockey scar on his left chin. "Hey, Curtis, just an update. Our investor, Mr. Pendleton, is still on his boat. The fog has lifted, but his pilot can't get clearance from Boeing Field to fly into town on his copter. He's trying to decide if he'll wait or take his Zodiac boat to the harbor and then have our people pick him up. I'll let you know as soon as he decides. Uh…" Thomas looked around the empty room through the camera above the screen. "Uh… it may be another forty-five minutes in case you need to get back to the lab."

"I'll wait here."

"Are you sure?"

"Absolutely!" came Curtis's confident reply.

"Can I have them bring you some coffee or snacks while you're waiting?"

"I'm fine."

"Okay." Then the monitor flickered back to darkness.

When Curtis entered the University of Michigan's medical school, he continued to excel... to a point. The limitation that governed the spin of his life was his social anxiety. He had never put it into those terms before, but, as he studied medicine, including psychiatric diseases, there was no question that social anxiety put a haunting damper over his entire life. Simply put, people scared him intensely, and he felt judged by them... almost to a state of paranoia. He had the insight to know that this was why he had been such a "good boy", because of his constant diligence to avoid giving anyone— including his mother—a reason to be critical of him. His father's deliberate rejection made this fear of criticism much worse. Would others walk out of his life, too, if they didn't like him?

The model of medical schools had started to change by the time he got to Ann Arbor. A greater emphasis was being placed on getting exposure to real patients much earlier in the student's experience. They were expected to take what they were learning over to the hospital during their third week of class, of their first year.

Previously they would have darkened the doors of a hospital until their third year of medical school.

Curtis discovered a real quandary in his life, patients made him feel very uneasy. He didn't like talking to people anyhow, but talking to them when they were in crisis and as an authority figure frightened him even more. Even though his knowledge of medicine was primitive, when he donned a waist-length lab coat, patients and their families looked to him as a medical professional. It was made especially worse by the fact that he—and all the medical students— had to pretend that they knew far more than they did. The sum of all of this was that he grew to loathe his clinical time.

Beyond that very silent and personal distress, he also noticed that other med students didn't carry his handicap. They seemed to enjoy their clinicals as if they were actors, pretending to be doctors in a hospital-centered soap opera. One of his friends chuckled and remarked how much easier it was to get dates if he was wearing his stethoscope, even if he didn't have a clue as to how to use it. By his last year of medical school, Curtis started to doubt his ability to be a doctor, especially a very public figure like a small-town family doctor. Then there was a pivotal experience that changed the entire direction of his life.

One Saturday afternoon he was working his emergency medicine rotation at the St. Joseph Medical Center. About five o'clock, just as his shift was starting, an ambulance backed into the ED (Emergency Department) bay. The medics had called ahead and spoken to the ED coordinator. The senior emergency medicine resident, Dr. Gary

Bowen, got the medics back on the radio so he could try to assess the seriousness of the injury. They had a young girl in the back of the truck who had a rollover on her four-wheeler and had injured her neck. She was taped down on a backboard with a hard collar on to keep her cervical spine properly aligned. She was squeezing the EMT's hand when they left her farm, but she seemed to be deteriorating just as they were arriving at the hospital. Dr. Bowen had already called the CT scan room, across from their trauma bay. He gave them a heads-up to be prepared for a stat, which was another word for urgent, neck view. But it was hard to determine the seriousness of the injuries because she was moving her extremities at the farm but now wouldn't even squeeze the medic's hand.

One thought, that seemed to be going through Dr. Bowen's mind, was that this progression of symptoms could be a severed spinal cord, where the bone fragments were gradually pushing through the soft-tissue in route, despite the precautions. That would be unusual because the medics were careful. It could also be a young girl with a simple neck strain who was starting to embellish her symptoms for the dramatic effect. The latter situation would certainly not be the first time he had seen such behavior in a teenager. There was simply no way to tell through a two-way radio.

The role of the medical student was to observe, to learn, to hold things, try new procedures, and to communicate with the families… but not much else. Curtis was nervous even though he knew he would not be making the crucial medical decisions.

8

The two big red doors of the ambulance burst open and the EMTs, who were moving rapidly, but with no sign of panic, gently jerked the gurney until the wheels fell and locked in place. "Where're we going, doc? I think this one is for real." They looked directly at Curtis (not realizing he was just a medical student) and he wasn't sure. He was in a panic until Dr. Bowen's calm voice came from behind him… "Let me look at her here."

Dr. Bowen was a black man, short, about five foot six, but very confident, as most natural-born leaders are. Nothing ruffled his feathers. He walked up to the girl. This was the first time Curtis caught the patient's face… which was sealed in terror. Despite her disposition, the mud on her navy hoodie, and the tape across her face, Curtis could tell that she was a beautiful girl. Her hair of a confluence of hues of blond and amber suggested it was natural, as were her blue eyes. They were squinting eyes that now held her fear tightly, like a clutched purse.

"Can you squeeze my hands, honey?" asked Dr. Bowen.

There was no movement in either. He quickly did a general survey of her, to look for any life-threatening problems or other injuries. From the bottom of her muddy jeans up to the ruffled hair, he examined her. He asked her questions about who and where she was. He checked her pupil response and looked closely for bruising around her head or scalp. He stuck his stethoscope in his ears and listened to her heart and lungs. He worked his way down to her feet for any gross trauma. He felt his way back up her body, looking for any soft-tissue trauma. He stopped to feel her belly, and it was soft as it should be. He listened to her bowel sounds, and they were fine. The complete preliminary exam was accomplished in less than two minutes in the ambulance bay. Then he tapped—forcefully—with the end of his index finger over her right patellar tendon. Her leg jumped abruptly. That's all he needed to know. He looked up at the medics, "We're going straight into our secondary trauma room."

As they walked into the hall, Curtis looked at Dr. Bowen and said, "That's a good sign isn't it... she has good reflexes?"

Dr. Bowen gave him a strange look. "What *are* they teaching in medical school these days? Brisk reflexes could mean that the spinal cord's communication to the brain has been compromised. Eisner, didn't they teach you that the reflexes arise in the spinal cord and are suppressed by the brain? Brisk reflexes may mean less suppression." Curtis felt stupid in response, although that was not Dr. Bowen's intention.

The major trauma bay (T-1), just across from the CT room, had just witnessed the consequences of a drunk-driver head-on collision. One fatality. It wasn't the drunk. The ED team fought hard to save the young mother but with great disappointment. Curtis felt fortunate that he had missed the terrible incident because blood still made him queasy. The cleaning team had just started the process of mopping up the puddles and getting things ready for the next case, when the call came in about the girl with the neck injury.

Dr. Bowen looked over at Curtis, "Hey, Eisner, I want you to stay with..." then he looked down at the wristband the ED clerk was attaching to the young woman's right wrist. He turned his head to a perpendicular position to read the words, "Uh… Erika, and let me know immediately if she's having any trouble breathing."

Dr. Bowen stepped to the side and spoke into a microphone on his lapel to the ED coordinating desk. Again, calmly he said, "Hey, Ann, we need the trauma team called with a cervical injury and… who's on call for neurosurgery?"

While waiting for a response, he continued walking behind the gurney across the hall into the smaller trauma room (T-2). A young nurse, with chopped blond hair and a tattoo of a spider crawling up the side of her neck, walked up and followed them into the room. Without any instructions, she put a pulse ox (to measure the oxygen concentration of the patient's blood) on Erika's finger. She placed an oxygen tube around her face and under her nose, carefully as not to disturb her head at all. It looked like she had done this delicate maneuver to the point of becoming routine. Then she pulled over an IV tray with the tubing and needles already available. Dr. Bowen looked at her, nodded, and smiled, "Great. D5W for now."

About that time, a woman's voice came back across the microphone/speaker. "That would be… Dr. Gibbs for neurosurgery and I've called her. She's up on the floor and will be down in a minute."

Despite Curtis's responsibilities being limited, he was feeling a physical shaking of his insides. His only assignment was to watch her breathing, but he was more aware of his own shortness of breath than that of anyone else.

The monitor in the conference wall flickered on again, jarring Curtis's mind out of its daydream. He looked at the clock on the wall, and almost thirty minutes had passed since his last interruption. His mind raced back from his Michigan days into the damp Pacific Northwest. This time Thomas was no longer wearing his sports coat. His shirt with bold blue stripes and solid white collar had its sleeves rolled up, showing his well-defined biceps. "Hey, Curt, uh… he's coming by boat. But now he's waiting on some shipping traffic… another forty-five minutes at least. Go back to the lab. I'll call you there."

Indulging in the tranquility of the setting, Curtis quickly answered, "No, I'll wait for him out here. I can work on things on my laptop."

"You're sure you don't need some coffee? Our barista is one of the best?"

"Any more and I may go into an arrhythmia. I've been here all night trying to get the presentation ready for Mr. Pendleton."

"Hey, man, take a nap. I can have a cot in there in two minutes."

"Thanks anyway, but I'm fine." Curtis allowed the silence to waiver in the air until the screen went dark again.

His mind was drawn back through the narrow years to the girl… the Erika that redirected his entire life. He kept one hand on hers and tried to hold it, but she couldn't reciprocate. It felt like limp rubber, but warm rubber. He vaguely remembers other team members coming and going, in and out, of the small trauma room. But many of the details his memory had been set adrift. The trauma team PA came in to look things over. A respiratory therapist dropped by to check on her and then the trauma surgeon. The surgeon had just been in the ED with the drunk-driver victim an hour earlier. He did an emergent burr hole in her skull as the last attempt to save her. Dr. Gibbs, the neurosurgeon, wasn't there, but it was her idea. She felt they had nothing to lose. Regrettably, it failed. The trauma surgeon told them that he was going home and if Dr. Gibbs needed him, he could be paged.

Dr. Gibbs arrived. She did a brief neurological exam, turned to the group, gave them a feeble smile, and dismissed the rest of the trauma team. She then directed them to take Erika immediately to the CT scan. She was going back up to the surgery suite, to get her team together, and to prepare. She would look at the images there. Unless there were immediate complications from her injury, like losing the ability to respire, she wanted a cervical MRI to follow. That way the images would be available to her in the OR. She had created a rapid response MRI protocol, which was very helpful in these situations.

As they rolled her across the brightly lighted hall and into the CT scan room, Curtis kept one hand on hers, watching her chest rise

13

and fall, rhythmically and rapidly. As he looked down at her, the checker-board tiled floor of the hallway passed beneath them. The CT room smelled, oddly, of Pine-Sol. From that day forward, every time he smelled the potent cleanser, it brought back vivid images of that room and that night.

Four of them lifted the backboard, with her on it, onto the CT table. The tech positioned her in the white doughnut by moving the table. There was a soft mechanical grind as the table inched forward. On the side of the doughnut was a large G E, in cursive. The tech asked everyone to clear the room. Curtis asked if he could stay. The tech grabbed a leaded apron and handed it to Curtis and went into the windowed-room next door. Curtis put the apron on like a sports jacket. He was starting to tie the closure strings in front. The tech rushed back out into the room with some irritation written across his face "Take it off!" he said sternly to Curtis.

Curtis slipped off the heavy, bright royal-blue apron. The tech spun it around and put it back on Curtis with the open end in the back. He tied it for him and hastily ran back into the CT control room.

Curtis put his hand back on her hand, which she of course could not feel. He continued watching her chest rise and sink, sink and rise. He took his duty seriously. He was not cognizant that the pulse oximeter communicated directly with the nurse station through a wireless signal. There, a vigilant nurse with a spider tattoo was making sure all was well. His assignment, Curtis later realized, was a token one.

The tech reappeared and told Curtis that Erika's scan was done. They carefully put her back on the gurney and opened the shielded door where other team members were waiting. Two new faces included the anesthesiologist and a neurosurgery PA. They spoke to her to make sure she was doing well, and she was… except for her crescendoing terror.

As instructed by Dr. Gibbs, they rolled her toward the MRI room, about fifty feet down the hall. Dr. Bowen rejoined them to check on the status of the process. Things were going per the plan.

As they were rolling her down the hall, she asked Curtis, "Why are they doing another one?"

Curtis was preparing to answer her, but he knew that he would have to be emotionally detached. He wanted to speak with the air of confidence that Dr. Bowen was such a master of. He increased the pressure in his lungs to keep his vocal cords from shaking, "The CT is quick and better at looking at the bones in your neck. The MRI looks at soft tissue, such as your spinal cord, better."

Tears were pooling in Erika's eyes, as her head was still held in a fixed position by the braces and tape. When her sockets were full, like small tarns, the water eventually spilled over and ran down both sides of her temples into her ears.

They rolled her into the room with the big, tubular machine. The radiology tech said to her, "It will take a couple minutes to set up and calibrate the scanner, but the actual test will be quick."

They gently lifted her, still on the board, and laid her into the MRI tube table. The technician asked Curtis for his help while he, methodically, kept her neck and head immobilized with foam bars and removed the hard-plastic brace. Her head was carefully cradled in a headrest with a coiled-antenna cassette placed over her face and head, from which the resonance signals would be collected. As the table slid into the tube, Curtis allowed her hand to slowly slip out of his. He rested the itinerant hand on her knee. While socially inept, he carried more than his share of empathy. Patients could feel his concern through his nonverbal graciousness.

"Where's my dad?" Erika asked while they were waiting, her voice echoing out of the long cylinder, just as a loud banging inside the machine began.

Curtis remembered a man showing up just as they were leaving the T-2 room for the scans. He seemed panicked in his presence. He was talking to Dr. Bowen right outside the room as Curtis and Erika left to go to the CT room.

"Was he wearing running shorts?" Curtis asked in a loud voice, above the thumping of the magnets.

"I'm sure he was. He was out on a jog."

"He's here. I'm sure he's waiting for you in the ED. We'll be going straight back there when we're done here."

During a pause of silence, she asked, "Doctor… I'm numb. Everything's numb. I can't move my arms." She took in a labored breath, "Am I going to get better?"

Looking inside the tube to the mirror above her face, Curtis spoke to the upside-down image. He tried to pull together a weak smile, to comfort her eyes. He spoke, "We need to wait on the scans to see what happened to your spine. Hopefully it's just a bruise or swelling. If it is, then… uh, then your feeling will start coming back as the swelling goes down. We can use medicines like steroids to help with the swelling." He stood in silence for a minute, until the banging resumed.

After the MRI was done, and the automatic table moved her back out of the tube, the door to the MRI room burst open. Curtis turned, expecting to see the radiology tech, however, it was Dr. Bowen. Curtis asked him, "The scans are done; are we heading back to the ED?"

Dr. Bowen hardly made eye contact with Curtis and, while ignoring his question, looked directly at the girl. "Hey, Erika, hon, how're you doing?"

Tears continued rolling down the sides of her cheeks. "I'm thirsty."

"Well, I'm going ask you to take your mind off drinking for a little while, sweetie. It looks like we'll try to get you into surgery as soon as we can."

"Surgery?" asked Curt. "Have you seen her scans?"

"Yeah, I was looking at it as it was loading, as did Dr. Gibbs."

Erika began to sob, "What's wrong with me. Why am I numb all over? Is my neck broke?"

Dr. Bowen answered, "Erika, it looks like you have a fracture of your fourth neck bone, and it is pressing on your spinal cord. It doesn't look completely cut, you seem to be breathing and speaking okay, but it has cut through enough to weaken your arms and legs."

She was sobbing uncontrollably, "Am I going to be paralyzed!?"

"Erika," said Dr. Bowen, "no one knows at this point. But you'll be in the hands of a damn good neurosurgeon who'll do her best to make you whole. Dr. Ashley Gibbs is one of the best." Then he flashed her a big, confident smile. "She's the one I would to want to operate on my daughter." He patted her on her lifeless hand and turned back down the hall.

Crying uncontrollably, she said more in a screech than a voice, "If… if… if they can't make me whole, please let me die!" She looked directly into Curtis's eyes and said it again, but this time more assuredly, "If they can't fix me… make sure I don't come out of surgery alive! Do you understand?" Then Erika began sobbing so hard that she wouldn't have heard a response even if Curtis knew what to say… and he didn't. However, strange words flowed from his mouth, words he seemed to overhear as if he were a third person, "I promise, you'll get better and walk again. We will save you."

Dr. Bowen, who was down the hall, but still within earshot, quickly turned and gave Curtis a very displeased look before continuing to walk away, shaking his head.

The burden on Curtis to react with follow-up words was suddenly relieved when Ericka's father came running down the hall, passing Dr. Bowen. He came right up beside her face and looked at her, "Oh, Erika. Baby, are you okay?" He pushed her muddy hair out of her eyes. He looked sternly at Curtis, "Can't you clean her up… at least a little? What's wrong with you people!"

"Dad… I'm paralyzed, and they are taking me to surgery," she interrupted.

Both were sobbing, and her father stooped down beside her stretcher, laying his head on her chest as if to feel her beating heart. Then he looked back up. "Why in the hell did your mom let you go out with those boys? They're always so reckless. I'm going to chew their little asses out! That Pearce boy, he's nothing but trouble. I don't know why the hell your mother…"

Erika, seeming to get some control of her own emotions, interrupted again. "Dad, it doesn't matter now! Just stay with me."

Curtis returned his attention to the massive fir table in front of him and its confluent areas of pink and white wood. He laid his face down on the top surface of it and looked down to the other end. Then he rested the corner of his right eye against the top edge for a clear line of sight, as if he were aiming a gun. He was looking for a flaw, somewhere. Just one small bubble in a thin veneer would give it away, proving it was a fake... but there was none. Sitting back up, he noticed something quite peculiar. The table, which he had always assumed to be a rectangle, now seemed to be a bit askew. Two opposite corners appeared to be less than ninety degrees. The other two opposing corners appeared to be slightly greater than ninety degrees.

Curtis jumped up and slid his closed laptop down the table to the end. He positioned the computer in the corner, overlying the edges precisely. The right angle of the laptop corner made it clear the table's corners weren't ninety degrees. He looked up and studied the sides, which did appear to be parallel. However, the table was not a true rectangle. It was indeed a rhomboid. But was it a carpenter's error? Curtis didn't think so. Being a little obsessive-compulsive himself, he couldn't imagine that a craftsman would produce such a beautiful table but neglect such an important detail as right angles.

He stood up and looked around the room and back at the table. Was the room itself a rhomboid? He walked over to the right corner of room where the wall apron of exterior glass met an interior wall. He laid down on the low-pile tan carpet and pushed his laptop up to the corner. A small gap appeared between the corner of the computer and the corner of the room. He stood, then walked down to the left corner of the room and laid down his laptop in that corner. This time the corners touched, but there was play between the sides of the laptop and the sides of the room. The walls of the room, like the edges of the table, also seemed parallel. Yes, so he thought, I was right. The table matches the floor area of the room, both being rhomboids. That's why the table looks like a rectangle. It was an optical illusion.

The speaker buzzed and the screen on the wall flickered on. Curtis felt embarrassed as he was still lying on his belly, on the floor in the corner. He sat up. Thomas Howell's voice blasted across the room, "Dr. Eisner... Dr. Eisner, are you still in there?"

When Curtis rose from the floor into a standing position, Thomas asked, "Uh, Curtis, are you alright?"

"Yeah, I'm fine... just taking a nap."

There was a hesitation and then Thomas continued, "Uh... okay. Hey, Mr. Pendleton is in the building. My staff's showing him around Lab 3, and then he'll be up to my office. I'll bring him down... say in about fifteen minutes."

Curtis, now fully standing in front of the monitor answered, "Okay, I'll see you then." The screen went black.

Curtis walked over to the wall of windows. It was now sprinkling, lightly, from just one puffy cloud directly above them. The remaining sky was a true azure. The drops hit the window, mostly glancing off. Here and there, small, clear ovals formed, which— after a brief hesitation—would coalesce and streak downward. He could still see clear skies all around and even Mount Rainer to the south. The snow-capped Olympics were visible to the west, rising above a blanket of fog in the lowlands. Was the answer to why this room was a bit askew, written in those distant escarpments?

He looked straight down the outside wall of the building from his twentieth-floor perch. He thought his eyes were deceiving him, but they were not. The shape of the building was simply conforming to the shape of the city lot, which itself was a rhomboid. He'd always assumed that Seattle's streets were set up on a perpendicular grid, but maybe not. He looked north and south, east and west. For the first time, he noticed that all lots were a few degrees off, being parallelograms but not rectangles or squares. Why? He asked himself that question again. Curtis was a fool for answers, especially when it came to questions of patterns. He could leave no query left unexplored. Maybe it was this drive that led him to his great success as a research scientist.

As he continued to study the layout of the city, he noticed that even the streets had a superior reference point. The streets and alleys followed natural ridges. It was hard to make out the primeval geography of the land beneath the man-made super structures, but he could see it. The hills were parallel to each other but not to the shore of the Puget Sound. His eyes carefully followed the hills southward toward the big volcano. He recognized, for the first time, that the north-to-south streets followed the lay of the land. However, the east-to-west streets intersected with the harbor at right angles. This is what caused the deviation at the corners. Curtis considered that the orientation of the south-to-north grid was the result of subsequent lava flows starting over 500,000 years ago.

Then they were ground down and polished by revolving glaciers over epochs of time. The glacier silt was then washed away, intentionally, by water cannons around the turn of the last century.

Curtis had a hunch. He opened his laptop and pulled up on Google maps the state of Washington. With his stylus, he drew a line down the apexes of the Pacific Northwest volcanoes, starting with Mount Hood in Oregon and ending on Mount Baker just south of British Columbia. Then he drew a line perpendicular and stretching to the west. Next, he drew a line down the eastern shore of Puget Sound, creating a drawing like a big H. He copied and pasted his lines into his CAD program. He clicked on the sides of the lines and used the program to measure the angle of interception. The angle of where the line perpendicular to the volcanoes met the line of the sound was ninety-eight degrees and eighty-two degrees on the opposite corners. This corresponded, as best as he could gather with his eye, the degrees of the corners of the table. The epiphany fully embraced him.

Curtis closed his laptop, just as the door to the room was opening. He tried to formalize his thoughts before the coming disruption of visitors. So, the shape of the table was determined by the major geographic features of the region, whose shape, in turn, was determined by the tectonic plates of Earth itself. The tectonic plates were shaped—perhaps—and moved per the rotation of the earth, which was controlled by the gravitation of the Sun and previous asteroid impacts. He knew that there was something to that deduction. A philosophical message was hidden there, but he didn't have the time to ponder its depths.

CHAPTER TWO: ANASTOMOSIS

Mr. Mack Pendleton was a big man, six-foot-three and barrel chested. His physique gave license to those close to him to call him, "Big Mack." He wore long white hair, usually in a ponytail, that didn't quite look right because of his frontal balding. His face looked puffy and red, like he had a perpetual sunburn or a touch of rosacea that spared only the circles around his eyes, which his sunglasses doubtlessly covered. His personality was even bigger than his frame, and it was typical for him to suffuse throughout any room he entered.

As Thomas introduced Mack to Curtis, Mack reached out and grabbed the doctor's hand with such force that Curtis felt like his metacarpals had briefly dislocated and then painfully slid back in to proper position. "What a privilege it is to finally meet the world-famous Dr. Eisner!" came Mack's booming voice infected with an Arkansas accent.

Curtis smiled sheepishly and then said in a calmer voice, "It's good to finally meet you, too, Mr. Pendleton."

Thomas motioned, with a stretched-out hand, for them to take a seat at the table. Mack stood behind his chair directly across from Curtis and faced the windows. Mack was squinting and looking toward the waterfront.

Thomas sat on the same side of the table as the doctor but with an empty chair between them, upon which he sat his briefcase. Thomas looked up at his assistant, a young man with a white shirt and tie, standing just inside the door. Then he looked back at the men, "Can I get you gentlemen a beverage?" Thomas's eyebrows were raised in anticipation of an answer. He pointed his index finger first at Mack then Curtis and back at Mack again.

Mack bellowed, while still looking beyond the window, "Hey, Tom, you know me... it's always a Jackie on the rocks." Then he slowly sat down. "I was just checking on *Lolita*... my boat. Damn thing's too big to dock in Seattle and had to moor her in the sound. Damn ferry better not hit her or Seattle will have hell to pay."

Thomas and Curtis sat in a solemn mood, until Mack smiled. He looked across the table at Curtis, looking him up and down again like he was steer in a livestock auction and Mack the buyer.

Thomas glanced at the clock on the wall behind Mack's head, whose hands now indicated it was 11:40 in the morning. He looked back at his assistant, who was carrying a baffled look, "Can you get Mr. Pendleton a Jack Daniels on ice please."

Then Thomas spun around looking to his right, "Curtis? Surely you're ready for something?"

He smiled. "Okay, I'll take an orange juice."

"Great!" He looked back at the young man still at the door. "Make that a fresh-squeezed orange juice for Dr. Eisner... and for me..." The young man answered with a smile, "Of course, Mr. Howell, a dry cappuccino, correct?"

Thomas smiled, "Make it wet" and winked at him.

Mack looked at Curtis intensely and continued to study him up and down in silence, making Curtis blush in awkwardness. Then the big man spoke, "So, I finally get to meet the goose that laid the golden egg?"

Curtis was speechless. He just smiled at Mack and turned to glance at Thomas.

"So, Dr. Eisner," asked Mack. "Do you mind if I call you Curt?"

"That's fine," he said, even though he hated to be called Curt. His father called him Curt, and he had no desire to be associated with that man or the memories of him.

"So, Curt, I've read everything there is to know about you, including all your research papers." He laughed. "I certainly didn't understand them all. So, son, I remember that you're from the other Jonesborough. The one they spell like the British, J-o-n-e-s-b-o-r-o-u-g-h, while I'm from the one spelled correctly?"

Curtis smiled again, "Oh, I knew you were from Arkansas, but I didn't know you were from Jonesboro."

"That's right, son." Mack paused a minute and then leaned toward Curtis. "So, tell me, if you are a Tennessee boy, where's your damn accent?"

"Well," said Curtis, being rattled a bit. "I guess it's from all those years I lived in Michigan, New York, and then here in the Pacific Northwest… I sort of lost it."

Mack made a serious look. "Well, hell boy, I've lived most of my adult life in places like the French Riviera, Hong Kong, and Italy and still speak like a damn Arkansan. But I'm proud of where I come from. We gave birth to the greatest retailer in the world, David McAllen, of the big box stores. He was a good friend of our family and taught me a lot about business. Believe it or not, he and my daddy played high school football together. My empire in telecommunications isn't anything to be ashamed of so what makes you so ashamed of your heritage that you would change the way you speak?"

Curtis had been nervously awaiting the meeting with Mack Pendleton, knowing he could be confrontational, but he never anticipated that the conversation would seem to take such a strange and negative turn before it even started. He looked serious and stumbled for words. "Well, my wife's from New York and she couldn't understand me when I spoke like I was from Tennessee... uh, I didn't change the way I speak because I was ashamed of something... it was more of a practical choice."

Mack smiled big and then winked at Thomas, "That's okay, you can speak with a damn Russian accent if that's what you want. It doesn't matter to me. I'm here for your brain, so tell me your story."

Curtis was honestly confused. "Like my whole life's story?"

"Hell no, son," Mack responded. "I mean, if you want to tell me that saga sometime over a beer, when I'm too drunk to even care, you can start when you came out of the womb for that matter. But for now, I just want to hear about your work. I've heard that you can make paraplegics walk again like a modern-day Jesus… and like with Jesus, soon the whole world's going to be beating your damn door down… I should say, 'our damn door.'"

Curtis had never been compared with Jesus before. He was starting to feel a little irritated at the man but tried to hide his emotions beneath a business persona. He opened his laptop and logged back into the company network. The big flat-screen TV flickered on, and you could see the desk-top screen of his laptop now projected on the fat screen. He then moved the curser around and clicked on a PowerPoint file that he had named "Neuro-anastomosis: the Neurogenics Story." He began to speak as if he had given this talk before.

"When I was in medical school, at the University of Michigan, I became very interested in spinal cord injuries. I changed my program in to a combined MD/PhD program, with my PhD in neuroanatomy and neurophysiology, with an emphasis on nerve regeneration. After finishing med school, I chose neurosurgery as my residency. I was matched to Apple Health Medical Center residency program in New York City in 2008. New York was one of my top choices because Dr. Lennard Jacobs, a PhD in neurophysiology, was one of the finest researchers in the world for spinal cord injuries and was at Albert Einstein School of Medicine in the Bronx. I arranged with Apple Health a schedule in the residency program that would allow me to spend some of my time with Dr. Jacobs. I commuted over to Dr. Jacob's lab, and he became my mentor. There were rumors that he was being considered for the Nobel Prize in Medicine in 2010, being beat out by someone who invented in-vitro fertilization."

Mack asked, "So he must have been this LK Jacobs that was listed as a co-author on some of your papers?"

"Exactly!" said Curtis with surprise in his voice. "Yes, in our original work, we severed the spines of the *Rattus norvegicus*, or common brown rats, and then coaxed them into healing and restoring function. As I was completing my residency in 2015, I reached an agreement with Apple Health to stay on as a staff neurosurgeon. But my agreement with them also allowed us to create a second lab for Dr. Jacobs in our facility. I was permitted to devote sixty percent of my time in this research. The CEO of Apple Health, at that time, was Linda Boylston. She was very excited about the possibility of the Apple Health facility in New York City being the first place in the world to offer a cure for spinal cord injuries." Curtis suddenly halted and looked up. "I'm talking about my own life again, aren't I?"

Mack nodded his head, "That's fine Curt, I'm interested in how you got into this work, but do try to get to the point of how it works and how the future of this technology is going to shape up."

"Okay," Curtis continued, "Oddly, about this time Albert Einstein Medical School and Montefiore Medical Center—where he wanted to do clinical trials with humans—were waning in their interest in his work. I think it was the result of a decade of supporting Dr.

Jacobs without any tangential return on their investment. So, it was a perfect fit for him to transition over to Apple Health."

Curtis paused again and fiddled with his PowerPoint, moving ahead to find a new slide and talking point.

"So, by the next year we were making a lot of progress. We also got to know a couple of outstanding biomedical engineers from MIT, Drs. Jones and Fahlner. They were very helpful to our work as well. But then we had a sudden turn of events. Dr. Jacobs was diagnosed with acute myeloid leukemia and got sick rather quickly. I had to take over the entire project by 2017, leaving me virtually no time for general neurosurgery cases."

Mack looked at his gold Rolex on his right wrist and then back at Curtis. "Okay, let's jump ahead to when you made the magical breakthrough with humans and how you ended up here."

Curtis rubbed his chin, with its typical day's growth of stubby blondish-gray beard. "Well, there wasn't a single breakthrough, and there's nothing magical about our work. It was more of a process... a process of trial and error. We also built on the work of others and, like Isaac Newton said, we 'could see further by standing on the shoulders of giants.' Often it was more error than success. We worked with rats, dogs, then primates, until we got it right. Then we had our phase I human volunteers."

Mack, nodding his head, said, "And Phase I is the very first stage to prove that it is safe in humans, correct?"

"That's right. The volunteers all had injuries that left them with severed spinal cords."

The door to the conference room suddenly opened, and the young man, who had taken the drink orders, returned with a young lady in a short, but professionally appropriate, cobalt-blue dress. They served the men their drinks. Mack seemed to be totally distracted by the young woman and Curtis could see his eyes looking at her from her black, shiny pumps, slowly up, to her face and back down again. Then Mack spoke to her, "Hey, you're a pretty little thing." Looking at the young man he asked, "Is this your squeeze?" Then Mack winked at him, with a broad smile.

Both smiled at Mack, and then the young man raised his eyebrows and asked in a professional way, "Gentlemen, can I get you anything else?" He looked back and forth among the three men.

Mack started to laugh out loud. "So, you aren't going to answer me, boy?" No one spoke, so Mack continued, "Hey, I will be ready for another Jackie on the rocks in about forty-five minutes." Then he winked at the two assistants as they turned and exited through the door, closing it behind them.

Mack took a sip of his drink and embellished the flavor for a second with a smile and sighed, "ah... that's so damn good. The first drink of the day is the best. I never get tired of it." Then he looked at the two other men and commented as he pointed at the—now closed—door, "Gentlemen, now *that's* one nice piece of ass." He belly-laughed and Thomas chuckled, while Curtis pretended to ignore the comment. Then Mack continued, "I had a girlfriend that looked like her once… in Aubagne… Aubagne, France. The French women aren't hung up on the age difference like here in America. There, they find success more attractive than youth. When I pull my boat, all 280 feet of her, into the harbor, girls like that would line up as far as the eye could see. Size does matter there," then he chuckled. "Those girls all say yes." Then he took another sip, savoring it for a minute, leaned over the table putting his face closer to Curtis and Thomas's faces and continued with a whisper, "And, when you're a billionaire like me… even their 'no,' is just them trying to look respectable to their mamas. They don't mean it." He sipped his drink again and his ear-to-ear smile morphed into a full belly-laugh after he sat back up and swallowed.

Thomas laughed again, along with him… in a gesture of politeness. Curtis tried his best to overlook Mack's comments, fiddling around with his laptop. Thomas had warned him the day before, "Mack can be something of an arrogant asshole, but that's just who he is. Try to be respectful to the man. We need this deal, and we need him if we're going to help people." But Curtis couldn't believe Thomas's level of accommodation to the man. After all, Beth, the girl in blue, was his niece.

Thomas knew that "helping people" or, even more precise, "helping people to walk again" was Dr. Eisner's weak point. He could almost get Curtis to agree to anything if he defined it in those terms. He had so framed Mack's visit, and his association with him, as a great conduit to restoring the suffering patient.

"So, Dr. Eisner," said Mack, lifting his drink glass into the air like a toast, "as you were saying."

Curtis, a bit befuddled, "Oh, yeah… uh, so we were able to perfect the technique to the point that we could create an anastomosis of the injured nerves or a re-anastomosis of the nerves we had intentionally severed."

"Anastomosis and re-anastomosis," interrupted Mack. "Now those words are a mouthful. He sipped his drink and seemed to digress once again, "Dr. Eisner, you're a famous doctor and about to be a rich man yourself. I bet you could line up for yourself some girlfriends like our little server girl. I mean, we're on the verge of making you a damn rock star."

Curtis, shaking his head in disapproval, said, "Please, can we get back to the topic?"

Thomas added, "He is a very happily married man to a beautiful and charming wife, Becky."

Mack sat his drink on the tabletop, but his big, rough hands still embraced it, "Really? Happily married? From what I understand your work is your wife. May I ask, when's the last time your little honey and you took a long romantic trip somewhere or even went out to dinner, or—speaking like a medical professional—had sexual intercourse?"

"Please!" stated Curtis emphatically. "Can we get back to the topic?"

Mack laughed out loud. Thomas spoke up again to defuse the situation. "Mack, Curtis does work hard, but we are hoping we can give him a nice long respite soon—like a sabbatical—so that he can have some personal time and come back to this project refreshed. Now, his work is nothing short of amazing, so just listen to his story."

Mack, leaning across the table in front of Curtis, said, "So you can regrow nerves? I understand that your technique is complex and unique, and, best of all, Tom here"—nodding toward Thomas—"has a damn patent on it?" Then he laughed again in his loud voice and lifted his glass in the direction of Thomas as a toast.

Curtis said, with an impromptu change in subject, "I see that you are a lefty."

Mack set his drink back on the table. "Damn right, a real south paw. Got me a pitching scholarship for Texas A & M baseball. Why do you ask?"

"I wasn't asking… I was just observing."

"I guess that makes you a regular Sherlock Holmes, then, doesn't it?"

"No… I'm just a humble neurosurgeon. Neurosurgeons are keenly aware of brain-side dominance. It impacts our work. But as I was saying, back on topic, yes, we have a patent on the technique, or more correctly techniques, as we have different techniques for different nerve groups. Our major technique, for rejoining injured spinal cords, is patented as the 'Erika Procedure.'"

Mack asked, "So what do those letters stand for, E-R-I-K-A?"

"It's a girl's name," answered Thomas before Curtis had the chance to explain.

Mack chuckled and leaned across the table again, looking directly at Curtis, "Old girlfriend of yours perhaps, Dr. Eisner?" then he winked.

For the first time Curtis looked visibly annoyed. Until now, he had been—successfully—hiding his disgust since meeting Mack. "No, it wasn't a 'girlfriend' but a patient. So, let's get back to the story before we run out of time."

Mack smiled and nodded his head in the affirmative. Curtis started jumping through his PowerPoint slides until he reached a colorful one of spinal cord anatomy.

"You see," said Curtis, "the spinal cord is a wonderful and extremely complex organ. It isn't like just a bundle of wires, as some lay-people would think. It's more like a living metropolis with a very complex array of avenues and circuits. The problem of healing these structures in mammals, especially primates and humans, is due to the great structural and functional complexity. It is far different from the spinal cord of a salamander, which can regenerate and heal on its own. For example, there're more than seven major neuron groupings of thirty-one pairs within the spinal cord, and those are laid down in complex layers called laminates. There are ten laminates." He clicked to several different colorful photos that showed a cross-section of the spinal cord's circuits, looking like abstract art of psychedelic butterflies.

Dr. Eisner continued, "These structures only include the major neurons. We have neurons running up to the brain, mostly carrying sensory information, and running downward, mostly carrying motor neurons. There are even autonomic neurons in these tracks as well. Then we have a very complex system of architectural and nutrient support for the spinal cord. It is a living organ. Like any living organ, it needs this kind of support. Even the blood supply can be complicated to fix or re-plump as some laypeople might call it."

Mack spoke up, "So it's complex. I get that. But somehow you figured out a way around that?"

Curtis was momentarily lost for words but then continued, "I was just talking about the structural complexities of the spinal cord. I haven't even gotten to the physiological complexities. I must explain some of these intricacies to make sense of our technique and the challenges that we faced and will continue to face. For instance," Curtis's eyes were lighting up as he was now in his element, "when a human neuron is injured, it doesn't just sit there like a cut wire that you can later put back together. No, it goes through a very active and multifaceted degeneration. Just one of these degenerative processes is called 'Wallerian degeneration.' It is as if the nerves, at least in mammals, are programmed to seal themselves up after an injury so that they can never be used again. There're also other

37

structural changes. While the proximal ends of injured nerves, those closest to the brain, can remain alive and functioning, the distal ends, those on the other side of the injury site, start to immediately atrophy and pull away from the connection. So, we always have a structural gap between the two sides of the wound to overcome as well as the physiological barriers." Curtis paused to see if Mack was listening… and fortunately he was this time. "The longer it has been since the injury, the more difficult it is to bridge these barriers because, over time, they scar up and move further apart."

The silence gave Mack another opportunity to speak. "Hell, I can't imagine how you could beat this. I was thinking that you just had to sprinkle pixie dust on it, and the damn thing would grow back together."

Curtis smiled for the first time in a while. "Well, we do have some types of 'pixie dust,' but it's just one part of a very complex process."

Mack sipped his drink, and his slurping sound made it clear that his drink was finished. He rattled the ice, pulling a small cube in his mouth, sucking on it, and spitting it back out into the glass. "Intriguing. So, tell me about this Katie Procedure."

Curtis responded, "It is the *Erika* Procedure, and yeah, I will explain. Previous researchers faced the same challenges as we did; however, they approached the structural problems in somewhat of a blind approach."

Curtis paused quickly to finish off his orange juice without giving Mack the opportunity to digress. "In the beginning, we were only able to cause a re-anastomosis in the spinal cords that we had freshly severed in the lab. That was a baby step. But then, especially when we got to our human models, we had to use old injuries. We did have the opportunity to try some of our early techniques with human hand transplant patients. Two, to be exact. So, with them we had fresh nerve injuries as they removed the old hand, at least on the recipient side. But with spinal cord injuries, they were usually old. There was no mechanism for getting a patient directly from the ED or operating room to our lab. Everyone wanted to give it time to see if the function would come back before experimentation, even if it looked hopeless from the beginning. It would be difficult for the ethics committee or Institutional Review Board to approve us trying an experimental procedure on someone who had some hope of natural recovery."

The young man in the tie returned with a second Jack Daniels for Mack. It was exactly forty-five minutes since he had departed, to the second. Curtis was still speaking as the young man served Mack.

The big man was acting more subdued, and Curtis was concerned that, by the time he got to the important part of the story, Mack would be too intoxicated to understand anything. Mack may have been thinking the same think as he spoke up, "So, for now, let's jump ahead to the actual technique."

Curtis scanned through some more of his PowerPoint slides, and then he paused. "Okay. So, different from our predecessors and colleagues around the world, we wanted to start with better mapping of the injured surface. When I look at these colorful, stained ends of the spinal cord, I see a beautiful pattern. Patterns, which can be translated into mathematical equations. Unlike the other researchers, I also saw a great opportunity in those patterns; a way to use what nature has given us. We just have to follow its lead. We didn't want to use a blind scaffolding system for the nerves, but a precisely created system for that injury.

A researcher at Mayo Clinic, Dr. Richter, had pioneered a system of biodegradable polymers as a superstructure. It had great promise, but we believed that the nerves needed to be directed exactly to their old axonal remnant on the other side, not just a randomly applied superstructure. The secret was in identifying the patterns of the nerve layout and working to restore the patterns to their original form. This is the direction we moved in, with our help from Drs. Jones and Fahlner from MIT."

There was suddenly a muffled vibration coming from under the table. Then it happened again. And again. Thomas stood up and grabbed his vibrating phone out of his pants pocket and stepped out of the room for a moment to take the call. He looked at them and said, "Carry on, gentlemen," closing the door behind him.

Mack, looking sleepy, responded, "Intriguing. Curt, I don't know if you knew it or not, but I am… or was, a man of science myself before I became a businessman."

Curtis, smiling, said, "I'm embarrassed to say that I did not know that."

"Yes sir. I have a master's degree in electrical engineering from Texas A&M and was accepted at MIT myself for a PhD program. But then, as luck would have it, I made a quick million dollars in my upstart cable company. I was twenty-seven and never had the time to go back to school as the millions continued to roll in faster than I could spend them"… chuckling he added… "and I tried damn hard to spend every dime."

Thomas re-entered the room and Curtis continued his presentation. "Drs. Jones and Fahlner developed—just for us—an implantable, micro-mapping tool for the nerve bundles. Our first step was to create a clear surface on the nerve ending, by debriding the ends"… Curtis could see confusion on Mack's face so he clarified… "you must cut cleanly or shave off the ends of the nerves to create a fresh injury and one that is flat. Then we did histological staining… using a chemical stain to differentiate the unique structures. It was hard to even find a stain that would not damage the—in situ—living nerves."

Mack's eyelids were slowly closing.

Curtis continued, "The Jones-Fahlner device is a disk that is like a high resolution, microscopic camera. It is a charge-coupled device, on both sides of a plate. Simple in design but produces incredibly detailed images. The generic name they used for it was the CCW for 'charge-coupled wafer.' You slide the CCW into place and lock it into position between the two frayed ends of the nerve. The device is hooked directly to a computer via a micro USB. The camera takes thousands of images in a second, and they are merged into an extremely high-definition digital representation. Then the computer creates a model of the micro-structure of the nerve endings for creating a bridging superstructure. This—very precise superstructure—directs the nerves where to grow to form anastomoses. In other words, if nerves are left to grow alone, they will end up looking like cooked spaghetti thrown on the floor, going in all directions. But when they have little man-made tubes to follow, they grow straight and connect to their old end on the other side of the wound. Different from others, our superstructure is tailor-made to match the actual nerves of each case."

Mack, raising his hand like in grade school, said, "Question… so is this the only difference between you and all the other people who have tried to do this before, observing the patterns and creating a better scaffolding?"

Thomas replied, "Curtis, if you don't mind I will try to answer him in laymen's terms." Looking at Mack, Thomas continued, "It is a triad of improvements that Dr. Eisner was able to perfect. The accurate mapping of the nerve endings was the first half of step one. The second half of step one was creating that scaffolding. With an accurate model in the computer, it wasn't that hard to reproduce an extremely accurate 'coupling' sleeve or supporting structure. That was achieved, again through our friends from MIT, with 3-D printing technology."

Mack was looking a little confused. Noticing that his glass was once again empty, Curtis quickly added, "A big challenge was finding the proper medium for the printer. Certainly, polymers were considered, but we found a better structure, carbon nanotubes. Jones and Fahlner may indeed get a Nobel Prize for their work in creating a 3-D printer that can print with nanotubes, and again, they did it—at least in the beginning—just for us. I think they are finding other applications for this technology even outside of medicine."

Mack commented, "I can just imagine the possibilities even in the world of electronics, but aren't nanotubes tiny?"

"Oh, they are ridiculously small. You can't put anything inside them. But the printer, which was created by our MIT friends, lays down a weave of a triple-walled nanotube in a cylinder pattern like a Chinese finger trap. Therefore, it can create a variety of larger-sized tubes, corresponding to the size of the neuron that it is directing. These tubes, just like their Chinese finger trap counterparts, can grip the nerve endings on each side and hold them securely."

Mack asked, "But aren't nanotubes very difficult to make and use?"

Curtis continued, "Yes, but these tubes were perfect for us because they were made of carbon, which is the foundation to human tissue. Nanotubes are extremely strong and small. The last part was that they are electrical conductors. We found that, in our experiments, if we are able to apply a constant gradient of around four millivolts along the web of nanotubes, it profoundly increases the growth rate and orientation of the neurons."

Mack scratched his head and said with a bit of surprise in his voice, "So that's it? This is Erika?"

Curtis shaking his head… with a touch of exasperation, "No… it is far more complicated than that. As Thomas said, it is a triad of advances, and this is just on the structural side. Let's start with just the electrical current. We created an ingenious way to supply the four millivolts that doesn't require batteries and very little implantable hardware."

Mack said, "Since my background is in electrical engineering, I can probably understand this part the best."

Curtis continued, "The normal spinal fluid has a pH of around 7.3, which means it is slightly alkaline. We create a biological alkaline battery with two tiny monofilaments of gold wire. One is electroplated with zinc on one end and the other is electroplated with manganese oxide on one end. The electroplated ends are fused together with a hot ceramic weld. The ceramic material also acts like an insulator between the two electroplated materials. You end up with a wire that takes a Y shape, with the base of the Y being where the two wires are fused. Does that make sense?"

Mack, nods his head, "I follow you so far."

"So, the loose—bare-gold—ends of the wires are attached to a carbon nanotube on each side of the wound. When you suspend this device in the patient's spinal fluid, the zinc-plated side becomes an anode, and the manganese oxide side becomes a cathode, sending out a corresponding dc current. We can adjust the current strength, based on the pH of that patient's spinal fluid, by varying the length of the fused plated wires. We start with a thirty-five mm welded filament. We quickly measure the patient's spinal fluid. If it is closer to the lower end of alkalinity, say 7.32, then we use the entire filament. If the pH is on the upper end, we trim the filament by around five mm per hundredth of a pH point. We have an algorithm, which tells us exactly how long the wire needs to be based on the square millimeter surface area of the coated wires and the alkalinity."

Mack, looking astonished and sitting back in his chair, remarked, "That's incredible!"

"It is pretty amazing. The whole thing is about the size of a human hair but creates our four millivolts for the whole duration that we need. Eventually, the plating on the wires oxidizes and the current ceases but not until the wound fully heals. We have a patent on that part, and other people are interested in our technology. We could also take an acidic area in the body, such as the stomach, and create an acid battery, but changing our plating from manganese to carbon."

Mack pondered Curtis's words for a minute, as he looked into his empty glass. He looked at Curtis and said, softly, "Wow, you guys *are* freakin' geniuses."

"Well," said Curtis with a blush. "I can't take credit for the biological power supply... that came from Bryan Rogers. Bryan's a surgical PA whom I've worked closely with during my time in New York."

"A PA?"

"Yeah, he's quite the virtuoso when it comes to physics, especially electrical stuff."

Curtis continued after sipping another drink of his orange juice, "The next part was creating the correct environment to stimulate neuronal growth. That was achieved with a, let's call it a 'soup', of precisely balanced ingredients. If there's a pixie dust, then the neuro-growth soup is it. Infused right onto the microtubes are Schwann cells, which have been coaxed into behaving like stem cells. We then immerse the tiny tubes, which themselves are made up of woven nanotubes, in a bath of the neuro-growth factor, or pixie dust, as you may call it. Specifically, the neuro-growth soup is made up of a group of substances called neurotrophins—protein growth factor. These impregnated micro tubes direct the new neurons to advance to their targeted attachment on the other side. The last part of the triad is the precise electrical current applied through the nanotubes, which I have alluded to. The current must be exactly 4.32 millivolts as neither 4.2 microvolts nor 4.4 millivolts achieve the same outcome."

Thomas spoke up rather hastily, "These things are all proprietary, and we couldn't even discuss them with you if we hadn't signed our mutual confidentiality contract."

Mack rubbed his sleepy eyes. "This complexity is mind boggling. Are you sure there isn't a simpler way? Why can't you just sew the spinal cord together, sprinkle your neuro-growth factor directly on it, and then it repairs itself?"

Curtis chuckled, "There's no way around this complexity. Sewing the spinal cord together was maybe something they tried during the Frankensteinian period of the nineteenth century. You must dive right into the middle of it and deal with it neuron by neuron. You must respect the patterns that nature has given us. That's the only way. That's also why we've done it better than anyone else."

Mack stretched back in his seat and yawned again. Looking at his Rolex once more, he added, "I think I'm still on Hawaiian time, and I got up way too early this morning."

Curtis's immediate thought was that two morning glasses of Jack Daniels didn't help matters.

Mack leaned forward as Curtis was closing out his PowerPoint program and shutting his laptop. He played with his glass and drank the few drops of the liquor-laced melted ice. He looked back up at Curtis, "So, was Erika pretty?"

Curtis just smiled and shook his head in disbelief, "Yeah, she was pretty cute."

"That girl must have stolen your heart."

"I guess you can say that. But it had nothing to do with her looks. She was the first patient I ever met with a new SCI."

"SCI?" asked Mack.

"Spinal cord injury."

"Let me guess," Mack added. "And the first one you saved."

Curtis looked down at his closed laptop on the table and then back up to Mack. "Nope... couldn't save her. She died at age 24 after getting a Methicillin-resistant staph infection from pressure sores, which she got in a nursing home."

"Damn! What the hell was a 24-year-old doing in a fucking nursing home! Couldn't her parents care for her at home?"

Curtis continued packing up his papers and stuffing them into his backpack. "She was a quad, ironically caused by a rollover on a quad. She couldn't help herself at all. Her mother blamed her father for buying it. Her father blamed her mother for letting her go out with irresponsible friends. They all blamed each other into despondency... yeah, until the whole family broke into pieces. Then, with just her and her mom in the house, she became more than her mom could handle, both physically and financially. I mean, her mother tried to sue the quad manufacturer. They lost because they couldn't prove a design flaw. The legal expenses, ironically, were the final financial blow that forced her mom to turn her over to state custody."

Mack carrying a perplexed look on his face asked, "So, how do you know all of this?"

Curtis, as he put his backpack over his shoulder, flashed a quick smile, "Because I visited her every Thursday while I was in medical school in Ann Arbor and called her every Thursday once I moved to New York. I was on the phone with her mother—at her bedside—when Erika drew her last breath."

CHAPTER THREE: MATURATION

Dr. Eisner took the elevator downward to his basement laboratory, known by the staff at Neurogenics as simply "Lab 3." It was not readily apparent why it had that name, as there were no labs 1 or 2, at least in Seattle. Thomas gave it that name, and as far as he could remember, he did so because Curtis referred to it as his third lab. The first lab being Dr. Jacob's lab in the Bronx and the second one being Apple Health in New York City. As soon as the elevator door slid open, he stepped into the middle of a whirlwind of chaos. "Dr. Eisner!" yelled Jennifer, Curtis's personal assistant in the lab. She was motioning for him to come as she stood in the doorway of his office, thirty feet down the tiled hallway. Before he had a chance to answer her or take one step in her direction, he felt a sudden tight grip on his right arm. He turned and found himself looking eye to eye with a thin, bald man in scrubs. "Hey, Curtis, I need you to come up to the operating suite for a minute. I need to talk to you about some changes that we need to make."

Curtis showed some signs of irritation, which wasn't his typical nature. He held up his hand in a gesture to quiet the man. He then spoke while shaking his head, "Hey, Clay, this isn't a good time. I've been up all night working on things, a presentation for our investor, and now I have a pile of work on my desk. Can you send me an e-mail about this matter?"

Clay didn't look happy, either. He rubbed his brow between his index finger and thumb while looking down at the floor. He was trying to hold back, or so it appeared. He took a deep breath.

Looking back at Curtis, he responded, "This needs to be a priority, so I would appreciate it if you would give this some attention… plus you never answer your damn emails anyway. That's why I'm here in person." Pausing for a moment to take another deep breath, he continued, "Remember, Curtis, what we do in that OR suite is the heart and soul of Neurogenics."

"Yes, yes of course it is!" Then Curtis spoke in an angry tone, "Everything in this damn place is a priority, but I am only one person, and I can only address one priority at a time!" Curtis paused for a few seconds. As Clay was turning to walk away, Curtis quickly reached and grabbed his shoulder. "Clay, hey, I'm sorry. Let me get caught up in the lab, and I will be up before the end of the day and…"

Before Curtis was done speaking, Jennifer, who was now standing right beside him, with a big, disingenuous smile on her face, interrupted, "Dr. Eisner, we were supposed to have had a virtual meeting with our electrical engineers a while ago."

Clay entered the elevator, disappearing from his view as the doors closed. Curtis mumbled, "Oh crap." Then he turned and looked at her. "I forgot all about the meeting."

They started walking in the direction of his office, and Curtis continued explaining, "Our investor was very late this morning, and I was sure I'd have been back by eleven, but what is it now…" pausing to take his cellphone out of his pocket and lighting it up. "Good grief, it's after two. Are they still online?"

She laughed, rolled her mahogany eyes, this time with a more genuine grin and said, "I told them that we would call them back."

Jennifer was 24 and studying "textiles" at the nearby Seattle Institute of Art. She was petite, with waist-length, coal-black hair, representing her mother's Japanese heritage as if her father's thick German traits had been totally restrained. Besides being an "artsy" person, she had an instinct in science like one of those bi-brain geniuses, who work from both the left and right hemispheres. Curtis fondly called her their Renaissance Girl. Besides knowing her way around the lab as a scientist, she was the one who would decorate it with her latest paintings or sculpture projects. Curtis had tried to convince her to go to medical or PA school, but she wanted no part of that. Her father had been a doctor, an internist, on Seattle's "pill hill", and that was enough for her. She got this gig as a part-time lab assistant because of her genuine interest in Curtis's work... and to help with her rent in the pricy downtown rental market.

Curtis walked into his office and looked around. At one time, it had been a big office, but now it was so full of stuff you could barely walk through it. His bookcases, situated on two adjacent walls, looked like they were about to collapse due to the weight of the books within them and piles of journals, files, and additional books on top. On the outside wall was a leather couch, but the couch was stacked high with boxes, papers, and even more scientific journals, these ones still in their clear-plastic wrappers. You couldn't see the top of his desk or his computer monitor due to two large, white boxes with "US POST OFFICE" stenciled on the side. They each were piled full of mail. "Oh, good heavens," he said to Jennifer. "This mail has to stop. If all I did was open letters and read mail, I would still have twelve-hour days."

Jennifer lifted the boxes off his desk and set them on the floor. "I think we need to hire you an office assistant who could do jobs like answering your mail. I really need to devote my time to the lab."

He looked at her, exhaling with a sigh, "We have a department secretary you know, but even Carolyn is overwhelmed these days. It would take a full-time helper just to deal with the mail. Now Thomas is saying we need to cut our budget by thirty percent, at least until we start to see money coming in. However, if Mr. Pendleton, the investor, supports us… maybe we could hire someone."

She smiled at him. "It would help if an assistant could simply divide it up into important business mail, letters praising your work… and of course the hate mail."

Curtis, frowning, responded, "I just can't stomach reading any more hate mail. My hand starts to tremble just picking it up."

Jennifer handed him a typed list. "Here's our to-do items for today. I've already scratched off the virtual meeting with the electrical engineers. I think it's too late to call them now. It is after 5 p.m. on the east coast."

Curtis was starting to feel dizzy and nauseated, probably from only having orange juice for breakfast… and lunch. He looked around his office. "You know, I'm sorry but I haven't had a wink of sleep in," pulling out his cellphone and tapping the screen, "in over thirty-three hours. I need to take a quick power nap, or I won't be able to make it through the rest of the day."

Jennifer seemed flabbergasted and a bit disquieted. "Uh, o-kay." She folded up the to-do list and carefully slipped it back into her lab coat pocket. "I guess these things must wait." She looked around the cluttered room and then back at Curtis. "Where?"

"Well, I thought about running out to my car, but if I exit the door, unless I'm wearing a disguise, I will be hounded by media people, or someone trying to sell me something or ask me for a favor."

"Oh shit!" said Jennifer.

"Oh shit what?" asked Curtis.

"Speaking of media, there's a guy down in the front office with Carolyn who's waiting to interview you for an investment magazine. He's been there over an hour."

"Really? I'm sorry, but I just can't do this right now. I must close my eyes for a minute before I start to hallucinate. I used to routinely pull all-nighters as a resident, but age must be catching up with me."

Jennifer nodded. "Alright, let's clear off your couch, and I'll go talk to Carolyn about not scheduling any more media people for a few days."

The two of them worked to restack boxes, files, charts, and even old Styrofoam food containers—some of which still contained food. Curtis opened one with a half-eaten, moldy eggroll, retched, and tossed it into the garbage.

"There you go, boss. Lie down here, and I'll turn out the lights and do my best to keep people away from the door."

Curtis lay down on the couch, which was a few inches too short to accommodate his frame, so he rolled into the fetal position. Jennifer wrote out on a piece of paper in marker, "Do Not Disturb!" She turned out the lights, closed the outside door, and taped the makeshift sign on outside of the frosted glass. She thought for a second and re-opened the door, reaching inside to drop the vertical blinds to block the light coming through the door's window.

The room was dark, but not dark or quiet enough. Curtis could hear conversations down the hall. He could hear a man mumbling, "But I've been waiting here for over an hour." Then he heard Jennifer's faint voice, too faint to make out.

He rolled over to face the back of the couch to shield his eyes from the light coming in through the door, but then his butt began to slide off. He rolled around once again, facing out but trying to lay his arm across his eyes to shield them. He could still see the boxes of mail staring back at him in the dim light. They were twisted columns like a row of Tower of Pisas. He heard the letters… figuratively of course… whispering his name.

Slowly, Curtis started to drift into this twilight world between consciousness and sleep where thoughts start to frolic in mystic fields without inhibition. He spent so much mental energy over the previous forty-eight hours reliving his past, preparing the historical record for Mack's visit, that now he could not pause the reminiscing. His mind journeyed to a place five years earlier. At that point in 2015, they were just starting to make breakthroughs, and his work seemed promising. He imagined, at that juncture, that by now, rather than him lying on a couch, in his office, exhausted and—at times—hating his own life, he would be traveling the world visiting spinal anastomosis centers.

He imagined that highly trained scientists and surgeons—using the techniques he and Dr. Jacobs had perfected—would be giving people the gift of walk and movement. He imagined a great atmosphere of happiness surrounding all the clinics. He let his mind meander behind one such imaginary clinic, perhaps in Delhi. There, somewhere near the clinic, local craftsmen would be recycling old wheelchairs—turning them into bicycles and skateboards. That was his dream. He allowed his mind to get silly for a moment, imagining a parade through the Indian streets with cheering and a long line of women in saris out front throwing down a bed of jasmine as ex-paraplegics or quads were marching, riding bicycles, unicycles, skateboards, being showered with brightly colored handfuls of powered chalk, and followed by highly decorated elephants.

Curtis then could see an image of him sitting beside Erika's bed and taking her by both hands, turning her and allowing her to put her feet on the floor. He could see her face with great clarity. He remembered the gathering of dark freckles around each cheekbone. She grimaces because she could feel the cold tiles on the bottom of her soft feet for the first time in years. Then she flashes a brief grin. With his assistance, he sees her standing on her own again, as a huge smile sweeps across her dimpled face like a late summer brush fire. She takes a step and begins to giggle, giggle and cry, "You told me I'd walk again and I didn't believe you… but now I can! You really did save me."

He peeked between his eyelids to see the boxes of mail, still stacked high, not moving, but perhaps leaning a little more. He asked himself, "How did things start to go so wrong? When did I get caught on this path that has led us to this moment? How did everything become so complicated and so damned difficult?" It wasn't at all as he had imagined.

He did remember his first full box of hate mail. It was right after he and Dr. Jacobs had published the paper presenting the study that used Rhesus monkeys as research subjects. The study described how they had to "surgically induce a severed spinal cord." It sounded sterile and scientific, but Curtis was there and did many of the procedures himself. It was hard. Very, very hard.

Curtis had been warned, when he first came to the monkey lab, to see them as lab objects and nothing else. The monkeys, by intent, had only numbers on their cages. But he named them all. He brought them treats, mostly dried banana chips. He spoke to them. He could look into their chocolate-brown eyes and see a soul looking back at him.

But the time finally came that rats would no longer suffice, and the first monkey had to be sacrificed. There was no way to go forward without it. There is no computer model sophisticated enough to come close to the data they needed. There were no robots to try things on. And the first monkeys were, indeed, sacrificed. All their early techniques failed miserably. The resulting quadriplegia or paraplegia... meant euthanasia.

He hated this turn of the process. He wished there had been monkeys with accidental spinal injuries that they could possibly help, but there were none. Maybe one in the world, but finding that one monkey would have been impossible.

Before moving to monkeys, they did have a period when they used dog models. Within the dog population they could find injured animals, mostly ones that had sustained spinal injuries from being hit by cars. They could work with that. They had hopes of returning the dogs to functioning, but the procedures didn't work, especially at first. Some animals were worse off afterward because to work on the spinal cord, they had to trim and debride it. Sometimes they had to take a partially severed cord and make it a completely severed cord so that their bridging apparatus would fit in the space.

Yes, he remembered now, the first hate mail came trickling in during the dog phase. It wasn't because they had made some dogs worse. It was the owners whose expectations far exceeded the informed consent. They let themselves believe that, by allowing Baily, Max, or Buddy to participate in the study, they would get their whole pet back on the other side. It just didn't happen... at least in the early days.

Curtis remembered opening his first angry letter. He, due to his social anxiety, always wanted to please people. When people said very angry things to him, it hurt. As soon as he saw the irate words on the page, he felt like a balloon of hot acid burst within the pit of his stomach. With each angry letter, he lost one, two, or three nights' sleep. Some of them said things that were very cruel. "Since you didn't help Buddy walk with his back legs again, like you promised, I hope someday you become a paraplegic, too. Bastard!"

But it was during the monkey trials that things got ugly. When their paper appeared in the *American Journal of Neurosurgery*, all hell broke loose, and he was ill prepared for those new developments. Somehow, he assumed that only scientists and surgeons like himself would read those complicated papers. But some of them must have had boyfriends and girlfriends, mothers, sons, and daughters... those who didn't see the big picture but only the cruelty.

The first full box of hate mail came to him within days of the publication of his paper. Then the volume increased. Maybe if he had been doing research somewhere else, such as Idaho or Alaska, no one would have noticed. There, animals are "harvestable" for human needs. But his work was in the heart of New York City. Sure, there were plenty of meat markets in the village and other parts of the city. There were also plenty of minks and furs around Midtown and the park. Most New Yorkers wore leather. But those people were so disconnected from the slaughter houses in the Midwest or Jersey that they had an intrinsic psychological insulation.

Curtis came to work one morning, and a group of protesters was trying to block his entrance. Then someone threw a plastic sandwich bag full of blood on his face. It was real blood. He could taste it... like a salty rust.

The protests eventually started to subside. The team of researchers was making progress, as they continuously fine-tuned their approach. Curtis remembers having an incredible amount of hope the first time he saw post-procedure movement in the feet of a Rhesus, one he named King Kong. He had given him that name because he was the biggest monkey. Maybe that is why the procedure worked with him first. But it wasn't a complete success, and the animal still had to be sacrificed, much to Curtis's consternation.

The next round of trials came after the introduction of the precise cross-injury current and the new optical sensor for mapping the spinal cross section. The next two monkey subjects regained their full lower extremity neuro-functioning within six months. They had a huge party in the lab that night, and it was one of the few times in Curtis's life he ever became intoxicated. Becky drove him home, and the next morning, save a nasty hangover, he was euphoric. Life, so he thought, couldn't get any better. He knew then that the cure would come to humans… it was all a matter of time.

He switched his research—now that they were past the primary discovery phase—into perfecting his technique by returning to the dogs. This time with hope. He put out an ad in *The New York Times* looking for dogs, or even cats with spinal injuries. He was looking for those who had a loss of function in their lower torsos. The response was overwhelming. Not thinking about the nationwide, or even worldwide, reach of the local edition of the paper, hundreds of requests came in from around the world.

A Saudi princess offered him a million dollars if he could restore function to her cat's rear legs. Apparently, its spine had been severed when her irate husband stomped on its back for peeing on his priceless Persian rug. Ironically, which gave Curtis a brief morbid chuckle in his half-sleep state… it was a Persian cat.

Curtis knew that his lab couldn't handle more than just a few of these animals. They wanted a cross section of young healthy animals, older animals, those with new injuries and those with old ones. He was rightfully warned to not do business with the Saudi princess. While the money could help support their research, a failed treatment could mean a political scandal. In the end, he selected seven animals. Out of the seven subjects, five returned to full-function within six months of the procedure, one had continuing neurological deficits, and one died during the surgery.

The owners of the animals with successful outcomes were deeply grateful. However, a new wave of hate mail came, this time from the owners of the thousands of pets which were rejected for the study, including the princess. Curtis even had a few death threats this time. He never imagined this kind of response. The animal rights advocates, protesting his use of monkeys, hadn't personally threatened him like the rejected pet owners had. The blood thrown onto his face, he thought, could've been a treat. It would have been an attempted murder if it was HIV or hepatitis positive blood. He had a colleague in another lab agree to do testing on the specimen he recovered from his face. It was real blood alright, but, thank goodness, not human. It was genetically proven to be chicken blood, a Jersey Giant to be precise. But where did someone get their hands on a cupful of fresh chicken blood? Curtis had no idea. He also had no idea why someone would consider it ethical to kill a chicken to eat but hideous to kill a monkey that could eventually lead to saving the lives of thousands.

Curtis rotated once more, trying to face the back of the couch so that he wouldn't face the boxes of mail on the floor and could get his mind off them long enough to allow sleep to flow into the crinkles of his tired brain. Then, in his side, he felt the poking of a button sewn into the seat cushion.

His mind started to fade again and then journey back, within the twilight of sleep, to that place a long time ago. His face was pressed so far into the back of the couch that he could barely breathe, but at least he wasn't falling into the floor.

He was remembering in 2017 when his team had accomplished ten consecutive treatments on six dogs and four monkeys. They were feeling confident enough to consider human trials. His team worked on their proposal for the Apple Health's Institutional Review Board (IRB). The IRB is a group of people from many perspectives: physicians, citizens, clergy, lawyers, and business owners. The purpose of the board is to assure the research on humans is worthwhile and done with the utmost safety and ethical concerns for the patient.

Curtis and Lennard were very excited to do their presentation. They were already several steps beyond all other spinal researchers in the world, and no one had experienced their level of success. They had done their homework, consent forms, protocols, inclusion, and exclusion criteria; they knew that their request would be a slam dunk. After all, there was so much at stake. There was an estimate by the World Health Organization that over 300,000 people worldwide suffered new spinal cord injuries each year. If their work was successful, it would bring a profound improvement of life to each of them.

But it wasn't an automatic approval. The IRB lawyer, Dan Brice, was concerned about the debridement part of the procedure. He was the lawyer representing Apple Health's liability concerns. He pointed out that spinal cord injuries have underwritten many of lawyers' yachts and mansions. If Curtis and his team were to take a paraplegic and turn him or her into a quad, it could be a suit worth tens of millions of dollars. Curtis's team reviewed with them the few animal cases where more harm was done, but they had a string of undeniable successes.

Curtis had to point out to the man that paraplegia versus quadriplegia wasn't an issue of the severity of the spinal injury but the location. In rebuttal to the general concern, he also indicated that if a SCI was worth—per Mr. Brice—tens of millions of dollars, then turning a quadriplegic into a restored, whole person should be worth tens of millions of dollars.

Dan said to them, with a bit of chuckle in his voice, "Okay in theory that's true. However, no patient is paying tens of millions of dollars for the procedure. I won't be surprised if many patients fought to pay us nothing. So, the equation isn't as balanced as you imply."

The most enthusiastic supporter on the IRB, to Curtis's surprise, was Rabbi Lewis. He was excited about the discovery, commenting, "Folks, do you realize that the hopes of thousands of patients, the dreams of families for centuries, is now here, and it is at our facility? We must support this with all of our beings."

That end of the table had three clergy sitting around it, and Rabbi Lewis was in the center. To his right was a Catholic Priest, Father Marino. He was a distinguished and quiet man. On his left was a pastor of the largest evangelical church in Manhattan, Pastor Ricky

Clawson. While Father Marino smiled, and seemed to agree with the Rabbi, the pastor had a disturbed look on his face.

Rubbing his chin between his right thumb and fingers, Ricky spoke. "Drs. Eisner and Jacobs, have you used any fetal parts in this procedure?"

Curtis felt a sense of pride in the fact that he had been prepared for this question. One of his early mentors had warned him that if he used fetal parts for his work, someday he might reach an impasse in his progress due to a political opposition. He looked at Pastor Clawson and answered, "We've tried very hard to avoid any tissue that was harvested from aborted fetuses. We do have cultures of cell lines that were created by the humanization of rabbit Schwann cells as well as neonatal cord blood and donated miscarriage fetuses. But none of these cell lines are from elective aborted fetuses and we can document that fact."

Pastor Clawson's eyes lit up. "So, you do use fetuses?" He stared with a pondering look and added, "When you say 'humanized,' does that infer that you use GMOs, too?"

Curtis was startled from his attempted nap on his couch by banging on his office door. He pulled out his cellphone to check the time. He had only been resting there thirty-five minutes. With his mind so deep in thought about his path to this point, he knew that he hadn't slept at all, at least no more than the twilight phase. *Bang, bang, bang,* came the noise from the door again. It was so hard that it caused the brass latch to rattle. He slowly sat up on the side of the couch as he felt dizzy. He looked at his phone again, for the first time noticing that he had missed thirty-two calls and had fourteen new voicemails.

Bang, bang, bang, came the knocking. He yelled, "Okay! I'm coming!" He was wondering what happened to Jennifer's promise to keep people away.

As he sauntered toward the banging noise, he stepped over the cartons of mail, tipping over one box and catching it just before the whole tower tumbled. He opened the door, and there stood Wilmer, one of Neurogenics' lawyers with a file under his arm. Apparently signs that say, "Do Not Disturb" don't apply to lawyers, at least in their opinions.

Wilmer said in a loud voice, "Must be nice, having a nap time when so much is going on for your sake upstairs, Dr. Eisner."

Curtis shook his head and rubbed his eyes, "Do realize that I haven't been home in well over thirty hours. I do have to sleep and pee sometimes. Who knows, maybe I will even get to eat something besides vending machine food someday, too."

"Turn the lights on. I need to talk to you now, and then you can go back to your nap."

Curtis reached over and switched on the lights. He squinted with the sudden brightness of the overhead LEDs. "So, Wilmer, what's so damn important?"

"I've been leaving messages with you for days that I need to talk to you. This couldn't wait any longer."

"What couldn't wait?"

"I'm trying to clean up the damn patent mess."

"I've turned over every patent that we had to Neurogenics. Did I miss something?"

Wilmer spoke as he pulled out a stack of papers, all legal-sized and with little pink paper arrows stuck on it in places. "You did turn over your patents but it wasn't that simple. Your process is complex."

Curtis chuckled out loud, saying, with a sarcastic flair, "Really... I didn't know that."

"Listen, I'm being serious here. Your patents cover the broad procedures and some of your specific techniques for imagining the nerves and spinal cords, but you have many other parts of this procedure that aren't covered well by the patent. I need you to sign these contracts ASAP so that I can represent your interest in getting patents on all unique procedures. Then we can sign those over to Neurogenics."

"Fine," said Curtis. He reached out and pushed some junk off his desk as a gesture of annoyance. The stapler, assorted files, and coffee mug all fell to the floor with a recalcitrant crash. Curtis placed the papers on—a now—flat place to write. He started to sign the contracts without reading them. His eye did catch one page that discussed the neurogenesis solutions that he had developed to stimulate nerve growth. This included the Schwan cell lines. He looked at Wilmer, "Actually, we are working right now to create our own line of these cell solutions so that we don't have to depend on an outside supplier. Then the cell lines and solutions will be completely ours."

"Fine," said Wilmer. "But sign these to cover us in the meantime."

As soon as Curtis was done with all the signatures, Wilmer gave a quick, "Thank you," and he was out the door, turning off the lights as he exited.

Curtis felt sick. No sleep, no food, and even before that, weeks of little sleep and surviving on candy bars, potato chips, and Red Bull. It was catching up to him. He walked out into the brighter lights of the hallway to the bathroom to relieve himself. He quickly returned to the solitude of his, now dark office, before anyone else spotted him. His office smelled of damp paper and something sour, like old milk. He glanced at his phone again and tapped on the voicemail button. He saw no less than five voicemails from Becky. "Oh, crap!" he mumbled to himself. He poked the "Call Back" button on the phone. It rang and rang with no answer. Then he punched the voicemail buttons.

"Curtis, it is nine o'clock, which is about the time you normally come home, but you're not here. I had a nice dinner on the table. So, can you call back and tell me your plans?"

He clicked the next voicemail from Becky.

"Curtis, it's 11 o'clock, I put dinner in the fridge. I have no clue where you are. Did you get killed in a car wreck on the way home?" Then she said with some emotion in her voice, "It is hard living like this. It would be so polite if you would tell me if you're not coming home so that I don't worry!"

He clicked on one more message, one that had come in at 10 a.m.

"Curtis, so you didn't come home at all. I assumed that you weren't killed last night because the police would've been here by now... uh... so maybe I'll see you tonight, unless you are staying with your girlfriend."

Curtis felt anger at those last words. Anger and guilt. He knew that Becky was having a rough time with his schedule, and he knew that he gets so distracted that he forgets to call her. But to suggest a girlfriend on the side made him angry. With his dad's history of infidelity, such joking... if it was a joke... lost its comic appeal.

Curtis's love for Becky was drawn from a deep place, even though he didn't act like it at times. He kept thinking, "Soon, this hectic pace will end, I will turn this work over to others and retire before age fifty. Then Becky and I will have the rest of our lives together to just have fun." But he realized that he was turning forty-four this coming summer and that he was quickly running out of time.

Curtis stuffed his phone back into his pocket and lay back down on the couch. This time, though, he went into deep sleep. He didn't wake up until the lights were dim in the hall. He looked at his phone again. It was 6:45 in the evening. He felt awful. He tried to call Becky again, but again there was no answer.

He sat up and rubbed his face. His bladder was about to burst and indeed that was what had awakened him. The Red Bull seemed to run through him like a sieve... yet not pausing long enough in his brain to enhance his alertness. He got up and opened the office door and made his way to the bathroom. He could see lights and hear machines running in the lab. On his way back from the bathroom, he went past his office door to the source of the sound. He looked in and saw two of his assistants hard at work. "Hi, folks," he said, startling the two young men.

"Hey, doc, we heard that you went home early. Are you back?"

Curtis replied, "Well, no... I never left. I have been passed out in my office for the past four or five hours." He had a bad headache, pulsating like a beacon light in the midst of a mental fog.

Cutis walked farther into the room containing work benches, centrifuges, refrigerators, vented hoods, and enough glass work for a mad scientist setup in a horror movie. "So, what are you working on tonight?"

"We are still working on the N-4 line [*meaning the Neurogenics culture line four of humanized Schwan cells*]. As you know, with this line we found that a partial exposure to a mycobacterium culture has caused a cellular regression toward a stem cell state. We have been studying ways to find the optimal exposure. We have found that, with a certain time exposure, we see a linear progression, but with a little more time exposure, it is like a quantum leap backward to a total stem cell behavior."

Curtis, nodding his head in agreement, said, "I was looking over your charts the other day and meant to say something to you. I've read the articles by our colleagues abroad on Schwan cell manipulation. Of course, we don't want total stem cells or the differentiation would be hard to manipulate. We want the cells as immature as we can get them, but after the differentiation into useful cells has already started. I noticed one variable with the mycobacterium-exposed cells, that they are very temperature dependent. You have to keep the culture at exactly 37.4°C to get the same outcome as a factor of time; otherwise, as Dr. Khoury found in Tehran, it is all over the map."

The two young men looked astonished, "Of course," said one of them. "We had assumed that that the cells had to be kept close to 37°C, give or take a few decimal points, but we didn't do trials with precise temperature controls."

Curtis smiled and said, "I bet if you go back and look at your charts, you will see the quantum leaps back to stem cells occurred when the temperature had risen." For the next two hours, Curtis, donned in his lab coat, struggled to get the incubators with the N-4 line precisely controlled at 37.4°C. They would fine-tune the thermostat and wait. The temperature would go to 37.6°C. Then Curtis would turn it down, and it would drop to 37.2°C. He made finer and finer adjustments. Concerned about a minor air leak, he adjusted the door seals until they got a consistent 37.4°C. Curtis then said, "Boys, I'm calling it a night."

Turning off his office lights and locking the door, Curtis headed down the hall and up one flight of stairs to the street level and then through a long tunnel that lead to the parking garage. Sitting in his Jeep, he tried calling Becky again. There was no answer. As he pulled up on to I-5, heading north, he let his mind, once again, go back to those early years in New York.

He remembered that it was during that time, the first wave of disillusionment fell over him. The FDA determined that they must file an IND (investigational new drug) application before they could proceed. This new development would take at least six additional months of work. Curtis and Dr. Jacobs had both assumed that they were exempt from this arduous process because they were not introducing a new drug, per se, but a new procedure.

It was about this time that Lennard found out he was sick. First it was just extreme fatigue, but then he poked his finger and looked at his blood under the microscope. The smear was flooded with immature white cells. He knew then that he had a serious problem and quickly made an appointment with a hematologist-oncologist. The timing—as if there was ever a good time to get cancer—was terrible for them.

The spinal anastomosis procedure was complex and did utilize several new biologics, including the Schwann cells and their neuron growth "soup." Within this soup were growth factors and nutrients for cell survival. The FDA also required them to give the whole procedure a name so that a license could be given for legal clarification. They could not deviate from that procedure without a new IND submission. At that juncture, Curtis, who was mostly working alone, picked the name "SRA-1", for spinal anastomosis type 1. It was in a subsequent IND application, after the last round of tweaking, that Curtis eventually used the name, the "Erika Procedure."

The hard thing for Curtis to figure out (and little did he know at that time that it was only the beginning) was the long and bumpy road to success. At times, it seemed like the whole world was against them when it should have been cheering them on. Rabbi Lewis seemed to be the aberration.

Toward the end of their Apple Health IRB review, about the time that Lennard started his first round of chemo, Curtis came to the meeting alone and delivered—what he thought—was a moving speech about the needs of the patients and how that must outweigh their other concerns, concerns of lawsuits, patents, and reimbursements. When he finished speaking, Lisa Braun, the Apple Health VP of Clinical Affairs, looked at him with a sweet smile. He assumed that he had won her over, but then she said, "Dr. Eisner, what you really need is to mature professionally… and to embrace the real world."

CHAPTER FOUR: BECKY

Curtis pushed the button clipped to his Jeep's sun visor as he approached his condo. The garage door began to open, and the lights came on inside. He started to squeeze in beside Becky's VW Beetle, but her balloon-tired Schwinn was parked on his side of the garage. "Damn it," he mumbled to himself before thinking, "I think she does this just to piss me off." He had to back out again because the door of the Jeep wouldn't open while he was idling halfway in the garage doorway.

His intention was to move the bike. He grabbed it, but when he looked around the garage, he didn't see anywhere convenient to put it that would leave enough space for his Jeep. He punched the button to close the garage, leaving his Jeep parked in the driveway. He walked back into the garage, ducking the dropping door, and up the steps and opened the entry into the kitchen. The house was dark... dark and quiet with only the soft hum of the dishwasher in its last cycle. The light of a quarter moon infiltrated the windows and skylights with just enough light for him to see where to step. He looked at the clock, and it was only nine. Becky had been known to go to bed early, but this was even early for her.

Curtis opened the refrigerator and peaked inside. He was hungry for good food and the voicemail—at least from the previous night—said that dinner could be found there. Apparently, she had thrown it out... maybe in spite. There were only condiments. He opened the cheese drawer and did find one big block of mozzarella covered in saran wrap. He grabbed the cheese, took it out, and unwrapped it.

He pulled a butcher knife from the wooden block beside the stove as he passed it. He sat at the table and sliced the cheese with the knife into thin layers. He jumped up again and pulled open the cracker drawer. The artisan crackers, which Becky was so fond of, weren't there—just an open box of Ritz Saltines. He tasted one, and it was horribly stale. He tossed the whole box into the garbage under the sink. Not finding any decent crackers, he simply ate the cheese by itself.

As Curtis chewed on the rubbery slices, he sat on a bar stool next to their kitchen island. He turned around, facing out toward their huge front window. Two blocks away, but in clear view, was the long Salmon Bay. While he couldn't make out the water in the darkness, he could see the lights of several boats making their way to the Chittenden Locks and out to Puget Sound... or going in the other direction, toward Lake Union. He thought about those people, the ones in the boats. He had no clue who they were, as he couldn't see them. But he could imagine. Maybe one of them was an Alaskan fisherman making his way home after a grueling season on the Bering Sea. He must be eager to see his family again. He could just envision the reunion at the marina with powerful embraces. One set of lights seemed to triangulate far above another area of the dark water, defining the stays and mast of a sailboat. He assumed that those on board were making their way home after a great day of sailing out in the sound or perhaps even out at sea. He imagined that it was two couples—lifetime friends—who were sipping wine and eating aged cheddar on good artisan rye crackers. Between bites and sips, they laughed about all their great times together. He envied them. He wanted to sail away too. Far beyond the boundaries of Puget Sound, he wanted to sail out to the Pacific and across to the other side. Maybe getting lost in coastal Alaska would suffice… if not there, then lost in the Sea of Okhotsk. He and Becky could go alone with time to talk again. He chuckled to himself as he imagined stopping off in Dutch Harbor for some good crackers and smoked salmon slices to go with his cheese. He visualized placing the smoky, pink fish and cheese on the crackers and feeding them to Becky, like they had done with dark chocolate morsels on picnics in Central Park. But those were their romantic years, of dating and the first year of marriage. He didn't know the woman anymore, who she was now or what her dreams were. He felt especially sad because he was losing her, and the loss was on his watch. With that thought, he started to tear up.

Curtis tried to understand the sadness, but it was complicated… and opaque. How could he be sad? That morning, one of the world's richest men referred to him as the "goose that had laid the golden egg." This would stroke any man's ego. But right now, in his kitchen, in the dark, eating cold mozzarella cheese slices for dinner, he felt afraid. He felt alone. He knew that he needed to speak to Becky that night, even if she were sleeping. His darkness was submerging their relationship like an insidiously rising tide. He was determined to stop the progression of the malignant march, before it was too late.

He had met Becky on his first day in the lab at Apple Health in 2014. He was struck by her wavy auburn hair, hazel eyes, and natural beauty that required no maquillage. But it was her confident way around the lab that sealed her allure. She had her own ambitions, hoping to leave that lab and to continue her graduate studies at NYU in biochemistry. Her goal was being a research scientist in nutrition. However, she had to drop out of school to get a real job to earn some money.

Becky's father promised to support her though all her studies. As he got older, he was replaced at his company with a younger, more computer-literate man. She knew he couldn't support her any longer.

Her father had been a Wall Street man, but not one of the millionaires that you hear about. He was, what some called, "the rat in the pit." Running numbers was almost like coal mining and working down in the colliery, only he shoveled sells and buys rather than coal. But he was just a pawn, un-commissioned and easily replaced when computers made him obsolete. In an ironic twist, while he was so busy bracing up the retirement funds of thousands of strangers, he didn't have one for himself. Becky had to get a job. Soon after coming to Apple Health, she jumped at the chance to work with Dr. Eisner's team.

Curtis had fallen in love with Becky during his first glorious spring in New York City, as she did him. He was working with her, alone, for a full day in late May. It was the first Manhattanhenge of the year. He remembered the evening vividly. The two of them walked out of the lab together at the end of the day, exhausted. Once on the sidewalk, they saw people standing and staring into the west. Curtis's attention was drawn in the direction of their collective gawp. The end of 23rd Street disappeared into a sky painted in a bright chili hue. But it wasn't just the sky. The buildings and even the street itself were being pulled into the fireball with an irresistible force. Becky, a native New Yorker, had to explain to Curtis what was happening, about how the streets were laid out in a true grid, north to south and east to west, creating a situation where, twice a year, the sun sets exactly in the middle of the west streets. For some in the Village, it was even a spiritual experience. A couple stood, dressed as Druids, with palms held up to the sky. Curtis and Becky stood together in awe as the brilliant beams of orange lit up the sharp corner of the Flatiron Building like Hecate's Torches.

Although not spiritual for Curtis, it was romantic. The milieu set the mood. They stood, spellbound, like a pair of Meissen porcelain figurines. The whole city, if not the whole world, seemed at halt. It felt as if their very heart beats paused in respect to the spectacle.

When the sun had finally succumbed to the Hudson, dusk decanted into the streets, drifting in from the east. Then, like the turning of a switch, life returned to the bustle of lower Manhattan. At that precise moment, before the scene had the chance to scatter, Curtis looked at Becky and asked her to have dinner with him.

By the second Manhattanhenge, on July 12th, they once again stood on the corner of 23rd and Park Avenue. This time they were intentional spectators with a boxed dinner and two plastic, screw-topped bottles of a cheap merlot. As the imaginary curtain began to fall at the end of the glorious show of nature, Curtis dropped to his knee and presented Becky with a diamond. While the courtship was brief, the confidence in the relationship was unwavering.

Now, just six years later, he felt no different about the woman, but something awful was standing in the way of that love. It was ambiguous. Did she still love him? He no longer knew. Within his subconscious, he knew that she had reasons not to. Maybe it was neglect.

Curtis looked at the clock on the wall and thought about the fact that it had been thirty-eight hours since he had walked out the door to go to work. The sad thing was that this wasn't an atypical day.

Becky gave up her dreams to follow his. She saw the same potential that Curtis had, a world without disabling spinal cord injuries. However, as Curtis's career started to entangle him in the snare of detail, it closed Becky out. She had given up her job at Apple Health after they got married. But she and Curtis were on the same page at first. Both envisioned the day when the Erika Procedure would be perfected, and Curtis could step back and play the role of advisor. They wanted to wait and start a family and then both work only part-time. Curtis's longing to be a father was only second to his dream of bringing healing to SCI sufferers. He imagined a day would come when fatherhood would be even more satisfying. He realized that part of his motivation was to be the father that he never had. He had to prove something. He could be better than that.

But Curtis, due to no fault of his own, became swept up in the harsh realities of trying to get things done in a complex world. It started with the animal rights protesters. That was just a taste of what was to come. Then came the resistance with the IRB and the requirement to go to the FDA with not just one, but several IND applications. That process seemed to take forever and meant writing proposal after proposal during late nights at the end of grueling days in the OR. They had to write papers clarifying their process and the development of their proprietary recipes for cell growth. Each paper he wrote was followed by more questions from the FDA.

The most despairing blow, by far, came with the death of his dear friend and mentor, Lennard. His last words to Curtis, accompanied with a soft smile, were, "Let them walk again." He was drifting in and out of consciousness, and no one knew what he meant… no one, but Curtis.

Curtis took his shoes off and left them in the kitchen. He sat them beside the refrigerator, next to a large, brown paper bag full of wine-bottle empties. They were all merlot. He tiptoed through the house, pausing to pet their cat Racer, who was half-asleep on the back of the sofa. She partially awakened, arched her black, silky back and extended her front paws in a long stretch. Then she scratched him, drawing blood.

"Damn it, Racer, what's wrong with you!" he said in a whispered shout.

Opening the door to their master bedroom, Curtis looked carefully in, not allowing too much light from the hallway to penetrate through the door opening. He could see the outline of Becky in bed beneath her grandmother's crocheted, lime green bedspread. He watched her breaths as they caused her body to slowly rise and fall in a slow, repeated pattern. He closed the door and tiptoed into the en suite. He closed the pocket door behind him and turned on the lights. He looked at the large mirror that covered almost the entire wall.

He turned on the clear, globe lights around the mirror and studied his face. "Curt, you look like shit," he whispered to himself. His eyes were red, like lazy—not glorious—setting suns over dark, baggy hills. Nothing like Manhattanhenge, that's for sure. The light above the mirror enhanced the thinness of his hair. He was feeling—acutely—the rapid passage of time. He was officially middle aged and he could see them, the years, written on his face. He felt old and tired. His little boy dreams seemed to have eluded him, and the chronic disappointment seemed to haunt him these days, hiding in every shadow and every dejected cranny that he passed.

He brushed his teeth, continuing to look at himself in the mirror. He could see his father looking back at him. He had tried hard to forget what the man looked like but could never erase the image completely. The reflection kept that image alive. He spit into the porcelain scallop-shell-shaped sink. He did his final routine of flossing and urinating, slipped on his pajama pants, and slid into bed. Becky moaned and moved away; then she was instantly slipped back into a deep sleep.

Curtis thought he would, likewise, drift into a coma-state, being cuddled by the soft memory foam below and the comforter and bedspread above. Sleep, however, shirked him. Oddly, it seemed as if his exhaustion was causing his insomnia. . . or perhaps it was his long afternoon nap. He punched his pillow to make it thicker in order to raise his head higher. He put his interlocked fingers as a makeshift second pillow, in which he rested the back of his head—elbows pointing outward. He stared at the ceiling. The ceiling was one of the few places that he and Becky had not finished painting when they first moved into the townhouse sixteen months earlier. They had applied a primer coat but never got around to the finish coat, as it was at about that time he started staying at work late. He could see the faint water stains of previous roof leaks. The leaky roof held up their purchase for almost six months, while Curtis lived alone in a hotel. This gave them more stress. Becky moved out to Seattle the day they got the keys to the condo.

Neither of them ever anticipated living in the Pacific Northwest. With his roots in Tennessee, where his aging mother still lived, and

Becky's in Long Island, they always assumed they would end up on the East Coast. He had dreamt of being at Johns Hopkins in Baltimore, but that didn't work out, as the timing wasn't right.

Curtis thought back to those last two years in New York City. He, and the ailing Dr. Jacobs, filed their first application for the IND to the FDA. It didn't go as smoothly as they had hoped. The first problem was getting past the pencil pushers, who needed the forms filled out exactly right. But the computerized forms forced them into boxes that they didn't belong. One of the hardest questions was, "Is the new drug a derivative from a natural source, from another branded chemical source, or created new from scratch within your own laboratory?"

Curtis literally shook his head, which continued to rest in his clasped hands above his pillow, as he reflected on that question. How could they have answered that query, since their neuro-growth soup was made up of many factors? Some of the factors were modified stem cells, some from natural nutrients such as a modified glucose, and some additional compounds that were proprietary and produced in their lab. It would be the same as being forced to answer the question, does your beef stew contain meat or vegetables, an "either/or" question without the possibility of an "and." Maybe when the FDA created this application process fifty years ago, this made sense, but now it was only an obstruction.

Never did Curtis think that such a silly application would hold things up for over six months. Each time he started to feel frustration, he would focus on Erika—the actual girl—otherwise he would've given up. He constantly asked himself, how many people died today, just like Erika? How many are suffering? How many see no hope? He also knew that Lennard's time was running out. Curtis didn't mind taking up the brunt of the work, but he wanted Dr. Jacobs to be around long enough to witness their success.

The other frustrating thing with the FDA was that he couldn't talk to a real scientist, one who would hopefully understand his dilemma. He couldn't speak to a scientist because he hadn't been assigned an IND process ID number. He couldn't get the IND process ID number because all his paperwork was being rejected by the government clerical people. These people knew how to follow rules and make sure blanks were filled in properly, but they didn't understand the science enough to appreciate the way he was writing in answers.

Eventually, Dr. Jacobs told him about an old grad school colleague, Luke Napier, who was working at the FDA. Dr. Jacob called Dr. Napier as an old friend the day after he had his first bone marrow transplant. Direct contact with a scientist as an applicant would be considered inappropriate if not illegal. Such a call would have been considered "influence" by the applicant. Lennard thought it was rather funny that Congress, full of prolific receivers of influence peddling, would write a bill that guards so closely the use of influence on the FDA. But it was what it was, and that is all that Dr.

Jacobs could assume. He did speak—very carefully—to Dr. Napier explaining that they wanted to apply but were running into this problem of definitions. Luke Napier started to chuckle (while Lennard didn't think it was a laughing matter at all).

"This is what it's like working with the government," came Dr. Napier's conciliatory reply. "I work within chemistry, mostly new industrial chemicals seeking approval for safety; however, I do understand your problem. I'm often called in to help sort these things out by our biomedical department. Really, the best way to file an application is to file three or four different applications, one each for each ingredient of your proprietary soup."

"Really?" came Lennard's annoyed reply.

"Yes, really… but it isn't as complicated as you may think. You do have to file all the paperwork for each IND, but once it passes the pencil pushers and the forms are correct, then you can file to create an IND "Grouping." This IND-Grouping is then processed through the FDA as a single entity, while each part is also considered unique. Does that make sense?"

"I guess so. But why couldn't the people on the front end have told us this?"

"Sadly," came Luke's reply, "we have a lot of new people as the turnover for those positions is quite high… and frankly this information is beyond their pay grade."

"This is absurd!" said Lennard. "So, you are telling me that the hopes of paraplegics walking again can hinge on a high school graduate's ability, or lack thereof, to understand the complex paperwork process?"

"Hmm… exactly," said Luke. "We live in a crazy world, a world built, brick by brick, by lawyers and politicians."

"Bullshit!" came a third voice that hadn't been part of the conversation until this point. Curtis was sitting beside Lennard's hospital bed, leaning over and listening to the cell phone, which was set on speaker. Lennard frowned at him and put his finger to his lips as a sign for him to be quiet. Dr. Jacobs had, rightly, assumed that if both (including Curtis who had no prior relationship with Dr. Napier) were to be part of a conference call, it would certainly be assumed to be an attempt to influence the FDA by applicants.

"Was that you?" asked Luke.

This time Lennard spoke, trying to imitate Curtis's voice, with the hint of southern draw, "Bullshit. I said bullshit! This's nuts, man. Can't you fix this mess?"

Luke Napier, seeming set back a bit, remarked, "Anything else I can do for you, Lennard? I mean, it was great hearing from you after all these years, and I compliment you on your work, but I think there's nothing more I can do."

Curtis and Lennard pulled their office resources together and were able, after two more months, to produce three acceptable IND requests. Fortunately, Lennard was regaining his strength at that juncture.

The process, from the time that they first approached the FDA until their INDs were approved, took a total of eight months. At that juncture, they then had to go back to the Apple Health's IRB three more times. The group only met once a month, so this was yet another three-month delay. The holdup was "Pastor Ricky," as Curtis called him. The lawyer, Dan Brice, wasn't much help, either. Pastor Ricky was still voicing concerns over GMOs and cord blood for stem cells that, according to him, may have theoretically come from elective abortions.

Pastor Ricky was replaced when he moved to Ohio to take over a large church somewhere near Cleveland. Rumors in the New York tabloids said it was a reassignment due to sexual misconduct, but that was another, and unsubstantiated, story. But just the thought seemed perplexing to Curtis. Ricky, who opposed them so much on obscure and precise moral grounds, didn't seem to have a personal standard of morality. Luckily, the replacement to Ricky's position on the IRB didn't raise any issues, clearing the way for them to move forward.

Dan Brice, who represented Apple Health, was concerned about someone dying or coming away with an even greater impairment, which could mean a multiple million-dollar lawsuit. The eventual consent form was five pages long, plus Dan insisted that they videotape the initial counseling session with the patient and the patient's family, including the signing of the consent form. Then they had to create a new consent form just to get permission for the videotaping.

So, what Drs. Eisner and Jacobs had envisioned as a six-month process became a ten-month progression. During that painful waiting period, Curtis continued perfecting his techniques and doing general spinal surgeries to keep his surgical skills fine-tuned. It was extremely frustrating for him to debride a spinal cord injury, knowing that the patient would be a paraplegic for life, when he had the skills and resources that could allow them to walk again... but wasn't allowed to use them. The rules and fears of litigation prohibited him from saving people. It was an absurdity. Curtis used to say, "Someday, in a hundred years from now, people will— hopefully—look back at the way we do things with disbelief."

His difficulty communicating with patients and families was still his Achilles heel. He resolved this problem when he hired a neurosurgery PA, Bryan Rogers, whom he had observed in the OR. Bryan not only had excellent surgical skills, but he was also very good at building rapport and communicating empathetically to patients and their families—a compassion that both he and Dr. Eisner shared.

Curtis heard Becky's soft snores pause. He took his hands from behind his head, which were now stiff. He rolled onto his side to look at her, thinking that she might be waking up and he could apologize. She opened her eyes and looked around, seeming startled.

Patting her on her back, "Hey, hon… it's me. I'm home."

She looked at him with disconcerted eyes, which seemed more brown than green in the dim light. She took a deep breath. For the first time, Curtis smelled the alcohol. "What time is it?" she asked.

Curtis rolled the other direction to look at the clock on his bedside table. "It's now two in the morning."

She rubbed her eyes. "What morning is it… uh… what day is it?"

Curtis had to chuckle. "I'm not sure if I know. I don't think it's Friday anymore." Pausing for a minute, he added, "Hey, I wanted to tell you that I'm sorry for not calling you."

Becky flopped back down on the bed and mumbled something, but Curtis couldn't hear her, as she was now facing the opposite wall. He rolled toward her in a spooning position and put his arm around her waist, "What did you say, hon?"

Without looking at him, but speaking very loudly, almost like an angry shout, she responded, "I really don't CARE anymore, so just go to sleep and leave me alone!" Within seconds she was snoring again.

Curtis rolled back over to face his bedside table. He contemplated what her answer may have meant and wasn't sure. With his digital clock shining in his eyes, he rolled onto his back again and put his hands under his head as he stared at the stained ceiling. There were concentric but irregular rings of beige and linen white against the pearl white ceiling. The primer paint had only diminished their presence but not covered them. It dawned on him that they probably represented successive periods of leaking, somewhat like the rings in a tree tell the annual seasons of growth.

His mother used to tell him that there was something strange about his brain that allowed him to see patterns wherever he looked, patterns that were not noticeable to anyone else. However, that gift may have permitted him to succeed in spinal anastomosis when so many brilliant people had failed. He took his mind off the ceiling and, in his insomniac state, let his thoughts return to how he got to where he was now.

It was also during the prolonged period of waiting on the FDA and IRB approvals that the new Apple Health CEO, Bill Turner, summoned Curtis to a meeting one morning. Curtis assumed it was going to be a "getting to know you gathering" between the two of them. Lennard had taken a turn for the worst, his body rejecting the new bone marrow, and couldn't make the meeting. But when Curtis walked into the executive conference room that day, he was caught completely off guard by the presence of six other people, including the lawyer Dan Brice. Next to Dan sat the new CFO (chief financial officer), Nicole McKinney. The others—as it turned out—were marketing people, an insurance contracting representative, and a member of the company board. Only as they were making introductions, when many had simple smiles seeming to mask much more serious demeanors, that Curtis knew that there was trouble.

Mr. Turner was a tall and stocky man with a big, square, Dick-Butkus-like head with a 1960s crewcut. He always wore dark suits with finely pressed, collarless dress shirts. He asked in a gentle voice, "So, Dr. Eisner, give us an update on your work."

The timing wasn't good as it was at the stage where they were struggling to get past the pencil pushers at the FDA. He did his best to fill the group in with his latest news. He and Lennard had just spoken to Dr. Napier a few weeks earlier, so there was some hope due to their new plan of action.

Bill, with a somber look, turned to a woman across the table and spoke, "I think you know Nicole, our CFO. She has some information that she wanted to share."

Nicole loaded her PowerPoint presentation onto her laptop and fiddled around with it until the first slide was projecting. The first slide simply read, "Apple Health's Erika Procedure." She glanced at Curtis and smiled, saying, "We're very happy to have you, Dr. Eisner, and your wonderful work here at Apple Health. Give our regards to Dr. Jacobs and our well wishes."

Curtis smiled back and nodded his head, "I will. I'm seeing him this evening. He went home yesterday."

Her smile quickly faded as she added, rather abruptly, "We do have growing concerns about the viability of the Erika program." Curtis opened the water bottle in front of him and nervously took a sip.

The next few slides were numbers, lots of them. They itemized the investment that Apple Health had made into Drs. Jacob and Eisner's program over the past four years. These numbers included his salary, the salary of Dr. Jacobs, and the consulting fees that MIT's engineers had collected for their work on the Jones–Fahlner device and the 3-D printer. Then she flashed numbers representing the studies, the animal lab, the main lab, and the lab assistants, including their benefits and salaries. Then she added the clerical staff salaries, the office supplies, and the rent based on square-footage within their facility. The total cost for the project, according to Nicole's numbers, was $10,745,332.45. Yes, it was down to the penny.

When Curtis saw the figure, he was a bit surprised, but not shocked. Then, on the next slide, she posted the "credit" side of the ledger. Credit items included income from the standard neurosurgery services that Curtis had offered during his spare time, and which were funded by patients' insurance. For the entire four years, it was a dismal $760,544.15. Then she added the National Institute of Health grant of $2,000,000.00 to the credit side. "So you see, Dr. Eisner, we are presently running a deficient of $7,984,788.30 on your program."

The panel stared at Curtis in silence until he spoke, "Well, I know that looks like a lot, but, as Ms. Boylston, the previous CEO, and I discussed, we didn't expect to see a profit for several years. And then there are the intangibles that aren't reflected in your presentation, such as the notoriety that having the world's only SCI cure program would bring us."

Bill, taking off his glasses and putting the end of the temple piece to his lips, asked, "Dr. Eisner, how far along are your competitors?"

"Do you mean the other scientists working on spinal cord anastomosis?"

"Yes."

"Well, their overall progress is slow. There are four, maybe five, major teams working on this around the world. However, unless they have something up their sleeves that I don't know about, they're nowhere close to our level of technology and breakthroughs."

Bill put his glasses back on and then looked down at some papers in front of him. He looked back up at Curtis and added, "Dr. Eisner, we have also heard rumors that your technique will never work, not on the general public, not in real-life circumstances."

"Rumors? Rumors from where?"

"I can't say."

"We have had successes. In our studies, we had twenty-one completed cases."

"Well, there's concern that those weren't good candidates—that their spinal cord injuries would have gotten better with more conservative treatments. I wasn't here then, so I don't know the details."

"I was here!" said Curtis with alarm in his voice. "We made them better and there's no doubt about that."

Then another lady spoke up after Bill nodded in her direction. "Hi, Dr. Eisner. I don't think we've met, but I am Linda Gross, and I am Apple Health's Director of Payer Contracts."

She was a tall, lean lady in her forties with short bleach blonde hair. She was wearing a pin-striped navy suit and a chain of pearls around her neck. Curtis could tell the pearls were real because they had a slightly irregular taper on one end.

She continued, "As you know, our core customers are our own HMO subscribers. However, we also provide care for subscribers for all major insurers. The model of being an HMO may have worked in the 1980s and 1990s; however, we're in the age that it's no longer sustainable. I can explain the complexities of that at another time. Our future will be moving in the direction of being health care service providers and not an insurer. We will become totally dependent on other private and government payers within the next five years. As we," and she looked around at the people sitting at the table, "have looked at the costs that we have incurred so far and the projected number of patients that we can serve in the future with spinal cord injuries, we have created a very reliable computer model. Then we added in the actual cost of doing the procedure, your team's time in the OR, which you said would be six hours, or longer, per case. We added the equipment that you require. We added the cost of the intensive care and prolonged rehab. Considering the total cost of each procedure, plus our need to recoup our $9 million that we have invested so far, we will need to bill each procedure out at about $800,000."

"Holy crap," mumbled Curtis. "I didn't think it would cost anywhere near this level. Previously we had figured about half that for each procedure."

Linda continued, "Well, algorithms don't lie. These numbers are quite reliable. Now, if we collect any money from the insurers, we would hope to collect a little more than half, so around $500,000. On those collections, we would not even break even. That's not even the real problem." Linda looked down at her laptop and moved the pointer around with the touch pad. She reached over and twisted opened her bottle of Perrier. She took a sip and sat it down, screwing the cap back on, seemingly to preserve the bubbles.

Curtis sat in a state of nervous deferment.

She continued, "I've met with all the major insurers in the northeast and discussed this procedure. While they cannot give me hard answers yet, most said that they would not cover the Erika Procedure... at all."

Curtis sat up in his chair, alarm written on his face, "This makes no sense! No damn sense! We're talking about the first time in history of that paraplegics will have real hope of walking again. This is madness. The insurers and Apple Health all have to look at the intangibles."

Nicole smiled and spoke up again, "Curtis, this is business... the reality of business. Intangibles don't appear in ledger books at the end of the fiscal year. So, the concern that Apple Health has is recouping our expenses. We are also concerned about how long we can continue supporting your work without seeing a return. If your procedure isn't supported by the insurance companies, there will be intense social pressure to offer the procedure as a courtesy. Can you imagine the PR disaster of having the world's only cure for spinal cord injuries and then charging more than a half mil, in cash, to treat people? Offering free treatment would eventually bankrupt us. So, rather than being the good guys who bring hope, we will be the bad guys who have hope but don't share it because of perceived greed. In business, as in politics, perception is more important than reality. Do you understand where we're coming from?"

Curtis was scratching his head as he nodded. He started to say things... very personal things... that he would later regret. But he was just speaking what he was thinking... and feeling. "I have given my whole life, my career for the simple goal of helping paraplegics walk. But it seems like the world is against me. I don't get it. Where's the enthusiasm? Where's the support? When did the world get so screwed up?"

Bill spoke again, with his perpetual—although artificial—smile, "Curtis, we all support you. Good grief, we've supported you to the tune of almost $10 million. But we're also realists. For Apple Health to survive, we must be good business people, and that's what this meeting is about. My background is in marketing and the public face of a brand is tremendously important. We would love to project the image of having the world's only SCI cure center. However, just think about it. Imagine a row of people in wheelchairs camped out on our sidewalk holding protest signs against greedy heath care corporations… like Apple Health? Yes, we can offer some charity work, which we always do. But, for each charity case, we must increase our fees on the paying patients. But who will pay? The insurance providers are saying they will balk at this. We will continue to support you and your team, but we must start to see some end to this hemorrhaging of funds. There must be a horizon where we will start to see the cash flow reverse in our direction. That's all we are saying. I'm proud that you got the NIH grant, but there must be more grants or something to sustain your work. Today I have come with a proposal, if we don't see income on the Erika Procedure by this time next year, we may ask you to buy out your contract."

Curtis had a contorted and confused look on his face as he looked around the room. "Buy out my contract… what does that mean?"

Linda answered the question, "Simply pay us back for our expenses, and we'll let you go. The ownership of your patents would revert to you and you would be a free man."

Curtis sat up in his chair, "You mean *me* pay you $8 million? You know that I don't earn half as much as the other neurosurgeons because of my limited time in the OR. How would I come up with that kind of money?"

Postulating that it was a rhetorical question, no one answered. Curtis looked down at the table in a state of despondency. Bill spoke again, "So, I think we've made our point. We're proud of you and are glad you are part of Apple Health." Looking around the room, Bill added, "Does anyone else have any items of business?" With his inquiry being met with silence, he adjourned the meeting. Curtis stayed in the room as he finished his Perrier… then reached over and grabbed Linda's half-drunk bottle, unscrewed the cap, and finished her Perrier too. He wasn't that thirsty, but it was a spontaneous, primal act of insolence. Then he sat back down and stared at the black wall.

Suddenly, Curtis realized that he was now staring at his own water-stained ceiling, and he was in Seattle, two years later. Becky was snoring deeply. It was a snore that he had heard before… coming from the back rooms of the emergency department where he interned. It was the place where they put the drunks at three in the morning, as they sobered up enough to be discharged home.

CHAPTER FIVE: SATURDAY

When Curtis awoke, he heard the song of a marsh wren sitting in a madrone tree outside the bedroom window. The light of summer solstice is intrusive even at night, so though the sunlight appeared all-encompassing outside, he knew it could still be quite early. But it wasn't. He turned his digital clock around, and it read "10:45" in bright red letters. "Holy crap," he said to himself as he sat up in bed. "Am I late for work?" When his question dissipated into the air and no sound came in response, he looked over next to him. Becky wasn't there.

He rubbed his face and tried to think for a moment what day of the week it was. He remembered coming home late, but the last three or four days had been such a blur he was chronologically disoriented. He grabbed the remote from the bedside table and turned on the TV, which was mounted high on the wall. He felt woozy from the disorientation and pulled Becky's pillow over, creating a raised area that he could lay back on as he waited for the screen to boot up. He flipped through channels trying to grasp some meaning to what was going on in the world to figure out the date. Was he late for work?

It took a few moments of listening to CNN before the day was mentioned. They were talking about a bombing at a mosque in Kyrgyzstan during Friday prayers that had happened "yesterday." But, being in Kyrgyzstan, was yesterday really yesterday, or, with the time change, was today still Friday on America's west coast?

Curtis got up again and opened the bedroom door. It was always stuck during the winter monsoons but opened so freely in the summer, so freely that it flew open with a bang. He stepped into the hallway and shouted, "Becky. Becky... hey, BECKY!" All he could hear was the returning, unaccompanied echo. He walked over to the window that faced the canal. His Jeep was still in the driveway, but he noticed the raised garage door. He walked into the kitchen and opened the inside door, which led to the garage, and looked in. Becky's Bug was still parked where he had seen it the night before. She couldn't have backed it around his Jeep anyway. But her Schwinn was gone.

Curtis started the automatic espresso machine and stepped into the shower. Being Saturday meant that no other people would be in the office, except for his faithful lab assistants. The pace of his day would be a little slower without the constant visitors and phone calls, but he had to go into his office seven days a week to have any hope of digging out of the avalanche of work.

It was noon before Curtis backed his white Jeep onto Canal Street, turned, and started heading toward the freeway. He drove slowly thinking that he would see Becky somewhere. She often visited the farmers' market on Saturdays, so he turned in one block toward the water. The market was set up in a large parking lot next to a waterfront business park. The park had a cluster of one and two-story buildings, all in the Northwestern tradition of cedar siding and roof shakes. Between them, there were rows of rhododendron bushes, which had only recently lost their blooms. On the large, paved parking lot was an assortment of pickups, vans, and tents. They were stacked high with fruits, vegetables, cheeses, cut flowers, and rows of salmon filets and Dungeness crabs spread out on beds of crushed ice. Between all the vendor stations were a few hundred-people strolling, carrying baskets of their culinary treasures, and there appeared to be one dog on a leash for each person. There were many people on bikes as well, and even some of them had dogs on leashes. He kept thinking he was seeing glimpses of Becky, but when he almost hit a woman pushing a stroller—and she greeted him with an angry look and extended middle finger—he gave up on finding her. He had never seen a new mom display such a hateful gesture.

The freeways in Seattle were always congested, like trying to shove piles of dead bricks through a pipe. Curtis could remember taking a red eye to New York to finish closing out his lab. He had to drive to SeaTac at three in the morning to make his five o'clock departure. Even at that ungodly hour, the driving was bumper to bumper, and he barely made his flight.

That was his last trip to New York. He didn't leave Apple Health on good terms. But he found himself in a position where nothing he could've done would have redeemed the situation. He had planned on packing up his last files, saying goodbye to the remaining staff, and then hightailing it back to Seattle without any more interactions with the executives. But it wasn't that easy. He had documents to sign with Apple Health lawyers and a message to see Bill Turner before he left town. To his shock, Dan Brice presented him with a

$45,000 bill to cover the tail coverage of the malpractice insurance. This tail coverage would guarantee that the insurance would cover him into the future if any claim rose out of the years he was in New York. This would usually be covered for a physician; however, in his unusual circumstances of being a researcher and clinician, it was not. Maybe if he had thought of it on the front end, he would have written it into the contract. But when he came to Apple Health, he was a neurosurgery resident, and malpractice insurance was part of the package. But after five years, he became staff, and at that juncture he failed to negotiate the tail coverage clause. Tail coverage to him wasn't even on his radar at that time. He imagined being part of the Apple Health system far into the future... maybe until retirement. He also never imagined that he would have to use the tail coverage policy against a suit, but he would eventually find out that was a mistaken notion as well.

Curtis exited onto University Street heading west toward the water. He drove down the hill, seeing the entrance to the parking garage in the distance. He noticed the same angles to the Seattle streets that he had noticed from 200 feet above. They appeared to be ninety-eight and eighty-two degrees respectfully at each opposite street corner. He pulled into the garage, which was almost empty, and found a spot near the tunnel entrance.

As Curtis walked down the hall leading to his office, it was peaceful. The only lights were coming from the lab, as was the familiar sound of Pink Floyd's *The Dark Side of the Moon*, which someone seemed to play on a continuous loop every Saturday. At first, he found it to be an insufferable noise. He put up with it, knowing that it helped his staff to focus and find some pleasure in the, otherwise, monotonous shifts in the lab. However, one day he started to notice the patterns of the drumbeat, the rhythmic—almost mesmerizing—seduction of the psyche. He felt the math of it all. It was a like a subliminal puzzle that his mind would play with as a distraction to the real-life puzzles in the lab that were not so playful. He started to like Floyd. One Saturday, as they were working on tough algorithms, trying to perfect their neuro growth factor, Curtis had an epiphany. He looked up at his team and said, "Musicians are simple mathematicians, acoustic geometers." The stares he received in return were unaccompanied by verbal responses.

He saw Jennifer's hand-written sign still on the glass, "Do Not Disturb!" He pulled it down, opened the door, and flipped on the lights. Shortly thereafter, a young man walked out of the lab, down to his office's open door, and stood there.

"Oh, good morning, Doc Eisner." Looking puzzled, he added, "Uh… I thought you were out of town?"

Curtis had a perplexed look on his face, "No, Randy. I'm here. I know I'm late, but I overslept this morning."

"No sweat, boss." He paused like he was going back in the direction of the lab but turned around. "Hey, boss, I got the message that the N-4 incubator must be kept exactly at 37.4°C. When I came in this morning, I noticed when I calibrated the thermostat to show two decimal points, the temperature was swinging between 37.37° and 37.48°. I wasn't sure what level of precision you wanted."

Curtis seemed to ignore him as he lifted yet a new white box of mail off his couch and sat it on top of the previous four boxes, gently stabilizing it before the whole stack inevitably tipped over. He looked at the young man, "So, how's medical school?"

"She's a bitch, boss. You know, I get the big concepts fine, but I was never good at memorization. Now I don't only have to memorize, but to memorize Latin terms… hundreds of them every week. Some people in my class can memorize like parrots but have no clue what they're talking about."

Curtis chuckled, "I know. And those last people, sadly, will finish at the top of their class. Then they will kill a few people during their residencies—the attending physicians covering for them of course—and then they will go on to beautiful and financially secure careers but won't know what the hell they're doing or help any patients in the process." Curtis smiled, as he could tell from Randy's face that he told him more than he wanted to hear.

Curtis didn't leave his office for the next five hours, except once to visit the vending machine. The only things left in it were two small bags of Bugles, which he didn't care for, but he was hungry. He purchased both. It was unusually quiet for a Saturday. He got much of his mail sorted, throwing out every letter that was written to either curse or praise him and his work. He did look for checks, as once Jennifer found one written for $12,000 in the recycling bin. It was a donation from someone who did it in the honor of their, now-deceased, mother. Neurogenics had created a nonprofit foundation and bank account for such checks; however, they were few and far between.

As the clock moved past five in the afternoon, the lab got quieter and quieter until he knew he was alone, but he kept working. He got his office organized a bit and tried to create a schedule for the coming week. Thinking of Becky, he was determined to leave the office "early" each day, around 6 or 7 p.m. He couldn't remember the last time they sat down at the table for a meal… maybe it had been months, if not a year. At the end of the day, he pulled out his phone. It now contained no less than eighteen un-listened-to messages. He sat down on his couch and played them one by one.

As Curtis was finishing up, he was proud of himself for meeting his self-imposed deadline of being out of the lab on that catch-up day before 9 p.m. He never could reach Becky by phone, except for one e-mail. He told her that he would try to get home so that they could have a late dinner, if she could wait until nine o'clock. Her response was, "Whatever."

As he was closing his office door his phone vibrated. Hoping it was a text from Becky, he was disappointed to see it was from Thomas Howell. It simply read, "Hey Curtis r u in the building?"

"Damnit," Curtis whispered to himself. He thought about ignoring it, but he figured that Thomas had already seen his car in the garage… otherwise he wouldn't be asking. Curtis texted back, "yes… why?"

Curtis was looking at his phone waiting for a text response when it startled him by playing Beethoven's 5th, the ringtone Curtis had assigned to Thomas. He answered, "Hey, what's up?"

"Curtis, come up to my office. I have some good cognac, which I hand-carried from Cognac, France. I also have some great caviar."

"Well, I was thinking about going home to have dinner with Becky."

Strangely, Thomas responded, "Well, she's not expecting you for dinner."

Curtis had a pause of confusion and then asked, "And how would *you* know that?"

Thomas replied, "I actually just saw your lovely wife when Ann and I went out to dinner in South Lake Union. She was sitting at the bar with one of the girls from the lab."

"Jennifer?"

Thomas answered, "No… it was one of your New York Sharks. I can't remember her name." The group of five lab people that moved out with Curtis from New York referred to themselves as the "Sharks" after the name of the Puerto Rican gang in *West Side Story*.

"Are you sure it was Becky with her?"

106

"Absolutely. Ann and I had to wait in the bar for a table to come available, and I spoke to her. I asked her if you were in the office and she said, 'I presume.' She didn't seem very friendly."

"Yeah, she is having a hard time right now… you know… with me working so much."

"Well, anyway, the girls said that they were waiting on a table, too, so I assume they are still out. So, come up to my office, I want to talk to you. I have a feeling that Becky isn't even home yet."

Curtis had to ponder those last words. He made his way up to Thomas's penthouse office suite.

The office was huge, approximately 1500 square feet, surrounded by glass windows, which now looked down upon a brightly lit Seattle. Along the wall were wooden book cases filled with business books on one end and travel books on the other. Along the shelves were assorted photos in gold frames of him and his family. His family consisted of his wife Ann, daughter Alisha, and his son Noah. Thomas's desk faced the south, so he had an incredible view of Mount Rainer on a clear day… and it was a very clear day, or at least evening. Now that the sun was low in the west, the Columbia Glacier, at the top of the massive mountain, was fully illuminated by alpenglow like a lavender moon. Thomas was sitting behind his polished basalt desk. On the other side of the room was a whole living room of furniture, a working fireplace, book cases, and a ping pong table. Thomas was a champion player in college, as well as a good ice hockey player, or at least that's what he claimed. However,

Curtis was starting to wonder if the man was a habitual embellisher, as some men are. Along the wall was a well-stocked wet bar and kitchenette. Thomas poured two drinks and motioned for Curtis to join him at the couch.

Curtis sat down and sipped the drink. "Wow. That's good. I'm not a big Cognac fan, but if they all tasted like this, I could be."

Thomas, raising his glass, said, "Cheers." Then, after sipping his own drink, he more fully responded to Curtis, "Well, most so-called 'Cognac' is from California or even New Jersey. While California may have mastered the wine industry, I think they're still behind the French in quality Cognac."

Curtis took another sip, put his glass down, and asked, "So, what's up? Did you hear from Mack?"

A big smile came to Thomas's face. "I certainly did. That's why we're celebrating tonight."

"That's great news! So, how much is he underwriting?"

"Our lawyers and his lawyers are ironing out the details, but his initial money investment will be $50 million. There's more to come. But in exchange, I must—temporarily—relinquish majority ownership over to his company."

"How does that affect Neurogenics?"

"Well, Mack having a fifty-one percent ownership puts him in the driver's seat. I personally would become more of a manager until we pay him off. Then we will write in the contract that the patents and controlling interest will revert to us. Yes, I will still be the CEO of Neurogenics, but I would have to answer to Mack as the chairman of the board… until I buy him out some day. Hopefully, that day will be sooner than later."

Curtis started to chuckle. "This is like some maddening game. I mean, I couldn't make the deadlines for Apple Health, so I was in hock for a nine-million-dollar payback. Then you came along to bail me out, which meant me relinquishing my patents to you. So now, to recoup your money, you are selling out to Mack. I don't feel like I'm a goose that has laid anything. I just feel like… well… Chaucer's *goosish*."

"Never read him or know much about him."

"Oh, I became a big fan way back in middle school. I think it made me feel special that I could read him and no one else in my class could understand Middle English."

Curtis took another sip of his drink and then took a cracker and scooped up the shiny black substance in a tin can on the serving tray. "Hum… that is good caviar. Let me guess, you hand-carried it from Russia?"

Thomas just winked at him.

Curtis continued, "Oh, as I was saying, Chaucer referred to people as *goosish*, or goose-like, because they were silly dreamers who never realized the substance of their dreams."

Curtis paused to take one more cracker full of caviar. Since he had only eaten two bags of Bugles all day, he was famished. Then he continued, "You know that my passion was to help people walk. We're on the edge of seeing this put into motion, and I just want to get there. I mean, I haven't seen a paralyzed person made whole since our last human trial, which ended over a year ago. People are suffering, and we are ready to go. This wait is driving me crazy. I have Clayton Emerson trained, and he is as ready as he'll ever be. I'll certainly scrub in on his first few cases. But he's young and a very good surgeon. It'll be hard to keep a good surgeon like him idle for very long. We've a list of patients who are eagerly waiting. There's a few bugs in the OR to work out. We need to hire the rest of our surgery staff, rehab personnel, and get our post-op suites finished. So, I think in four months, we should be starting our first cases."

Thomas smiled and looked down at the coffee table in front of them. He looked back up at Curtis. "Yes, I hope. But again, we must get credentialed by the state as a specialty hospital to do the procedures here and that requires a lot of work. I'm thinking that we will spend Mack's $50 million rather quickly."

Curtis added, "Yes, plus we need to get the Erika Procedure and our facility credentialed by the insurance companies to start the prior authorizations, and that alone can take three months."

Thomas sat up straight in his chair. "I will be direct with you, Curtis," he said, pausing to sip his drink, before adding, "it ain't gonna happen."

Curtis, feeling a bit startled by that statement, asked, "What do you mean it's not going to happen?"

"I know, I promised you when I recruited you, or should I say, *saved* you, from Apple Health, that we would include all payers in our program. But now Mack is in control, and one of the conditions of his grant was that we become a high-end, cash-only facility."

Curtis—sensing a deep sense of betrayal—lashed out, "Like hell, Thomas! I would never have accepted your offer if you hadn't promised me that we would be giving care to all walks of life, not just the wealthy."

Thomas, looking solemn, "Okay, Curtis, if you want to buy your way out of this project, as our contract dictates, simply pay me the nine million, plus interest, and you are a free man. However, you'll never do the Erika Procedure anywhere because we have rightful ownership of the patents. But," and he chuckled, "I'm sure that in another decade you could create another way of doing this that would not infringe upon Erika."

Curtis fell back into his chair and spoke to the air, "I feel some days like I'm living in a freaking nightmare."

Thomas let the silence play out for a few minutes, then he pierced that stillness again, "Hey, man, I know that it's your passion to help as many people as you can help. But we must be realistic. We have debts to pay. But once those debts are paid, and the price of Erika comes down through our greater efficiency, we will approach the insurance companies again. But this is out of our hands now. My man, Raymond Erickson, has done an excellent job in talking with the insurance companies and has struck out. They're not going to pay for the procedure even with your FDA approval and even with the great hope of helping cripples walk."

"None of this makes sense to me." He looked back at Thomas, still with some hostility in his voice. "And, as I said before, please restrain from using that term. Paraplegics and quadriplegics don't like it. 'Cripple' is a state of mind; an SCI is a state of body."

Thomas, obviously wanting the conversation to end, looked at his watch. "Well, Curtis, it's ten thirty, and I bet Becky might be home by now."

Curtis, shaking his head, said, "It may be too late for her, too."

Thomas looked puzzled. "Ten thirty is too late?"

Curtis exhaled slowly. "I wasn't talking about time... but it doesn't matter."

Thomas stood up and put away the Cognac and remaining caviar into his office's bar refrigerator. He got his jacket off the back of his office chair. Curtis walked over to the windows and looked down at the streets of Seattle. The street lights and moving cars, with their white headlights and red taillights, gave the city the look of some exotic festival of lights. He walked around to the other side of the room, facing north. The top of the Space Needle was all aglow in Mariner's teal. This caused him to, reflectively, walk back and look south again. Safeco Field was still radiant even at this late hour. He was surprised how many of the neighboring buildings still had office lights on. He knew that they weren't just left on without occupants. He could see people moving in them. Now, below the buildings, everywhere he looked, north and south, east and west, he saw the city as rhomboids. He said audibly, "Did you ever notice that Seattle, unlike New York, isn't built on a true grid?"

Thomas was so confused by the statement that he chose not to answer. Flipping off the lights and opening his office door, he said, "Curtis... let's go home."

As they walked down the hall to the elevator, Thomas looked at Curtis, who was obviously subjugated by the developments. He put his hand on his shoulder, "Hey, I want to set up a meeting between you and Raymond on Monday. He's very knowledgeable on the payment structures. He's also an expert on health insurance companies. I don't know if you knew this or not, but I recruited him away from Sparta Insurance Company. He was truly an 'inside man' and will explain things that you'd never hear directly from the insurance companies. He started his career as an actuary and is quite good at it. He has some amazing stories to tell."

CHAPTER SIX: ACTUARY

The early July sun was just capturing the peaks of the Olympics to the west. The snow line had climbed the sides of the mountains with each passing week, and now only the tops were iced in. The big green and white Washington State ferries were crawling across the dark Puget waters from Bainbridge and Bremerton like figeater beetles, loaded with sleepy workers for Seattle's hollow and, now, dark offices. Curtis made his way out to his Jeep, with its cloth top down. Leaving it outside and uncovered made sense the previous night when he had parked it under a brilliant firmament of stars. In the summer, showers are rare, but as he sat on the seat, he could feel the chill of wetness seeping in around his buttocks. "Damnit!" he screamed as he punched the steering wheel with the palm of his hand. Sometime during the night, they must have had a brief rain, coming in and then slipping away with the morning owls, leaving no trace in the perfectly clear skies of the new day's dawn. However, now in the dim light, he could make out a few small puddles in the street. He felt guilt for punching his car. He used to be known as a man of patience who never had a temper. Now his fuse was stubby at best.

Curtis contemplated which course of action to take. He turned the key until the clock light came on, at which time—unfortunately— the blaring radio did, too. He quickly turned it down, but within a minute an upstairs light came on in the bedroom window across the street.

It was a quarter to six. He had a scheduled breakfast meeting with Raymond at eight; however, he wanted to check out the new operating theaters, as he had promised Dr. Emerson. Apparently, there were some issues, at least in Clayton's mind, about the way things were coming together. Now Curtis realized that he wouldn't have time to go back into the house to change pants, dry out his seat, and reach downtown before the traffic turned into a sludge. "Damnit!" he said again. Then he turned the key further until the engine fired up and headed to the freeway. He had the choice of going south on Highway 99, across the lofty Aurora Bridge, or taking Interstate 5 south into the city. The distance was equivocal, so it depended on traffic patterns. That morning, I-5 seemed best.

As he drove up onto the six-lane freeway, he thought back to the reason he bought the Jeep in the first place. He and Becky had been penned-up in the city of New York for over six years. Neither of them owned a car, and there was no point. City transportation was adequate, and they never had the time to venture beyond the reach of subways or ferries. But, coming to Seattle, they thought things would be different. Curtis imagined them discovering the North Cascades every weekend… with a tent. He wanted a Jeep so that they could take the longest and most rugged roads into the mountains to get access to the best trails. Yet, now it was two years later, and the Jeep had never seen a dirt road and never had its four-wheel drive engaged, not even once. There was simply no time.

Arriving at the Neurogenics building, Curtis darted from the parking garage to his office. He needed to grab a lab coat off the coat rack behind his office door to cover the wet seat of his pants. He had texted Clay the night before to confirm the time.

When Curtis arrived on the tenth-floor operating area at 6:30, Dr. Emerson was there waiting. He always wore scrubs, even though he wasn't cutting on anyone, at least at their facility. Curtis studied the man as he walked in his direction. The man had almost no body fat, which was perplexing to Curtis. He knew that Clay didn't work out more than walking his Newfoundland each night. He had gone to dinner with the man, and he ate like a horse. Yet he looked like a world-class marathoner. The two men shook hands. Clay was cold toward Curtis, a coldness that was born in the impassive fields of long delays and silent frustrations of the previous three months. This was why Curtis made it such a priority, despite an overwhelming demand on his time. He knew that Clay wasn't happy, and, as Curtis had told Thomas, he knew better than anyone that you cannot keep a brilliant neurosurgeon idle for very long.

They toured the suite, including the two operating theaters, marked "A" and "B." It was Thomas who decided to use the term "operating theaters" rather than "operating rooms." To him, as a nonmedical layperson, "room" gave the impression of a simple and sterile place where things like appendectomies were performed by a simple surgeon with a scalpel, a nurse, and a basin. But Thomas wanted to project something much grander, where bigger performances would ensue, with many characters.

Within these theaters would be surgeons, surgical technicians, electronic technicians, 3-D printer technicians, scrub nurses,

116

anesthesiologists, and a host of other high-skilled individuals making up a well-orchestrated dramatis personae. Above and around each theater was a balcony behind glass, where as many as thirty people could observe each case. Curtis imagined it was where neurosurgeons from around the world would sit and observe before being invited to scrub-in on other cases, learning the hands-on skills needed to bring healing to the remote places of the globe. His hope was to eradicate spinal cord injuries once and for all.

Thomas seemed to cringe when Curtis talked about sharing their secrets with the world. Thomas's imagination ran in a very different direction, seeing news reporters and even TV cameras in the viewing balcony. He wanted them to have enough of a view to be amazed but not enough to see the details that they could duplicate. This was just one of many areas of contention between the surgeons and the business side of Neurogenics.

Indeed, some of the logistical problems that Clay's surgeon's eye had caught were structural flaws that had originated with Thomas's design team. His team, while talented, had the hearts of artists and marketers and didn't appreciate the technical side of the procedure.

The pre-op area, for example, had 20-foot ceilings. It gave the grandiose feeling of being in a museum or ballroom. It also gave a viewpoint from the surgical observation balcony's side windows. Thomas thought that guests should not only be able to watch the procedure but also see the care that goes into the preparation for surgery.

117

The only problem with this arrangement was that the lighting from such a high ceiling cast shadows that made it hard for them to do their work. The scene looked good from above, as was intended, but was not functional for the staff. The operating theaters had the same layout but had surgical lights just above the table, and the surgeons would also be wearing headlamps. This was not true in the pre-op area. Clay pointed this out to Curtis and asked him, "How in the hell can we even start an IV in here, not to mention all the preps we must do?" He rubbed the top of his slick head as he always did when he was stressed.

Curtis kept a list of glitches as Clay pointed them out. He promised Clay that each one would be remedied before their opening day, even if it meant a total remodel.

Curtis sensed that Clay was satisfied with his visit and his pledge to help. They shook hands. Curtis glanced at his phone to see that he had missed six voicemails already, and it wasn't even 7:30. He turned away from the surgical suite, studying the voicemail numbers as he walked. His phone indicated that four of them were from his mother. While waiting on the elevator (which seemed to be stuck on the basement floor), he punched the voicemail button and began listening to the first message. Clay suddenly reappeared at the elevator door. Curtis put the phone down and looked at him with raised eyebrows.

"Hey, Curtis. I wanted you to know that I have interviewed at Harborview."

Curtis felt a punch in his gut. He slipped the phone back into his lab coat pocket. "Come on, man. I'm sorry about how busy things are for me and the long delays in getting started, but you are key to this endeavor. You'll never be on the ground floor of something like this anywhere else in the world. Not at Mass General, not at Johns Hopkins, Mayo, and certainly not at Harborview."

Clay, shrugging his shoulders, said, "Well, they have a fantastic package… they, too, are doing some exciting things in Parkinson's surgery. They even showed me a new prefrontal procedure that might cure severe depression and anxiety for some patients. They will be starting trials later this year."

As the elevator door opened, Curtis stepped in, and he turned around and looked Clay in the eye. "Please, can you give us four weeks to fix things?"

Clay seemed to be nodding in the affirmative as the door closed.

Curtis briefly considered what a nightmare it would be if they tried to get the program off the ground and he was the only trained neurosurgeon on the team. He texted Thomas: "Think about giving Clay a raise. He's considering his other options."

Rather than meeting on the Neurogenics campus, Raymond wanted to meet in the downtown Sheraton's lobby restaurant called the Daily Grill. It was a four-blocks walk from the Neurogenics campus. Fortunately, it was on the downhill side.

Curtis walked briskly toward the waterfront, still wearing his lab coat to cover his wet ass. Once again, he felt the asymmetry of the street intersections as he crossed each one. It was so plain to him now, while for almost two years he hadn't noticed.

A homeless man—apparently a near quadriplegic—sat in an old, beat-up wheelchair at the edge of one of those abstruse corners. Curtis observed him carefully in his peripheral vision as he crossed the street. The man was wearing an army surplus jacket with a German black, red, and yellow flag on the sleeve. He was smoking a cigarette in a silver cigarette holder, which was wrapped— corkscrew-like—in the end of the coat hanger wire. The other end of the hanger wire was folded into a handle, like that of a flyswatter. He manipulated the cigarette to his tarred lips by holding the handle end between his thumb and forefinger, which lay on the arm of the chrome chair. The rest of his hand and his tattooed arm were quite atrophied. Strangely, on his lap was a dark oak offering plate with a green felt bottom, obviously commandeered from a church. A few coins were laying in it.

He saw Curtis's donning of a lab coat as being advantageous to his needs. "Hey, doctor, give me some dough, man! You've got plenty," the panhandler shouted.

As Curtis passed in front of the man without making direct eye contact—except for an accidental glance—the man mumbled audibly, "Selfish asshole!"

A block away, Curtis entered the main doors of the hotel. He paused to ask a bellhop where the restaurant was located. The man in the red coat pointed down the hall. Through the glass doors he could see Raymond seated and sipping coffee from a white mug. Raymond was a short man with a thick head of brown hair, more so than you would expect for a middle-aged man. He was heavy, carrying most of his weight in his torso. His face had a perpetually oily appearance that gave the impression he was an animated wax figure. Curtis never figured out if this was caused by him using an oily lotion as part of his morning ritual or if his appearance was from a natural adiposity.

Raymond wore designer suits with gold or diamond cufflinks and brash—almost clownish—ties. He had a reputation, as a numbers man, of being extremely punctual. Curtis looked at his watch: it was seven minutes after eight. He walked in and greeted him, "Good morning, Raymond."

"You're late," Raymond said without making eye contact.

In a moment's flash, Curtis felt an anger brewing in his chest but quickly suppressed it with a pretense of gratitude. "Oh, thanks so much for agreeing to meet me here." Then he gently lowered himself in the chair across from the big man.

Raymond looked up with a sour face. "Well, this is where I have breakfast every morning and read the *Journal*… the *Wall Street Journal*. I guess I'll just have to read it later."

121

Curtis didn't know how to take this, as an unprejudiced statement or complaint. The waitress came, and he ordered food immediately from the menu. He decided to order something healthy and filling because he had been living on junk food for weeks. He asked for two scrambled eggs, three slices of Canadian bacon, tomato juice, and a bowl of granola.

Raymond sipped his coffee and looked sternly at Curtis and asked, "Do you know what an actuary does?"

"Well, I have an idea. It's someone who looks at statistics and tries to predict risks."

Raymond rolled his eyes a bit and smiled. "Well, that's the superficial understanding of the field; however, it's far more developed than that now. It's a true science, just as much as medicine, and it's an important branch of mathematics. Going back to the Greeks and then Romans, financial interests were always tied to risks. If the math could have figured the probability of a shipment of olive oil reaching Egypt or the likelihood of an individual dying and not being able to pay his debts, it would have been of great value. However, the forecasting of risks wasn't married to the science of statistics until John Graunt did so in 1662. He showed that there were predictable patterns of death in certain groups of people based on previous death and mortality statistics. This was a profound change for the insurance companies." Curtis was silently staring, so Raymond asked, with intensity, "Are you listening to me?"

"Of course."

Raymond continued, "Prior to this, insurance was like playing the roulette wheel in Vegas. Once the field of actuary science was perfected, it became a virtual gold mine for insurance companies. Nothing happens by chance in the companies anymore, or at least not the good ones. Everything is highly calculated. Insurance companies after that point knew exactly what to charge someone for life insurance, knowing with absolute certainty that they would make money. What was previously a game of chance became a game where the house always wins." Leaning into the table, he added in a hushed tone, with his fork pointed at Curtis's nose, "and I mean *always*."

"Okay," said Curtis as he leaned back and way from Raymond's Tabasco breath. He was starting to think that the man was making points about his distinguished profession because he felt intimidated working with doctors, and he wanted them to know that he was highly trained as well. He decided to ask directly, but tactfully, "Raymond, I know that your time is valuable, so why don't we get to the information that Thomas thought that I should know."

"I'm getting to that point, but it is important that you know where I'm coming from first."

"Okay," said Curtis, as the small Asian waitress served him his food. He smiled and thanked her. She smiled back before turning and walking away. Curtis took this phase of listening as an opportunity to eat… and he was hungry.

"As I was saying," Raymond continued, "actuarial science became extremely important to the insurance industry. This new science was what allowed these companies to move beyond insuring payloads of ships coming from the Far East, and the chances of someone dying, to creating health insurance. Once they could predict not only when someone would die, but when they would get sick and—most importantly—the cost of treating that sickness, they could offer a guarantee of payment based on a set of premiums."

With a piece of whole-wheat toast in his mouth, Curtis nodded and mumbled, "Sure," as crumbs tumbled down his shirt. He dusted them off with his hand and continued to listen.

"Because we knew the risk ratios, meaning the risk of payment for care as a ratio of income from the premiums, the health insurance companies became one of the richest and most powerful industries the world has ever known."

Raymond paused for a moment to check his cellphone for messages and then looked back up. "The first major use of computers wasn't putting people on the moon, but figuring out exactly—in real time—people's chances of getting cancer, or MS, or emphysema. A lot of things we know about disease states came from insurance-funded studies. While that information was helpful to public health epidemiologists, the original purpose was to increase revenues for the insurance companies."

Curtis cleared his throat and spoke up. "But how does this relate to us? Are you going to tell me that the insurance companies will see the Erika Procedure as too risky for the premium?"

"It is more complicated than that." Raymond sat up in his chair and finished off his coffee. He looked at the waitress and held up two fingers and mouthed, "Two checks." Curtis let it go, although he was prepared to pay the bill for both.

Raymond leaned forward onto his two elbows, which were firmly planted on the table. He put his face close to Curtis's again. He spoke in a quelled voice, just above a whisper, "So, you know that Thomas is a world traveler?"

"Sure."

"I bet you didn't know that he was fascinated with Russian history, especially the reign of the Tsars."

Curtis was shaking his head.

"Did you notice the set of Matryoshka, or what some would call 'nesting' dolls, on the shelf in his office?"

"No, but we had some fine caviar from Russia the other night."

"Insurance companies are like those Matryoshkas with layers upon layers of confidentiality. I was the chief actuarial officer at Sparta Insurance, which is the fourth largest in the US by subscribers and, I am proud to say, by profits. I was with the innermost figure of our Matryoshkas, the baby carved from a single piece of wood. We—

the baby at the center—were a team of six or seven executives who had a contractual allegiance and a singularity of intention. We were sworn to our secrets for life. I have violated that agreement by the things I've told Thomas and the things I'm about to tell you. If they knew that I was talking about this, they could sue me for millions of dollars. So, I am asking you to promise that what I tell you, you tell no one. Not any of our staff, not your wife, not your priest… not anyone."

Curtis, sipping his last swallow of tomato juice, hesitated for a moment but then said, "Sure. I hope this doesn't mean that you must have me killed after you tell me?" Then he flashed a broad smile.

Raymond didn't reciprocate with a show of humor at the corny statement, instead continuing, "Well, this is a serious issue. Our inner circle, and I'm sure all insurance companies have such management teams, met in private. We didn't keep records of our conversations. We never communicated electronically or by paper. You could hack us and come up blank… not a trace. I mean, it was a rather cloak-and-dagger existence."

For the first time, Curtis was becoming interested—genuinely interested—in this topic. His curiosity was expressed in his body language, laying down his spoon, resting his chin on his fists, and looking directly into Raymond's eyes beneath their oily lids.

Raymond eased back in his chair. Noticing Curtis's elevation in level of attention, the big man continued with slightly more vigor. He looked around them, as to make sure no one was within an eavesdropping range. "We were renting time on supercomputers to run large models of patient populations. Our innermost group, like the baby in the middle, worked carefully with these models. We had one goal and that was success, and success was defined by profits. It wasn't defined by better health for our subscribers or even their satisfaction. At the same time, the outermost doll was a facade, carefully generated by our marketing people, projecting a kind of not-for-profit altruistic society devoted to good health. We were to portray our corporate selves as the loving mothers who wanted our subscribers to wear a scarf when they went out in the cold and to treat the first signs of a sniffle. At the center, we hoped that they didn't treat their sniffle, unless it would save us money in the end, and we didn't care if they died. If the subscriber became chronically sick, we hoped they died and died quickly. That's why most health insurances don't offer a death benefit because it would be a 'conflict of interest'."

Curtis asked, "But none of this is too surprising for me. I knew that insurance was a business like any other."

Raymond sighed, closed his eyes for a few seconds, and continued, "I'm not finished yet, Curtis. You can't begin to imagine how finely-tuned the models were. Based on statistics, we knew who would get sick, what sickness they would have, how much it would cost to treat it, and how much it would cost us to ignore it."

"Were your models ever wrong?" asked Curtis.

"Damn right they could go wrong. I wouldn't be here today if it wasn't for one huge mistake."

Curtis was assuming Raymond had made the mistake and was fired. He was surprised that the big man with the even larger ego would be so humble as to share that story. But he would soon learn that it wasn't Raymond who made a miscalculation.

Raymond continued, "I was an assistant actuary at Sparta in 2008 when we started negotiating, along with all the other insurance companies, with the Obama Administration. The administration knew that it couldn't implement a pure government program because the powerful insurance lobby would never allow that, even if the people wanted it... and I'm not sure they do. A socialized, single-payer health care system would be too radical for them to accept at once, and that was a political problem. But this involvement of the insurance industry was mostly to appease the Republicans who wanted only a purely commercial program with no government role, except for Medicare and vouchers for the poor. But both the Democrats and the Republicans needed money for their re-election campaigns, and that year the insurance companies provided about $200 million to sit at the table. Sparta alone invested almost $5 million. So, we were invited to the table, too."

"In the developing world, that would be called a bribe," said Curtis.

"Well, it is the M.O. of getting things done in Washington, the other Washington. My boss believed that we could come out ahead if we participated in the government-sponsored health care program, as did all the actuaries. The models predicted that mostly it was the young and healthy who were uninsured. If we could bring them into the ranks of the insured for $500 or $600 a month, we figured that in the end our profits would increase by 25 percent. I was skeptical. I ran the numbers myself. The models they were using didn't account for those young people who were sick but untreated and that, as soon as they had insurance, would become big users, playing catch-up. I had people in my ex-wife's family who were in this situation. The models projected their future use on their past use, and I thought that would be a huge mistake, and it was. In the end, I was correct. The bill was signed in 2010, and by 2013, Sparta had lost $300 million on the program." Pausing to wink at Curtis, he then continued, "or at least that is how they portrayed it to the public. The truth was, they still made a profit, but had only increased their profits by five percent, not the twenty-five percent that was predicted. They wanted the other twenty percent."

He gazed at Curtis for a moment to weigh his level of captivation. Curtis seemed to still be listening.

"Their only recourse was to tighten the noose around all subscribers and all providers of care, trying to wring out of them the dollars we expected to make, but didn't, under the Affordable Care Act."

Raymond finished paying his check and signed for the credit card. Curtis noticed that it was a Neurogenics corporate card and pondered why Raymond hadn't offered to put his breakfast on it, too. It wasn't a big deal, just a curiosity.

Raymond continued, "With a $300 million profit unrealized, my boss was forced to take an early retirement, and I stepped into his shoes. Because I was right, I got his office and his salary… and ironically," he had a soft chuckle, "I ended up with his wife, too, but that's another story." Raymond seemed a bit surprised at the words that had just come out of his own mouth, and he paused to recollect his thoughts. "It was because I had such a high position that I caught Thomas's eye when he needed someone like me. I, too, was sick of it."

Curtis was squinting like he was thinking hard. "So, how does that involve me and Neurogenics? I'm having a hard time making the connection to Erika."

Raymond continued, "So, like I said, the outer shell is what we project to the public. The next two layers are innocent suckers. These are midlevel managers who honestly believe in the company and in the mission statement. We need these suckers, and our inner group called them the 'suckers' behind their backs. They were necessary to keep the facade propped up. But, behind the scenes, we were looking at things from a purely for-profit perspective, and we had the tools, the super-computer models, to do just that. So, we determined which subscribers were salvageable—meaning economically salvageable for our company alone. For example, the models told us that if one of our subscribers was diagnosed with MS, and there was a treatment available that would greatly enhance the patient's quality of life, allowing that treatment may not be the best for us. If this subscriber with MS has a higher quality of life, they'll continue working, paying the maximum premiums allowed, which is around twelve hundred a month, but we would still lose severely. The cost of their drugs alone would be five thousand per month. So, our strategy was to get them off our insurance. By law we could no longer just drop them. We called these people 'Deficits'. We had two ways to get them off our insurance enrollments. The first way was to deny the care they needed, hoping that they would either deteriorate to the point of becoming disabled… or die. If they were disabled, they wouldn't be working any longer and wouldn't be subscribers for our insurance. They would become Medicare's responsibility at that point. If they died, that would be a good thing for us because we don't offer death benefits. Of course, some would just be fed up by our poor customer service and find another insurance company, which would be good for us, too. It was a win-win."

Raymond paused to fold up his newspaper, then continued, "Our poor customer service was no accident. Having poor service was highly calculated. In some ways, it became an art form. We had to pretend we were doing the best we could, and those employees on the front lines thought they were doing the best they could. However, we made sure they didn't have the resources to succeed. We didn't want a good customer service, especially for Deficits. Do you see why this group had to be so secret?"

"I do," said Curtis, "but how do you control policy without subscribers getting suspicious?"

"I was hoping you would ask that. That's where the next shell of our corporate organization came in. These were the vice presidents, who were in charge of different regions and represented the inner-most doll outside our group, the 'baby' at the core. They weren't privy to our inner group plans and frankly weren't even sure we existed. They also didn't totally believe the full story, and neither did the midlevel managers. They were our conduits of policy and information to outer shells and the public. So, say in the example of the MS patient where there is a new treatment that is very promising, we would find ways to discredit the treatment. We could often get away with just saying that it was 'still experimental.' Our PR people were highly skilled in framing this in the most positive light. They would describe how Sparta was deeply concerned about our members' safeties and wouldn't support any treatment that wasn't proven to be safe and effective beyond a doubt. We redefined it as caring for our subscribers, just like that Jewish mother and the chicken soup. At the same time, at the inner level, we were plotting—thanks to our models—the demise of that person, which meant either getting them off our rolls, or a more literal demise."

It crossed Curtis's mind that Raymond, who was short on personality to start with, maybe was just a disgruntled ex-employee and embellishing the story, so he asked, "This story sounds quite cynical, Raymond. Did other team members see the company in this light?"

"Are you kidding me? Who gave a damn? Our CEO was making almost $100 million a year in salary and bonuses. We were each making more money than we ever dreamt of. Greed is the great equalizer. There were no Republicans, Democrats, atheists, or Christians in the group… meaning that those labels took a back seat to the money driving the car."

He leaned over and said, in a whisper, "Dr. Eisner, once you've had a taste of money, real money, the appetite for it becomes insatiable. The dollar is more addictive than crack cocaine." He sat back up, sipped the last of his black coffee, sat it down, and then leaned back over the table, only farther this time with his face inches from Curtis's. "I remember the first time I saw two commas in my portfolio." Then his mouth morphed into a little smirk, "I started to get an erection." He winked at Curtis and sat back up, wiping drops of sweat off his upper lip with his napkin. Then he added, "One day, and maybe one day soon, you're going to find out for yourself."

Curtis moved farther back in his chair to create more personal space. Then, shaking his head, he added, "I'm sorry, Raymond, but I have a hard time believing the entire insurance industry is built on greed."

Raymond was taken aback and sat up in his chair. "Well, I'm not saying that all the low-level employees were out to just make a buck. The financial gains rested mainly at the top tier. But to be fair to the insurance companies, if they paid for everything that worked, they would be forced to charge everyone a few grand a month for premiums or go bankrupt."

He then looked intensely at Curtis, leaned back over the table, and continued, "Now, before we run out of time, let me make this very personal. Your Erika Procedure came across our desks and was reviewed by our team as a new treatment for spinal cord injuries while I was still at Sparta. This, of course, was along with many other new drugs and procedures. We debated the choice if we should get involved with you or not. We ran models that showed that we could save some money at the beginning if someone went from a high-maintenance quadriplegic to a fully functional human being who continued paying premiums for years to come." Raymond pointed his finger at Curtis's nose. "Now remember, these models are on supercomputers using the latest data and facts. These same computers are used for complex and long-term weather forecasting. In other words, they're smart, damn smart... like doing a billion calculations per second... or something like that. Our models showed us that, in the end, Erika would be a net loss for us. So, if we paid $500,000 for the procedure and rehab, and considering a five percent total failure rate and a thirty-seven percent chance of complications, the average cost per patient came to $680,000. This means, to break even, that patient would have to pay premiums at the high end, say—for the sake of convenience— $1,000 per month, for"... Raymond looked up into the air to his right and mumbled numbers, using his fingers to carry the imaginary numbers from one side to another... "forty-eight and a third years. Now that's just to break even. Plus, if you add to the equation the regular health problems that a normal—healthy person—would experience in that time, twisted ankles, flu, annual check-ups, you would have to add six more years to the equation. Next, the models show us that if someone suffered a SCI at age 28.7—the average age of a spinal cord injury—and then the Erika Procedure worked perfectly, that person would then be closing in on seventy-seven years of age before we recouped our money. Only then could we move them out of the deficit category. However, they would be leaving our insurance at age sixty-five anyway when they went on Medicare. The numbers get skewed even more because the patient, in their final decade before Medicare, enters the high health care consumer years. During that period, their health care costs start to rise dramatically. Because they already had a SCI and are at the top of the premium payment schedule, as allowed by federal law under the Affordable Care Act, we cannot use a graduated premium scale like we can for other people. So, we could raise a healthy man who was paying $600 per month to $800 when he turns forty-five and then $1,000 per month at age sixty. But these SCI patients are already at $1,000 per month."

Curtis, literally scratching his head, asked, "But, you didn't include the dividends of not having to maintain a quadriplegic, which can be very expensive."

Raymond sat back in his chair again and smiled big. "You are mostly correct, Dr. Eisner. However, there is one caveat. The average duration that someone keeps a health insurance policy is 4.8 years. This is from moving, changing jobs, going back to school, and a host of other reasons. So, if we were to spend $580,000 on one of your Erika Procedures, there is no way in hell we would recoup half of that money by reduced medical costs. There would not be enough "credits"—meaning people who pay premiums that are well above their cost—to make up the difference. This may sound horrible, but this is business—profitable—business. Wall Street and our stock holders loved us, but they didn't know and didn't want to know what happened within our core group. The politicians loved us, too, both Republican and Democrats. They loved our contributions to their coffers. All of them chose to believe the same propaganda that we were telling the rest of the public. We knew that if we allowed the disabled to lay in their own urine and feces—to be graphic—that eventually they would go on Medicare and the feds would foot their bill. It was a win-win situation for us to reject the Erika Procedure."

Curtis looked shaken and disturbed. "But Raymond, how do the insurance companies get away with this behavior?"

"It's easy. We hired the best PR people in the world and had highly skilled midlevel managers. Step one, as I said, was simply to say that the procedure wasn't proven to be safe or effective, which we knew was a lie. But we also used more discursive approaches as well."

Curtis, looking down at his clock on his phone then back up, said, "Hey, why don't we walk back up to the office together and finish this conversation along the way?"

"Sure," replied Raymond. He grabbed his briefcase, which Curtis hadn't noticed was under the table, before struggling to go from sitting to standing as if he had bad knees. The two men exited the restaurant and, while walking through the lobby, Raymond continued his conversation. "As I was saying, we had other ways to discredit treatments that we knew wouldn't be in our best financial interest. If we wanted to cast doubt, we would assign someone for this sole purpose."

They came to the revolving glass door leading to the street. Curtis, realizing that they wouldn't both fit in one section, paused to let Raymond go through on his own.

Curtis could see Raymond continuing to talk outside the door while he was still inside, unable to hear him. Curtis hastily walked through the revolving door and caught up with him. They walked across the porte-cochère, turned the corner, and started to walk up the hill on Madison. With a surprised look in his face, Curtis added, "You would invest that much energy into discrediting treatments?"

Raymond grabbed him by the elbow to halt his walk. "Listen, you still don't get it? One biologic immunosuppressant, if we had covered it, would cost us tens of millions at least. So, hell yeah, it was worth the investment."

"But how would you go about it? Just by putting out bad PR?"

About that time, Curtis's eye caught the eye of the man in the wheelchair, who was still panhandling at the corner. Curtis flashed him a smile. The man, now with a new, long, white cigarette in his makeshift holder, slowly and awkwardly raised his weak right arm, still clasping the coat hanger holder between the thumb and forefinger of his atrophied hand. Curtis now noticed the braces on both wrists. The man struggled and slowly extended his middle finger toward him. The intent was clear. That was the second *finger* that he had been given in one week. Rather than feeling offended by the hateful gesture, Curtis was thinking of the man's cervical anatomy that would allow this limited use of his hands in this way... probably a C5 or C6 SCI.

Raymond's voice faded to the background of Curtis's mind. He instead reflected on his mentor, Lennard Jacobs, as he had cautioned Curtis that SCIs impact the entire spectrum of humanity. They don't make hateful and dysfunctional people out of nice people. The nice people seem to stay nice and do the best they can do with what they have. He would often point out that the late Christopher Reeves was the architype of such decency and courage in the wake of a severe SCI. Those who were angry assholes before their injury often remain assholes afterward—only now they were bitter assholes. He remembered Lennard chuckling and saying, "It's like marriage. A woman who has a jealous and abusive boyfriend... if she marries the bastard... then has a jealous and abusive husband. Marriage didn't make him that way and it didn't—despite her hopes—save him, either."

Raymond was oblivious to the brief interaction between Curtis and the man in the wheelchair. He didn't see the man. He looked over at Curtis and smiled, "Yeah, but drafting the PR wasn't exactly step one. Our man, or woman, assigned to this project would dig up dirt. They would go through every study that had ever been done, published or not. They would look at every adverse event, every failure, and use that data to support the finding that we can't cover that treatment. We would frame it as because we had 'concerns' for our subscribers, which was pure bullshit."

Curtis said questioningly, as he paused at the next crossing waiting for the pedestrian light to change in their favor, "The public would accept that verdict from an insurance company?"

Raymond laughed and added, "We had our own, so-called 'experts' on the payroll who would make the final decision. They were usually someone in the general field with no expertise in the specific treatment under consideration. For example, we might have a carpal tunnel surgeon review the Erika Procedure. These physicians would create the illusion for the public that it was a thoughtful, expert opinion that the procedure should not be covered. While it would be illegal to pay them to recommend denial of treatments, these hired guns understood that it was in the best interest of their employer to recommend denial of the procedure. We would never ask a neurosurgeon who actually was an expert on SCIs for their opinion. It was too damn risky. They might, and probably would, recommend that we cover the treatment because they knew what they were talking about."

They came to a covered, purple bus stop and Raymond put his briefcase on the bench and leaned on the post to catch his breath. After a couple of deep sighs, he continued, "It wasn't unheard of for us to protect our vested interests by doing our own studies as well. When you read about a study that concludes a cheaper treatment is as effective as a costlier one, for example, physical therapy being as good—or better—than back surgery, I can guarantee that an insurance company footed the bill for that study. Well, unless it was a group of physical therapists who were looking out for their own interest. The insurance companies would also carefully design the study to end up with the conclusion they wanted. If the study started to show the opposite, they would shred it and pretend it never happened. These studies would never be conducted independently by back surgeons because they, too, have a secondary gain." He picked up his briefcase and started to walk up the hill again.

"So, basically, you're telling me that the Ericka Procedure is dead in the water when it comes to reimbursement by insurance companies?" asked Curtis.

"Dead as a cod fish in the Sahara. They will fight you tooth and nail to the end. Eventually, an insurance company might cave in… but even that's not the end. The computer models were also very effective in showing us how to avoid paying for something even if we agreed to cover it."

Curtis looked over at him and gave a contorted smile. "You lost me there, Raymond."

They were turning the corner as the Neurogenics building came in to sight. Curtis was feeling short of breath himself after the four-block walk up the hill. It was hard for him to imagine that he used to be a runner. But then he looked at Raymond who was sweating profusely, as if he were toying with a myocardial infarction.

As they approached the side entrance to the building, Raymond stopped walking again to catch his breath. He pulled a handkerchief from his pocket and wiped his brow, now dotted with drops of a cool perspiration. "Remember, we used numbers and supercomputers. We created a 'prior authorization' process that gave the appearance of coverage but would never allow to occur. Maybe, for PR sake—and if the treatment wasn't exorbitantly costly—we would allow one or two to go through just to prove that we indeed covered it. But, to keep most out, our 'prior auth' process had flaws and complexities… by design." Raymond winked. "The failures were intentional. Do you get it?"

Curtis, shaking his head, said, "Actually, no. I don't get it."

Raymond continued, "Our computer models showed us that, if we had a limited number of personnel processing those prior authorizations, we wouldn't only save money on salaries but save much more through intended errors by overwhelmed staff. We would increase the paperwork burden on the providers, be they hospitals or individual medical providers. They would finally give up or go broke. It was our fantasy that every doctor, every PA, every NP or other medical provider in the country, would go bankrupt. Without medical providers, there could be no medical care provided… and therefore nothing for us to pay for. But that was just a fantasy. Our frontline staff were so overwhelmed that they would usually quit after a year, creating more shortages in our favor and more new replacements who had no clue what they were doing. I know this sounds sinister, but this tipping point was well-calculated. We had no financial incentive to streamline the process… none whatsoever."

They walked through the door into the first-floor hallway of the Neurogenics building, not far from Curtis's office, which was one floor below. Curtis looked both ways and saw quite a few people passing by, some he knew and greeted, a couple he didn't know. Fortunately, no one interrupted them with some new crisis that Curtis was supposed to immediately fix. Then he said to Raymond, "Hey, would you mind coming down to my office for just a minute? I'd rather talk in private."

Raymond looked at his watch. "Okay, for a minute. I do want to finish this discussion, but I also need to get up to my office as I have a conference call with the state of Washington at ten."

They took the stairs down one flight and turned down the basement hall. Curtis unlocked his office door, and they walked in. Raymond, being a man of order, seemed astounded at the bedlam of the place. "Uh, Curtis… where do I sit?"

Curtis took a new box of mail off the sofa, pointed, and said, "Here."

Raymond took out his handkerchief freshly damp from his brow's sweat and dusted off the couch. He moved with an awkward stiffness, like he was afraid to touch anything. Then he laid the handkerchief down and sat on it. His heavy weight caused the cushion beneath him to compress so much that the tower of US

Post Office boxes next to him on the couch toppled over into the floor. Curtis said hastily, "Just leave them."

Raymond sat up straight, so his back would have no contact with the back cushion, as if it had unknown microbes on it. He looked up at Curtis, who was sitting three feet away from him at his desk. The big man continued, "So, our models showed us how to incorporate interferences into the prior authorization process. I will be more specific." Raymond took a deep breath and gathered his thoughts once more. "With limited personnel available on our side, the provider's office would call and be on hold for ten minutes, thirty minutes, or even an hour. The poor suckers in our prior authorization office had no clue they were pawns in a very sophisticated game built on well-thought-out algorithms. This game had been well-orchestrated and rehearsed thousands of times within our computer models. We knew exactly how many personnel to have. We also knew exactly how many minutes they would stay on hold and repetitive attempts an office would make before they gave up."

Raymond cleared his throat, leaned further toward Curtis, and continued, "Our computer models say that most people will hang up after twenty-five minutes on hold." He chuckled and added, "We could even shorten how long the caller would remain on hold by playing bad country music anywhere outside the south and Hammond organ music—show tunes to be exact—in the south."

About that time, Carolyn knocked on the office door and opened it. "Oh, I'm sorry, Dr. Eisner. I didn't realize that you had company.

We do have several people in the office wanting to talk to you. I've been putting off Dan Mitchell for a couple of weeks. He is the journalist with the biotech journal."

Raymond stood up. "I think we're done here anyway… right, Curtis?"

Carolyn added as she was leaving, "Okay, just let me know when you are ready, and I will send him down." She left, closing the door behind her.

"So, Raymond, what you're saying is that it would be very, very difficult to get our procedure covered by insurance companies, and therefore it would be out of reach for most normal people?"

"That's right. Business is a cruel world." Raymond smiled, gave a quick wink, and exited the room.

CHAPTER SEVEN: JENNIFER

With the door closed, Curtis, in his office alone, was contemplating if Raymond was being honest with him or embellishing the level of cruelty for dramatic effect. He knew that even within the insurance world, there had to be some people of compassion and Raymond's view must come with a bias. However, he was starting to feel the greatest sense of loss that he had felt in a long time. He gazed into his screensaver, an image of two old Italian men with coffee, sitting on the hull of their royal-blue fishing boat, on the waterfront, with the village of Riomaggiore as their backdrop. Within the silence of the moment, he coveted their lifestyles with great passion. He wished that he too, only had to be concerned with the migration of sardines.

In a way, he was glad that Lennard had not lived to see this day. His own disenchantment had been building for months, but his meeting with Raymond seemed to be the nadir of that progression. As a physician, he kept telling himself not to listen to those inner voices of despair. He had always been a self-starter, but the mental fatigue was getting the best of him. When he moved to Seattle, he thought he saw the light at the end of the tunnel. But now he felt that it was only the taillights of the train ahead of him, grinding deeper and downward into the dark abyss. *Deflated* was the word that kept coming into his mind. He felt lonely, and it was a concentrated loneliness. He missed Lennard and felt the grief of the wife and two sons, whom the great man of science had left behind.

Becky, the love of his own life—growing more aloof—was also part of Curtis's grief. His, solitude of the soul, was no different than what an early American solo explorer would have experienced in the western wilderness. But at least they had their privacy as their friend. Curtis felt intensely alone but within the context of a suffocating crowd and crushing responsibilities. There is a way that a mob of people can leave you isolated—at least isolated from people who care for your soul.

He sat on the couch and rubbed his face. He pulled out his phone only to see two more missed calls from his mother. He had forgotten about the previous ones. He was hoping to see something from Becky. A text message would be fine, a voicemail even better. He was worried about her and their derelict romance. They had rough spots before, but never this serious. Curtis felt a lot of guilt about that.

But, in some ways, his entire life had been a river of shame. Those who knew him professionally would never have guessed he carried such guilt. At times, his culpability was like the mighty Amazon, with thousands of tributaries flowing from dark and convoluted places. These streams let through an incursion of black waters into the core of his being. He often wondered if his father left them because he didn't want children. Maybe if he had never been born into this miserable world, his father would have never left his mother, and they would have been forever happy. What kind of father would leave without saying goodbye to his only son? Only a father that despised the boy.

One haunting tributary was the one that had directed his life's work. It was an unfulfilled promise to a teenaged girl. If he had never made that ludicrous promise, would his life be better now? Would he be spending his days trying to fix unfixable, broken backs for piles of cash with no concerns about tomorrow? Maybe he would be living in Jonesborough, as his mother wanted, and be the town doctor. Maybe he would be living with her and giving her the kind of care and company, she deserved. He felt horrible leaving her in the hands of strangers.

The thought that something could be seriously wrong with his mother, and maybe that was why she was continuously calling, now intruded upon his flow of random thoughts. Closing in on eighty, she was in a state of remarkably good health. He pushed on her highlighted name his phone, and it started to ring. In a moment, he heard her familiar voice. "Hello."

"Hi, Mom."

"Curtis… thank heavens you're okay."

"Why wouldn't I be?"

"I haven't heard a word from you in a month. You used to always call me every Sunday. Is everything alright?"

"Yes, Mom. I've been busy."

"Too busy to talk to your mother for a few minutes? You know you're all I have in this world, and if something were to happen to me, you're the only person I could call."

"Mom, as I said before, I set up the alarm system for you. All you have to do is push the button on your bracelet, and they'll immediately talk to you and send help if you need it. No one can break in without the police getting a notice."

"Curtis, do you still love me? When you were a boy you loved your mother so much."

"Of course I do, Mom! That's a silly question. I've always loved you and always will. Why would you even ask something crazy like that?"

There was silence on the other end of the phone… then she spoke, "It's been over a year since I've seen you. When are you coming out?"

"I don't know, Mom. I hope soon. We need to get our program going again. Mom, we are about to bring hope to thousands of people who can't walk."

Those words didn't bring her any comfort, and Curtis didn't receive any praise from her as he had hoped. Her voice continued to be sour. "Curtis, did you forget my birthday?"

Curtis sank into the couch and put his head down with his left hand over his eyes. "Mom… I'm so sorry. It completely skipped my mind."

"Oh, I guess it doesn't matter. Women my age shouldn't be celebrating birthdays anyway. But it was the first time in seventy-nine years that I spent my birthday alone without a single call, without a card… nothing and…" her voice began to break a bit, "I just feel lonely."

Curtis, feeling even more guilt-ridden, said, "Mom, if it makes you feel any better, I feel lonely, too."

With a distorted kind of chuckle in her voice, she responded, "I don't think so. You have your important job and go to work every day. You have that beautiful and sweet wife of yours to come home to every night. So, why would you say that you're lonely?"

"Mom, you can be surrounded by people and still be lonely."

About that time, a knock came on his office door. There stood Carolyn and a short, balding man in black jeans donning a black Grateful Dead tee-shirt and a green sports jacket. Carolyn, not seeing his phone in his right hand, spoke, "Dr. Eisner, this is Mr. Dan Mitchell with the *Technology Investors Journal.* He had an appointment with you, actually it was last week, and he's back." Carolyn, now getting a glimpse of his cellphone in his hand, quickly added, "Oh, sorry boss… are you on the phone?"

Curtis put the phone back to his ear and heard his mother saying, "Curtis? Curtis? Are you still there?"

"Yes, Mom. I'm here. Mom, there's someone here to see me, and I need to go. I promise I will be down to Tennessee to see you within a month."

"Really! That would be great. Is there any special food you are missing?"

"Mom, I must go. We can talk about that later, bye-bye," and he stuck his phone back in his lab coat pocket without waiting for his mother to say goodbye.

The timing seemed terrible for Curtis to do an interview about the future of his technology with an investment journal. Honestly, on the inside, he felt quite pessimistic having just learned that the insurance companies would never be on board. Maybe in a week the cloud of discouragement would have lifted, but he couldn't stand the man up again to hold out for a better personal disposition.

He had to speak with caution. He knew if he said anything wrong, Neurogenics' reputation would plummet and their value would be diminished. He knew he had to put on a face of optimism.

Mr. Mitchell had the type of enthusiasm that you would expect when you are talking about a cure for spinal cord injuries. If anything, he was taken aback by Curtis's diluted zeal. Curtis reassured him that he was simply tired from working ungodly hours leading up to the launch of their program. Then came the poignant moment when Mitchell asked him, with his open tablet on his lap and his fingers poised to start typing Curtis's answer, "When will you do your first case?"

Curtis knew that he had to be honest because wrong information would come back to haunt the company with "they missed the mark" reactions from the market observers. He was hoping that they could eventually go public, raising enough money to pay back Mack and regain control.

He thought carefully and answered, "I really hope to have our first case here in two or three months. We're still finishing our state-of-the-art operating rooms and waiting for the state to certify us, then we can go."

"Do you have patients lined up?"

"Yes," responded Curtis. "We have a waiting list of about twenty screened patients."

Mitchell seemed surprised. With raised eyebrows, he typed for a moment and looked back up. "I thought with something like restoring paraplegics' abilities to walk, you would have a waiting list of hundreds, if not thousands."

"Well," Curtis said, "yeah, you would think." He paused to catch his thoughts, and added, "the holdup is the reluctance of some patients to be the 'guinea pig.' Now, we do have inquiries from thousands, but they haven't signed up yet to be screened."

There was a moment of silence while the reporter typed. Curtis added, "As soon as people see our successes, I'm sure there will be a flood of interest."

"I thought you had some successes already?"

Curtis smiled. "Sure. Yes, in our study, we have twenty-one completed and successful cases. I will comment that the last five went flawlessly. We have treated people who had severed cords seven years previously, but we are hopeful that we can extend that timeline even further back. However, we want to start with acute injuries, as the rehab would be less intensive. So, we're screening our first patients very carefully."

"Any other reasons for delays?" asked Mitchell.

"Well, like I said, we have a very complex operating suite that needs to be finished and the state needs to certify it."

"Why not start tomorrow at Harborview while you are waiting?"

"Really? It would take up to two years to start a whole new program at another hospital. I came out here a year and half ago, and we've been working day and night and are still a few months away from starting."

Mitchell typed for a few seconds and looked up, "Any other complications or delays?"

Curtis wanted to say something about reimbursement, but he decided not to mention it. Too much information could be a Pandora's Box for the investment community. But then Mitchell asked a direct question, and Curtis felt he had no choice but to answer it.

"So, what about getting the procedure paid for? How're the insurance companies reacting to footing the bill?"

Curtis hedged, "Well, that isn't clear yet."

"Not clear? Who are the twenty patients in line? Have their insurance companies approved the procedure for them?"

"Uh, not really" answered Curtis.

"Who's footing their bills?"

Curtis answered, "Well, the first twenty are cash-paying patients."

"Really!?" said Mitchell with a bit of alarm in his face. Then he continued, "I remember seeing that article in *People Magazine* about you… wasn't that two years ago?"

"Three."

"You were saying in the article that you're determined to bring the Erika Procedure to everyone on the planet who has a SCI. Have you changed your ambition?"

"No, that was… and still is my plan. We must start with the cash-payers until the insurance companies get on board. I hope that'll be next year." He pulled that last comment out of thin air and immediately felt regret about it.

Finally, Mitchell seemed satisfied with the interview. After a few more minor questions, he asked if he could come back in a few months, after their first case, for a follow up. Curtis, with hesitation in his voice, agreed, and Mitchell left.

By the time the interview was over, it was almost 11 a.m. Jennifer came into his office with another large box of mail. "Good morning, boss. Got some mail for you." She snickered.

Curtis had cleared enough space on his desk that he could set up his laptop and get busy working on things, finally getting past the screensaver of the Italian men, who were still sipping their coffee in the rapturous Cinque Terre. He responded without even looking up. "Hi, Nef. Yeah, there should be space on the couch. I had to clear it off for people to sit."

Nef was a name that Jennifer's father called her to distinguish her from the *Jennifer* and *Jen* in her class. When her father and mother talked about her, using the nickname Nef, they would be clear they were talking about their daughter and not one of her friends. When she told Curtis the story, he asked her what she wanted to be called, and she said, "Nef is fine." From that moment forward, that is the only name Curtis used, sensing that she viewed him as a father figure. He felt honored.

He heard her set the box down and thought she had left his office. He was concentrating deeply on the message in front of him. He was startled when he glanced and saw Jennifer standing beside his desk, completely silent like a lingering shadow. "Oh… hi. Did you need me?" he asked.

"Well, there's always stuff we need you for, but I was wondering if you needed me. I mean, you look haggard these days. Is there something more I can do for you?"

Curtis sat back in his chair and took his reading glasses off. "Well, that's nice of you to ask. I'm catching up on about 200 emails this morning… oh, and filing a new report for the state of Washington. Did you reschedule the meeting with the MIT people?"

"Not yet. I think they were a little put back that you didn't show for their meeting last week. But, if you want me to, I'll work on it today."

"Yeah, Nef, that was very rude of me. These guys, after all, are deeply respected in their fields, and who the hell am I to have stood them up? But I really do need them." He paused for a moment while he strummed his fingers on the desk top. He looked back up at her and added, "We need to work on a new charge-coupled wafer, and they are developing a prototype."

She seemed surprised. "I thought you were very happy with the one you have?"

"Oh, I am, but I'm looking ahead. Once we perfect our spinal cord anastomosis program, we want to branch out into smaller nerves. The cranial nerves would be our next area."

Jennifer smiled. "So, like my grandma with a droopy face from a stroke... you might be able to help someone like her?"

Curtis shook his head. "No, sorry. That's related to a brain injury, and we have nothing for brain injuries. However, if someone had a droopy face from having their facial nerve severed... that we could fix."

Jennifer blushed. "Of course. I don't know what I was thinking. But wouldn't working on smaller nerves be even more complicated?"

Curtis put his glasses back on and returned his attention to his computer on his desk. He answered her without looking at her.

"Not really. While they're smaller and harder to isolate and map than the spinal nerve bundle, they are far simpler from a neurophysiological standpoint." Then he glanced back at her and continued, "But the first step is creating a CCW that is much more appropriately sized that we could use to map the cross-section of the cranial nerves. We still have the hurdle of finding ways to create the X-Y-Z axis for the mapping. In the spine, we can anchor mapping magnets to vertebrae, which have been mechanically fixed in position. The cranial nerves are roughly two to three millimeters in diameter, and the spinal cord, depending on where it is cut, is about ten to fifteen millimeters in diameter. So, we also need a much smaller device."

Jennifer sat on the edge of his desk. "Curtis are you doing okay? I'm worried about you."

He looked back at her and smiled. "Yes, you're worried and so is my mother."

"Your mother?" She asked with a perplexed look.

He turned his chair to look directly at her and took off his glasses again. Her long black hair spilling over her left shoulder was still damp, apparently from her morning shower. She smelled of jasmine, probably from her shampoo. Curtis, for the first time, noticed the intensity of her natural beauty, like a twenty-something version of Lisa Ling. Maybe it was the way the tangential light was coming in through the door and striking her on her left, like an oil portrait in a chiaroscuro form. He took his eyes away from her and

156

regained his thoughts. He answered, "Yes, she's been calling me for a week and thought I had croaked or something because I hadn't called her back. To make it worse, for the first time ever I completely forgot about her birthday."

Jennifer asked him, "I've never seen anyone burn the candle at both ends like you. Do you ever go home?"

"I went home this weekend… at least to sleep. I mean, I always spend my days in the office or the lab."

"How's Becky?" she asked.

Curtis seemed surprised by the question. He picked up his glasses again, putting one of the temple pieces against his mouth, and looked back up at Jennifer. "Why do you ask?"

"Well, do you ever see her? I mean, as a woman, if my husband was rarely home… well, I would have a hard time with it."

He was surprised by her intuition. "As a matter of fact, she *is* having a hard time with it. I haven't spoken to her, more than a word here or there, in several weeks. We seem to be orbiting separate planets right now."

"I know that when you first came out here, she was orbiting your planet," added Jennifer with a broad smile across her perfect teeth and lit-up eyes. "I mean, if anyone really understood the significance of your work, they wouldn't hesitate to orbit that dream. I know that I would."

There was an awkward silence before Curtis broke his concentration and added, "I don't blame her. I've neglected her. I've ignored so many things, my mother included. So many people are mad at me right now that I've lost count. I guess I should add my name to the tech people's shit list at MIT, now that I stood them up," he added, chuckling tiredly.

"Boss, you seem especially down today, is there anything else eating you?"

Curtis paused for a moment to type on the computer and then looked up again, "Nef, you know my story."

"What story?"

"How I had this intense desire to bring healing and a new life to the SCI community. However, the journey is so damn uphill. I feel like I'm trying to climb a mountain alone when the world should be in front of me clearing an easy path. I just don't get it. I don't understand. Something is wrong with my approach, or maybe something is wrong with me altogether. I mean, I think someone else could have done this better."

Jennifer left her half-standing, half-sitting position on the desk corner and eased herself down to a full sitting position on the floor. She leaned back against the wall. She turned her head to the side and shook it, so her long hair fell beside her, out of the way. She appeared willing to listen with intently as she looked up at him. Curtis took advantage of her ear, swiveling his chair around to face her more directly. He laid his glasses back on his desk and rubbed his face, then continued, "Yeah, I'm really down right now. I'm realizing that we'll be a cash-only facility. Thomas has made that clear. That means only the wealthiest people with spinal cord injuries will be able to afford Erika. Who else would have half a million lying around?" He looked at her with the question written into his facial expressions.

She responded, "What's so bad about helping just the rich? They're suffering, too."

"There's nothing wrong with it! I will find joy in helping those people. But I feel terrible for those who can't afford it. Erika, herself, couldn't have afforded it. There are those, maybe a few, whose injury resulted in a multi-million-dollar lawsuit and may have sufficient cash, but many more became poor after their injury who weren't already poor before."

Jennifer then asked what she thought was an obvious question, "Curtis, why not go out on your own? You're a brilliant and kind man. You could call your own shots and treat whoever you wanted. I would be happy to go with you and work for you there. I think the entire lab would come with you, especially the Sharks."

Curtis leaned forward, placing his elbows on his desk, seeming a little upset. "Nef, I appreciate your support, but I don't think you understand. I'm a slave here… a real slave… indentured to the hilt. I have no choice. I'm owned by Neurogenics, and I mean *owned* in every sense of the word. I can't be emancipated until I pay them back my purchase price of $9 million. Then, I would need at least that much more as seed money for my own facility."

"How can they stop you from walking away? This is America; there's no enslavement of anyone."

"Nef, you are young and naïve, like I was. I've told you before what happened in New York. I signed a contract with Apple Health to do research and practice as a neurosurgeon. We had great hopes that we would become a world center for spinal cord injuries. They supported my research to the tune of $9 million over four years. Then I started running into problems, not with the science, but with the politics. We were nailing the procedure, but not the bureaucracy and paperwork. As Apple Health took on new leadership, it quickly became impatient with my financial deficit. Finally, I was given orders to adjust my schedule to spending ninety percent of it on routine, billable neurosurgery and just ten percent on my research. That was impossible. I had just lost Lennard Jacobs and had to run the whole project myself. It needed every ounce of energy that I had. So, I sent out feelers. Mayo Clinic was interested in my work, as was Stanford, the University of Paris, and several others. But then the lawyers at Apple Health made it clear that—per my contract—I couldn't leave until my indebtedness was paid off. How could I come up with that much money? None of the other institutions were prepared to make that kind of investment on an unproven procedure. I was a bound servant, and there was no other way to put it. It was only when Thomas read about my work in a magazine and heard that Apple Health was cutting back my program that he came to the rescue. He wrote a check for $9 million to buy me and his lawyers helped to disentangle me from Apple Health. Do you see, unless I win some mega lottery, I'm stuck here."

They both sat in silence for a while until Jennifer seemed to perk up. "Curtis, one thing that I don't understand is why you haven't approached any of the patient organizations. I had a friend in high school who was a paraplegic, and she was involved with a patient advocacy organization. She even participated in a wheelchair marathon. It was a true marathon race that was only open to people with spinal cord injuries. They raised a lot of money for research. Surely, they would want to work with you, the one person in the world with a possible cure. I have seen your mail. I have read some of the letters. I thought these were junk letters until I opened them. I had assumed they would be letters asking you for a donation. However, they have all implied that they would like to work with you, and the one thing they can bring to the table is money. Why not work with the Reeves Foundation? These organizations have reached out to you and you throw those letters away. I bet they could buy you out, and you could set up a clinic, maybe even a free hospital like Saint Jude's Children Hospital. I don't get it… why do you turn them away?"

"Nef, that goes against everything I've stood for. These people have suffered enough. It would be unthinkable for me to go to them to ask for money. I want to bring them help, not ask them for anything. They've 'given' enough through their suffering."

"I'm sorry, boss. I must disagree with you here. That kind of thinking is warped. If I had a spinal cord injury, I would work like hell to help myself, and finding a cure would be part of that. I think you are denying them the privilege of being part of the solution of their own dilemma. I don't think you have the respect for the SCI patients like you think you do. You don't like people speaking of them as if they are invalids, but in this case, you are treating them as such." Jennifer was appalled at her own words… and quickly regretted them. She added, "I'm sorry, I mean, I know you care about them, but let them help you. You can't do this alone."

Curtis sat back in his chair, sticking the temple piece of his reading glasses back in his mouth and looking at the open door behind Jennifer. He watched as people passed back and forth, hard at work to make his dream come true. He was silent. Finally, she spoke again, "I guess I better get back to the lab."

Curtis continued sitting, silently pondering.

Jennifer stood up. "I'm just worried about you, and I want to be by your side to help you through this." Then she did something she had never done before—she hugged him and gave him a light kiss on the top of his head. Then she walked out the open door… closing it behind her.

CHAPTER EIGHT: MOM

As the weeks drifted into the twilight, and the blue skies of summer gave way to monsoon drizzles and abbreviated days, Curtis saw his prize closing in. The operating theaters were getting their last modifications per his and Clay's wishes. The hope of making a real difference in people's lives gave him some satisfaction, yet it felt distant.

Curtis had recruited Bryan Rogers, the surgical PA from New York, to join his team. Bryan didn't want to move out with Curtis the previous year because he had a girlfriend in the city. The girlfriend was trying to make it as an actor on Broadway (without success). However, since Curtis's departure, his relationship with the girl had fallen apart. He no longer felt anchored to Apple Health or the city, so he submitted to Curtis's persistence and moved out to Seattle. Curtis had sung Bryan's praises for many months. He wasn't just Curtis's right-hand man in the OR but his second set of intuitive eyes.

Curtis and Becky continued living different lives under the same roof. They no longer ate together and hardly talked. It seemed to him that Becky intentionally was absent the few brief waking moments he was home. The tectonic plates moved even farther apart the morning he felt the bed empty. He got up and walked through the dark house and was shocked when he found Becky sleeping in the guest room. She simply didn't want to talk about it, and Curtis couldn't muster the energy to pursue the matter. He suspected that she was drinking too much wine, but that conversation also required far more than he had to give.

He, of course, didn't keep his promise to his mother to visit her within the month. It was over two months later, as they were in the home stretch just about to do their first case, that he took a week respite to make the trip. But those seven days off—the first days off in two years—were met with a lot of criticism. The most critical were the lawyers at Neurogenics, who were still tidying up their paperwork.

One day during the deluge of daily mail, Jennifer pointed out that she had signed for a certified letter that morning while he was up in the surgery suite, and he better read it first. She was hoping that it was a huge donation. She had personally sent out letters to the different patient groups without Curtis's consent. It was only wishful thinking on her part, as the letter turned out to be a notification that Curtis was being sued.

On top of all the other things going on, Curtis found himself in the center of a time-consuming and frivolous (in his opinion) lawsuit. One of his patients who he had successfully treated at Apple Health was suing him for malpractice. Curtis couldn't get his head around it. He wouldn't take it seriously, at least not at first. Thomas said that it wasn't an issue for Neurogenics because it happened at Apple Health, but that Curtis needed to deal with it and deal with it quickly.

Curtis had to open old wounds by going back and working with the Apple Health lawyers, including Dan Brice, as well as the attorneys representing the malpractice insurer.

The patient was a forty-seven-year-old diabetic man. He was a— almost literally—starving artist living in the Village. His wife had just left him, and he was losing his studio space, which he shared with other artists, because he hadn't paid his share of the rent on time, multiple times. He decided to end his life by jumping off the Brooklyn Bridge. When he hit the water, it caused a violent twisting of his body, severing his spine at C7, leaving him paraplegia and some upper extremity weakness. The NYPD Harbor police quickly fished him out of the water and rushed him to a trauma center, saving his life.

Curtis felt sorry for the man and chose him for his study. He chose him because of several factors. One reason was that the injury was new. Another was because it was a challenging type of injury. Rather than a clean cut by a broken vertebra, it was a twisting and tearing-type of spinal wound.

The procedure went flawlessly, and the outcome was better than expected. That is why Curtis was so surprised by the suit. But the man was an angry man before he ever met Curtis. One of his first comments to Curtis was, "I can't do anything right it appears… including killing myself. Next time, I will use a damn shotgun! If only I had the strength in my hand to pull a trigger." It was also the reason that Curtis selected the man, thinking that by curing his infirmity, it would bring him some happiness again. Looking back,

Curtis realized that his thinking might have been a little Pollyannaish.

The malpractice claim was that the surgery, while giving the man full use of his legs again, gave him an unbearable, burning pain in his feet. The claim of malpractice was that Curtis's team hadn't warned him of this possible outcome in the consent. The consent form did list pain and even death as a possible outcome, but it didn't specifically mention burning pain in his feet.

During the "discovery phase" of the lawsuit, Curtis had asked his lawyers to procure the man's full medical records, including exams by neurologists, spinal MRIs, and nerve conduction testing. Curtis carefully reviewed the records and tests himself, and his suspicion was confirmed. The man was suffering from small nerve fiber disease, precisely diabetic neuropathy, and the pain wasn't being generating in the spinal cord. It had nothing to do with either his spinal cord injury or the surgery, but rather his diabetes. He thought that would settle the case. It didn't.

The plaintiff's attorney came back with a modified claim. Yes, the pain was indeed being caused by diabetic neuropathy—and they would not challenge that fact—however, the consent didn't warn him that, when his spinal cord healed, he would start to feel the pain from the diabetic neuropathy for the first time. Previously, the severed spine prevented him from feeling anything from the waist down.

The Apple Health attorneys believed that the case was weak; however, juries tend to look with compassion toward the ill, especially the pitifully ill. As Dan Brice coldly said, "People in wheelchairs always win their cases, the only variation is the amount." The man had started using his old wheelchair again for no other reason than to see sympathy, practicing for a jury. Curtis emphasized once again, "But the man was in a wheelchair before we did the procedure, and we did the entire treatment for free. Now he has full use of his legs. Is there no fairness left in this world?"

Mr. Brice once again looked at Curtis through the virtual conference screen. "Curtis, as I've told you many times, this world isn't aligned with justice… it runs on money. One of these days you will see that… one should only hope."

The plaintiff's attorneys requested a deposition in New York, and all parties had to be there, including Curtis. A virtual deposition request was denied.

As Curtis planned his trip to New York, he decided to add a detour on the way back via Atlanta and Tennessee to see his mother. He invited Becky to come with him, but she wasn't interested. However, to his surprise, she booked her own flight to New York to visit her parents the same week that Curt was going to be there. He asked her, "Can't we at least have dinner at one of our old favorites, like the Manhattan Grill?"

Becky texted, "If I have time." The act of her going to the same place but on a different plane seemed a little passive-aggressive to him, but he was trying to give Becky the space she wanted. He was afraid that any day she was going to ask for a divorce or at least a legal separation. He just wished she would talk to him. Maybe talking about a divorce would be a starting point, even though he loathed the idea of such a conversation. But even a difficult conversation was starting to feel preferable to total silence.

The deposition was held in Apple Health's main conference room. Curtis had been in that room many times meeting with the executive staff about his research and their IRBs. Now he was a fish out of water. Neither Dan nor the other Apple Health attorneys were in his corner. They were only defending Apple Health's interests. Certainly, the plaintiff's attorneys weren't in his camp. He sat, rather passively, alone, watching in disbelief as the men talked for hours about suffering and semantics surrounding consents.

Once in Tennessee, Curtis rented a car at the Tri Cities airport and drove down to Jonesborough. His mother made his favorite dessert and had it waiting for him: rhubarb pie and vanilla ice cream—real vanilla ice cream. It was good to be home.

Despite being in his forties now, he felt a strange type of comfort sleeping in the same bed he had used from the time he was three until he turned eighteen. It was a simple, single bed with a wagon wheel design in each end. The bed sagged more than he remembered. Maybe it was getting old. Or maybe he was getting old and heavy. As he lay in that old bed, he remembered that he used to hide things between the mattress and box springs. Out of curiosity, he reached between the two to see what he could find, if anything.

Toward the foot of the bed he felt a piece of paper with his fingertips. He was able to pull it out, gently, without tearing it, treating it as if it were an archeological artifact or ancient papyrus. He laughed himself silly when he unfolded it and it was an old black and white glossy photograph torn out of a 1960's *National Geographic*. It was of a native girl on a South Pacific Island wearing only a palm-leaf skirt with bare breasts. He figured that he must have torn it out of the middle school library's issue of the magazine when he was about thirteen.

At breakfast, Curtis noticed that his mom looked much older than he remembered… and frailer. She walked with a limp and a little unsteadiness. After oatmeal and sausage, they strolled through her rose garden, the petals now lost to the season. "Mom," he said. "The garden must've been beautiful this year. You've done a wonderful job with it."

"It's my life. I have absolutely nothing else to do. I can either work with my roses or watch old TV shows in the dark house, where I just feel depressed."

He took her hand and squeezed it and led her to the old bench swing that still hung between two old elm trees amidst the rose bushes. They sat in silence looking at the barren trees around them. They were just starting to develop their buds, within which the leaves of the next summer were being contrived.

"Mom, when you were a little girl, did you ever expect that life would turn out the way it did?"

She thought for a while and then looked at him. She let go of his hand and hugged herself to ward off the chill. "I don't know. When I was born, everyone was still talking about the end of the war. There was a great optimism, not just with me, but with everybody. We felt like there was no problem that we couldn't overcome. I guess I dreamt of being swept away by a handsome man." She thought for another minute and added, "I thought we would travel the world and live in a fine house overlooking the hills and mountains where people raised sheep," she said with a big smile on her face. She added, "And I wanted a daughter." She realized how bad that sounded and quickly added, "I mean, a daughter after you."

It was hard for Curtis to even bring up, but the moment seemed to demand it. "Do you still miss Dad?"

Without a pause, she responded, "Every day."

They sat in silence as each gathered their wayward thoughts. His mom spoke again, "You know, I was older than your father. That was frowned upon in those days. He had come back from Vietnam shaken up and I was one person that would listen to his war stories. I was almost thirty and he was, I think, twenty-five or six. I don't know if he saw in me his mother or a wife. But I really wanted him to ask me to marry him. He was very handsome, and I was afraid that I would never marry. Then he did ask me. He asked me on a fishing trip on Douglas Lake. I said yes, of course. We both wanted to have children but had a hard time. You weren't born until I was thirty-five. Wayne worked hard to provide for us at the insurance office. He was a good father and husband."

Curtis, his curiosity being stirred a little, asked her, "Do you have any clue what became of him? I mean, you knew his sister, do you ever hear from her?"

"As far as I know, he's still alive, living in California... I think. But once he left, I never heard from any of his family."

"Why were they mad at you? You didn't do anything wrong... did you?"

"I must have. I mean, a man doesn't leave his wife for no reason... not unless she's boring, or ugly as a goat, or just getting old."

"Mom, you're too hard on yourself. We all get old and we're all boring at times. I'm sure Dad was, too."

She leaned into Curtis's shoulder, and he put his arm around her. She looked up at his face and asked, "Do you remember him?"

"I'm sure I do... if I allowed myself. I try to never think about him. Whenever I see his image in my mind, I quickly think of something else."

She pulled away from him and looked down at the ground. "Curtis," she said, "You know, he really was a very good dad."

Curtis looked down at the ground, too, and shook his head. "No, I don't think so. Good dads don't just run off with some young woman leaving their son and wife alone."

After sitting in silence, Curtis looked over and noticed big tears tumbling down his mother's face. She wiped them off with the sleeve of her sweatshirt, which she was now wearing over her hands like mittens. Curtis put his arm around her again and pulled her closer to him for warmth. His mother spoke again. "I don't think his family is mad at me. I just think they were too embarrassed to have contact with me. You know people do strange things. Avoiding talking about things that shame them is typical human behavior."

Curtis responded, "I don't know why they feel so much shame. Dad wasn't the first business man to run off with his secretary."

She began to weep even harder, so hard she could barely talk. After a while a few words slipped out, "Curtis…"

"Yes, Mom?"

"Curtis… Curtis… there's something I need to tell you. I mean, who knows how long I will be on this earth."

"Oh, good grief, Mom. You're in great health." He looked at her with a serious eye. "You're not sick, are you?"

"No, not as far as I know. However, so many of my old friends are gone. Cancer has taken several, and any day my number might be up. But just listen to me. This is very hard for me to talk about, but you should know. I'm afraid that this is going to hurt you even more."

For the first time, Curtis's interest was really drawn to the surface. He looked at her with raised eyebrows and took a deep breath.

172

What crossed his mind was the notion that his mother may have been unfaithful first. "Mom… what do you need to tell me?"

"Curtis… hmm… you see, son," She paused to wipe her face again. "I know this will be hard for you to understand. Your father. Your father's secretary…"

"Go ahead, Mom, and tell me! I think I've heard everything bad I could possibly hear for one lifetime. Just spit it out. The suspense is killing me!"

His mother looked at him with red eyes. "Son, I don't know how to tell you this… but your father's secretary was a young man."

CHAPTER NINE: PRELUDE

The winter months were passing, and Seattle was shedding her damp gloom as early spring seeped back through the cracks and passes down from the towering North Cascades onto the Puget Sound shores. It came first as episodic days of brilliantly blue skies followed by days of light drizzle. Soon the good days outnumbered the wet. The monsoon rains eventually retreated back out over the Pacific, losing their scuffle with the summer's drying sun.

The years of hard work were coming to closure. The Neurogenics Specialty Surgery Center was complete and retrofitted to the two surgeons' expectations. An area on the twelfth floor was created as a pre-op hospital stay. These were luxury rooms that would rival any executive suite of the best hotels in Seattle. All suites had incredible views of the waterfront and the Olympics to the west. They were carefully planned and laid out by a group of three architectural designers, each, themselves, with spinal cord injuries. Thomas searched for this special team by Curtis's request and recruited a couple of them as contractors from two different firms. The third one was a freelance designer from San Francisco. When they understood the gravity of the work that was going to be done at Neurogenics, they did much of their consulting for free.

Curtis wanted the designers to go far beyond the state requirements for "handicap access" rooms with widened doors and handicap toilets. This team had a personal eye for detail, as wall electrical, cable, and USB ports were installed three feet off the floor, making them easier for someone sitting in a wheelchair to access. The rooms had multiple choices for entertainment with the best movies and TV shows that anyone would want. However, they also offered complete solitude with soundproof walls, including the exterior, glass curtain walls. The suites had a second sleeping area for family members or guests who wanted to stay overnight. The décor, wall art, and color schemes were all carefully chosen to evoke a hopeful feeling and aid in creating a climate of optimism. The floor also had a commons area, where they planned on having live music several nights a week.

While it was now officially called the Neurogenics Building, Thomas had bought the whole thing for nickels on the dollar during the big real estate bubble crash of 2012. However, they didn't occupy floors three through eight and floors thirteen through twenty. He wanted a building of this size for their anticipated growth. They leased out part of the old bank building to other entities with an occupy rate of about seventy-five percent. The rents from these spaces were very valuable during their early lean years.

Thomas hired RNs for positions that they called MPAs (medical personal associates). One was assigned to each patient. Once hired, they were specifically trained in the Erika Procedure, so that they could answer any question asked of them. However, their role went beyond nursing to acting more like a personal host and patient advocate. They wore business attire to avoid giving a "clinical environment" for those waiting on surgery. Their job was to make the transition from street life to the day of surgery as easy as possible.

Neurogenics also hired a full surgical staff, including the technicians to operate the charge-coupled wafer (CCW) devices, helping the surgeons to position them and then making sure they were collecting accurate data from them. From a single cut through the spinal cord, the devices could capture the image on both sides simultaneously. If there was more than a five mm gap, the wafer had to be repositioned, one for the proximal cord and one for the distal cord cross sections. After the imaging was complete, they would then be responsible for running the very complex CAD translator program, taking a visual microscopic image collected by the CCW and rendering it into a mathematical scheme that would run the nanotube printer. They practiced until they could get a final bridge matrix within twenty minutes of opening the patient's spine. It took two such technicians per surgical suite. To anticipate vacations and other missed days, Neurogenics had to hire and train six.

Neurogenics hired two excellent surgical nurses per surgical theater suite. They were trained for six weeks before FCD (First Case Day) using virtual-reality software and a headset, where they had a very real 3-D world they could work in, much like a pilot using a flight simulator. That program and equipment cost Thomas $80,000, but he felt like it would be a good long-term investment. Curtis and Clayton thought it was silly and a waste of money because good OR staff learn through hands-on experience. Additionally, it meant that Bryan Rogers and the two surgeons had to spend countless hours programming Thomas's toy, when they thought they had better things to do.

Each surgical theater needed one surgical assistant and one anesthesiologist. They decided to "farm out" the role of anesthesiologist to a company in Seattle that supplied such services to area hospitals. Eventually, they planned on hiring their own.

Bryan had arrived from New York a month before FCD as the last of the Sharks. He had been a neurosurgery PA for six years. Before going to PA school, he had finished his undergraduate combined degrees in Philosophy and General Science while—at the same time—completing all his premed requirements. With his wide spectrum of studies, he still graduated summa cum laude from New York University. He then had to serve the army back for his tuition. He was trained as a medic and did two tours in Afghanistan. It was there he became interested in neurosurgery when he had the opportunity to scrub in and assist the field trauma hospital. He eventually lost his drive to be a physician because he figured he was doing it for the wrong reasons: prestige and money. He still had a passion for patients and the love of medicine. When he returned to the states after discharge and enrolled in a PA medical school. He shared a kindred heart with Dr. Eisner, seeing the great hope that Erika could bring the world. Having worked together for four years in New York, Curtis had learned to trust Bryan's keen eye for each facet of the procedure. In New York, Curtis trusted his judgment even more than some of the other neurosurgeons. He brought

Bryan in, not just to his third and fourth hands in the OR, but to help him manage all the cases as his "Assistant Medical Director."

On the ninth floor, they set up the intensive, post-op area. This required them to create an expensive post-surgical ICU, with a great deal of sophisticated monitoring equipment and a nursing station, where there would be two highly trained critical care RNs per patient. Curtis and Bryan had designed a recovery bed, which held the patient in a fixed position for one week. Yet, it would flip, every hour to avoid pressure points. The patients were expected to spend at least four days there for close monitoring. If they started with two cases per day, it would mean the ICU would have eight patients at a time. However, if they worked up to four cases per day, when new surgeons were added, the ICU would have sixteen patients or more, especially if some had delays on moving out to the floor. They were poised to reclaim the seventh and eight floors as their own and to expand the rehab unit downward from the ninth.

Because they couldn't chance having a patient being aggressively moved or even going home to their own bed, they devoted the entire ninth floor to their rehab unit, right from the start. But rather than using the term *rehab*, they decided to call it their NLAU for "New Life Assimilation Unit." To make it easier, they arbitrarily decided to pronounce NLAU as "Now," or "Now Unit." This unit had nurses, a physical therapist, and an occupational rehab specialist who would reintroduce them to working and social activities.

The stay in the NLAU would depend on the patient's progress. However, with typical, uneventful cases, you could predict the duration of stay based on the number of millimeters of spinal cord that needed bridging and the location and age of the injury. If a patient had a cervical dermatome six injury—meaning the lower part of the neck—and the injury had been within the previous two years, their stay could be as short as two weeks. They would then go home with external fixation (external metal braces with pins penetrating the skin into the vertebra). But older and higher injuries could require a longer stay, up to two months. When they got to full capacity, doing four cases per day, they could have as many as 120 patients in the unit at one time, requiring three whole floors, at least. That number was mind boggling for Thomas. By that time, he would have to reclaim the other floors in the building from the lessees for the expansion. They would eventually train other surgeons and move beyond spinal cord injuries into treating all major nerves.

Besides all this medical-centric infrastructure, Neurogenics had a business office to support, including a legal team, marketing team, and others. Mack Pendleton's fifty million dollars was almost exhausted before they had even started the first case, so they needed to move quickly before they went into the red.

Thomas met with Raymond and his team for a week to establish the price that they would need to charge to cover their expenses. They arrived at $350,000 per case for the actual surgery, and another $500,000 for the peri-surgical services, including rehabilitation. At the end of deliberations, they held a virtual conference call with Mack, who was living, at the time, on his yacht in Singapore. When they informed him of the price, he fired back rather quickly, "Uh, boys, we're going to charge $450,000 per case for the surgery and another $800,000 for the peri-surgical services. We will require $100,000 cash deposit before they ever get on the list. The full amount must be paid in full by the day of surgery. Our patient contract should account for complexities. For example, if one of our patients was to contract a flesh-eating bacterium—God forbid—we would have to be able to charge for those extra expenses."

Raymond asked Mack, "But excuse me, sir, I have crunched the numbers carefully, and a total price of $850,000 would cover our expenses, represent a decent payback for our stockholders, and keep our services marketable."

Mack started to belly laugh before Raymond was even done speaking, "Stockholders? You mean stockholder... me."

Raymond added, "Well, someday, sir, we should go public."

"We'll see," answered Mack. Then he added, "My people have crunched the numbers, too. Did you know that a damn lung-heart transplant costs two and a half mil? Just a heart transplant alone costs $1.3 million. I had a company run the numbers, and the quality of life gain for a heart transplant is a factor of 2.7, and for a spinal injury repair is estimated to be about a 4. The reason for this higher gain for our patients is that the transplant people stay sick, and they must take bags of medicine every day to avoid rejecting their new organ. Our patients will be back to completely normal with no drugs within a year. That's a damn freakin' gain that is worth something. People would pay millions for that… and I'm damn sure going to make sure they do."

Thomas, in a conciliatory tone, said, "Well, if those are the numbers you have arrived at, then we will go with those."

Mack then added one more surprising twist. "My folks have looked at other marketing strategies. One idea is to sell our rights as a license for about a million dollars a pop. Then keep the patent on Curtis's pixie dust. We would then become a pharmaceutical company and make most of our profits from selling the actual neuro-growth factor rather than doing the surgeries ourselves. Did you know that big pharma is the largest donor to American politicians? The government is in their pockets, and they can do whatever they want. That's where we can go after the mega dough. We figured that our lab spends about a grand to make enough for one procedure. We would charge about $50,000 per unit. Once hospitals around the world are using the Erika Procedure, they would have to buy their neuro-growth factor from us and us alone. There's no other business like the pharmaceutical business, in the world, where there is a 5,000 percent markup."

Thomas was scratching his head, literally, as he mulled the idea over. "Well, I think Curtis would like that idea as more patients would have an opportunity to get help if more facilities were offering it. And, of course, they would have to be trained here and would have to pay for that training."

"Absolutely, they would pay for their training," said Mack. For now, though, we are going to focus on doing the procedure for profit and keep this other model on the back burner. We need to build our brand now with success stories."

The price for the procedure was out of everyone's hands except for Mack's. The following week, Thomas summoned Curtis up to his office. He had poured him a glass of rum, which he had just purchased on a trip to Cuba. "Good stuff isn't it, Curtis?"

They sat down on the office couch. Thomas asked him then, "So, how's it going these days? Aren't we about three weeks away from FCD?" Before Curtis could answer, Thomas added, "I can feel the electricity in the building as we ramp up. Aren't you excited?"

Curtis smiled. "I am."

Thomas gave him a strange expression and added, "I thought you would have more enthusiasm that that, man. This is your life's dream and work."

"Oh, I am. I'm very excited. I'm tired… but excited." Curtis took a sip of his drink and then leaned toward Thomas, "So, what's the damage? What's the price we're talking about? I know that's why you brought me here, and the fact that you're beating around the bush… well, I hope it's under a half of a million for the procedure."

"Now, Curtis, we have to be reasonable. Mack's people have given us the final numbers. For the whole thing, including the procedure and the rehab, we will collect one and a quarter million dollars."

Curtis felt the remaining life drain out of him. He thought back to those early days at Apple Health, when he estimated that they could someday heal a severed spinal cord for two or three hundred thousand dollars. Even with a decade of inflation, he never thought it would exceed five hundred thousand. Curtis put down his drink and rubbed his face. "So, Thomas, this means that we'll never have the chance to get the insurance companies on board?"

Thomas had to chuckle. He sipped his drink and said, "I'm afraid not. I think the CEOs of insurance companies would crap in their Desmond Merrion's to even consider something this expensive."

Curtis looked puzzled.

"Desmond Merrion makes $50,000 suits for men," added Thomas.

Curtis's puzzled look morphed into shock.

Pointing to his pants, "This is a Desmond Merrion," added Thomas.

Curtis gave him a bug-eyed look and shook his head in disbelief. Then he stated, "After my enlightening conversation with Raymond a few weeks ago, I wouldn't be surprised if the insurance companies are working behind the scenes to discredit us."

Thomas, shaking his head, said, "Probably. But the savings for us will be a lot less hassle from not having to deal with those bastards."

They sat in silence until Thomas spoke again, "We have already informed our first patients on the schedule about the price. They didn't blink. I think money is no object for them… I'm telling you this to make you feel better."

Curtis got up and walked over to the window. He looked down at the streets. No longer seeing the grid of squares, he saw parallelograms spreading out in all directions. He looked over at Thomas. "Have you ever noticed that Seattle isn't set up on a perfect grid?"

Thomas looking confused answered, "Uh… no, not really. I think I heard you say that before. It looks like a grid to me."

Curtis continued, "No, the streets conform to the geographical world that was here from ancient days. The hills and the coastline aren't parallel. They all have an outside reference point that aligns them just the way they are. New York, on the other hand, was built on a true grid because they were not following any geographical reference points when they laid out the city in 1811."

Thomas asked with a perturbed expression, "Well, why does that bother you, and what does that have to do with anything we're talking about?"

Curtis finished his drink, walked back over to the couch, and put his empty glass on the coffee table. "I don't know. Nothing, I guess. It was just an interesting observation to think that the shape of the streets, the shape of our building, and even the design of our furniture within our building can be determined by something in the cosmos."

Thomas rolled his eyes as a gesture of incuriosity. He looked up at Curtis who was still standing. "Sit down; I have one more story to tell you."

Curtis slowly took a seat back on the couch. Thomas looked at him and continued, "I talked to a friend over at Scandia Medical Center. He is the chief financial officer there. I asked him about their high-ticket items: heart transplants, liver transplants, cancer treatments, etc. How do they offer these services to anyone but the wealthy? Of course, most insurance covers at least part of cancer treatment—which can run into the millions of dollars. The insurance companies fight like hell to avoid paying for the transplants. Most of them pay a small percentage. But there's other funding. They end up writing off a very large percent, making up for it by charging a hundred dollars for each plate of tasteless meatloaf and peas served on the floors or ten dollars for a Band-Aid. But these days, patients themselves find other funding."

Curtis was quiet. Thomas had that look on his face when someone feels they aren't connecting to their listener. He sipped his drink, finishing it off and sitting the glass on the table next to Curtis. Thomas looked into the empty glass like he was looking for words. He picked up his empty again and held it up to the light. Looking back at Curtis, he added, "Have you ever seen the jars in the convenient stores raising money for burn victims or cancer treatments? They could do the same for spinal cord cures." Then he winked--a gesture that he had apparently picked up from Mack.

"That would be a damn lot of pennies and nickels," replied Curtis.

185

For consolation, Thomas added one more thought, "Curtis, our estimates are that almost fifty percent of spinal cord injuries are due to litigious injuries. I know that many of the patients have already received payments for their injuries and have probably spent the money on useless crap. However, our lawyers said, if a cure was found, the patients' lawyers could possibly go back and sue to get enough money to buy the cure. They could present it as true justice. Even if they had blown the first money on lotto tickets and whores when a cure wasn't available, they could go back and make the case that they need more money. Now that a cure is available, it would make a second trip back to court reasonable. In the future, the initial lawsuit would include monies earmarked for the procedure."

Curtis's composure seemed to brighten just a bit as he seemed to be in deep thought.

Thomas added, "Curtis, if Erika had her four-wheeler accident today, I bet a good lawyer could raise the money from somebody... the manufacturer of the four-wheeler, the land owner, or even the kids she was riding with—if they were being reckless—to cover the cost of the treatment. If they had been drinking, they could even sue the joint that sold alcohol to underage kids."

"They weren't drinking," said Curtis in a soft voice.

The two men sat in silence, and Thomas was waiting for more of a response from Curtis... but none came.

"Curtis," Thomas asked, "are you familiar with the 'implied humanitarian social contract'?"

186

Curtis looked puzzled. "I could guess what it is, but... no... I haven't heard of that term precisely."

"Whenever a medical provider, hospital, or other human service provider has a humanitarian service, it is considered unethical to withhold that from the needy." He paused for a moment, looking up at the ceiling, then spoke again. "The best case I can think of is where a town is hit by a hurricane, and there's no running water. At first, the local grocery stores might try to gouge people with inflated prices for their bottled water. However, if the situation gets desperate, there is an implied social contract that the grocery store must offer the water at no cost."

Curtis just looked at him.

Thomas continued, "So, Curtis, the people at Scandia Medical Center brought that to my attention. They said that they must offer some heart transplants at no cost whatsoever. These are more like token, free procedures. Of course, they couldn't offer it to too many or they would quickly go bankrupt. But they will do a case a year. They try to redeem some of that money by highlighting the case in their public relations. So, it's not purely altruistic in motive. What I am saying that you will have at least one case a year we can give away for free to someone with no means."

Curtis asked, "So how does Mack feel about that?"

"We haven't discussed it yet. But it's a part of reality that he will just have to accept."

"Maybe you have a point there," responded Curtis again in a soft voice, just short of a whisper. Then he stood up, stretched, and walked to the door. "I need to go down to the lab and finish up some paper work. I have to sign off on an agreement between Apple Health and the plaintiff in that stupid lawsuit."

"Did they settle?"

"Yes, for $500,000."

"That sucks," said Thomas.

"Tell me about it. We took a guy who was wheelchair-bound and gave him a normal quality of life; we did it for free and in the end, *we* must pay *him* $500,000. There's really no justice in this world."

"This world runs on money… not on justice." Thomas winked at Curtis again and added, "When're you going to learn that, son?"

"That's what I keep hearing from everyone. When you call me 'son' you start to sound a lot like Mack." They both laughed.

"Speaking of Mack," Thomas added, "he told me that there really was a whorehouse in Reno that catered to cripples."

Curtis shook his head. "I guess he would be the one that would know." Curtis walked almost out the door and stepped back in. "Thomas, I am concerned that Mack is starting to wear off on you. Please don't talk about our patients like they're a novelty or commodity… and please, once again, never, ever refer to them as cripples!"

Thomas, smiling, said, "Curtis, you're a good man. Probably the best man I've ever met. I wish I could change the world for you, but I can't. It's like evolution. You've evolved beyond this world and are better suited for an improved one, a world that doesn't exist yet. You're like a fish that grew lungs in a world where there's no air. Maybe your world will never exist. But you have to adapt to the reality of the world in which you live, or you'll go nuts."

Curtis did have a growing concern that Mack, and others, were having a negative influence on Thomas. He had been a decent man too, when Curtis first met him. He loved his family immensely. He had great compassion for his kids, especially Noah, who had Down Syndrome. He loved the boy so much that he had absolutely no regrets about him coming into his life.

Still standing in the doorway, Curtis changed the subject, saying back to him, "Now I want to move ahead and focus on those patients who are coming to us in a couple of weeks to be made whole. That's why I still get up every morning."

Leaving, Curtis took the stairs down to the basement. He came into his office and flipped on the lights. Neurogenics, in its build-up toward being fully functioning, had finally created a mail room. Its job was to screen the mail, starting with the ten boxes in Curtis's office. He asked that the hate mail not be forwarded to him anymore. He was no longer writing apology letters. He always felt compelled to write long, three or four-page letters where he tried to explain his actions. He felt compelled to justify his use of animals in their research or why they couldn't accept everyone into their treatment studies. But now, he didn't have the time or emotional energy to respond to or even read those letters.

He sat at his desk and opened his laptop. It was dead in the water, as the charger plug had wiggled out of the wall socket. "Damnit," he mumbled to himself. He plugged it in and just sat and thought for a minute. He used to be a easy-going man, but now the slightest addition to his daily grind left him irritable—even just sitting and waiting for a laptop to recharge enough to boot up.

His mind took him back to his mom's rose garden and the porch swing suspended between the two elm trees. When his father first hung that swing, the trees were barely big enough to support it. Then, over the next decade and a half, they became mighty stalwarts, standing guard and offering shade to the despondent and tired. But then the trees themselves succumbed to despondency as Dutch elm disease stole their glory and strength. This left them half-dead stubbles of wood. He considered taking the swing down when he was at home, so it wouldn't collapse someday as his mother sat upon it.

He then thought of the conversation which they had shared three weeks earlier. His mom was so worried that the new information about his dad would cause more pain for Curtis. But it hadn't. He felt nothing. But more than nothing, he sensed some peculiar peace or closure, and the reason was ambiguous to him… at least at first.

After his visit with his mother, he had returned to Seattle in a firestorm. The days were counting down to their first case, and so many new problems were coming to the surface, not the least of which was the state not certifying their diagnostic lab. This meant that they would have to outsource all their lab tests until it was resolved.

His personal life seemed no better. Becky had gone to New York the same week he had been there, somewhat to rub their distance in his face. She never called him while they were both in the city, and she didn't return his calls. She was back in Seattle before Curtis because she flew directly back.

With Becky still sleeping in the guest bedroom and emotionally distant, Curtis used this time as a license to practically live in his office, especially with the countdown to FCD rapidly moving forward. One morning Curtis had confronted Becky and asked her point blank, "Do you want a divorce?"

"Is that what you want?" she asked.

"No. It has never been what I wanted. But I just can't live like this anymore."

"Like what? This is the way I've lived for the past two years… alone in this house. How's it any different now?"

"You used to talk to me. Now I feel like I'm living with a stranger, a visitor from Bhutan, whom I don't understand and who doesn't speak to me because…" He paused to collect his thoughts. "They don't speak English, and I can't figure out their nonverbal clues because I'm not familiar with their culture and customs."

Becky started to laugh as she was combing out her wet hair while looking in the bathroom mirror. "Curtis, you just don't get it, do you? How many times did I try to talk to you? I bet I left hundreds if not thousands of voicemails on your stupid phone that went unanswered. You're the one that went silent first. I just gave up. I don't want to try and communicate anymore. Why try? I'm guilty of fatigue, if that matters."

He looked at her in the mirror. "Becky, I still love you as much as the day I first met you. I fell for you when I watched how much you enjoyed the simple setting of the sun into the Hudson. Nothing has changed. How many times do I need to tell you that I'm sorry? Let's start over. We can fix this."

Without making eye contact with Curtis, still looking in the bathroom mirror, she added—with a bit of hesitation in her voice— "I've heard rumors that there's someone else, another woman in your life."

Curtis felt rage at such a suggestion and tried to filter his words very carefully, so as not to make a bad situation worse. But, with a lack of discipline, he shouted, "That's bullshit, Becky! Who in the hell told you something like that?"

She turned and looked directly at him and didn't say a word, just stared. Then she grabbed her backpack off the coat hooks in the hall and headed for the door.

"Where're you going?" asked Curtis, with his hands held out, palms up. "You can't just say something like that and leave."

She looked back at him as she opened the door into the garage. She pushed the button to open the outside garage door. As the hum and whine of the door filled the air, she spoke, "I'm going to be late for lab. I'm starting school today… to finish my own PhD… as if you cared." Then she closed the door behind her as Curtis was mumbling, "But I do care."

Curtis listened as the VW Beetle started and backed out of the garage. He watched out the window as the car sped up the street toward I-5.

CHAPTER TEN: FIRST CASE DAY

Curtis held his arms in front of him, his elbows bent at ninety degrees, and his palms in front of his face. This position allowed him to examine his hands thoroughly as well as let the sterilizing soap drain after one last rinse in the large, stainless, sink. He used his knee to operate a stirrup valve to turn the water off.

Beside him stood Clay who, like him, was wearing a surgical hat and mask plus surgical goggles, was still scrubbing his fingernails with a povidone-iodine soaked plastic brush. He was operating his sink, which was designed just for him, with a foot pedal to control the water flow.

The two men were handed sterile towels to carefully dry their hands in a methodical way to avoid contamination. Then a sterile gown was held in a carefully choreographed way. They each put their arms into the sleeves and then handed the technician a tab that held the sterile tie. The technicians rotated the straps around them and tied them. The surgical technicians, one for each man, carefully held surgical gloves, fingers pointing downward. The surgeons slipped their hands into them, one at time. Next came a second sterile glove over the first.

They walked toward a set of stainless-steel doors that separated the air-locked gowning area from the main surgical room marked "Surgical Theater #1." As they approached, the doors automatically slid into pockets on each side, like something from a James Bond movie. Already in the room was—what seemed like to

Curtis—a crowd of people. The patient was lying face down on the special spinal surgical table that Curtis had designed. Bryan had supervised the positioning and draping of the patient, as he knew, from experience, exactly how to optimize the patient's position for visualizing the particular area of the spine. The patient was covered in a way that made them look like a pile of towels that were over their back with one eight-inch by six-inch section exposed. The anesthesiologist was behind a sterile drape, surrounded by electronic monitoring equipment. The room was silent except for the very low whish of the ventilator as it breathed for the patient, rhythmically in and out.

Bryan stood across the table facing them as they entered the room. He was in surgical attire with a short, clear visor over his eyes and a halogen headlamp on his head. He was a stocky man, about five-nine, with lamb-chop side burns beneath his surgical mask and thick, curly hair beneath his surgical cap. While he may have intended an Elvis look, his musical hero, his muscular frame evoked mental images of Wolverine. Around the Apple Health OR, they had called him Logan. Some of the younger patients called him—fondly—Mr. Wolverine. He was asked, more than once, if he performed surgery with his adamantium claws. He went along with it but didn't necessarily like the comments. But this combination—in an odd way—made him a strikingly handsome man, so much so that his New York girlfriend wanted him to try modeling, as a macho character, to pay his way through med school. He thought that idea was ridiculous.

Poised in his right hand was a scalpel with a pointy, number 11 blade. Bryan's hands were crossed, with his right hand—and the scalpel—resting comfortably on his left.

Curtis took a position directly across from Bryan. Because this was Clay's first real case, he took the position as the second assistant, standing next to Bryan. He had protested that role at first, but Curtis reasoned with him that, despite being a skilled surgeon, for this procedure, he could learn from Bryan. Bryan, after all, had more experience in the Erika Procedure than anyone in the world, save Curtis himself.

To Curtis's left was Brenda, a seasoned neurological scrub nurse. She had jumped at the chance to come to Neurogenics when she heard that Curtis was starting a spinal cord repair program. Her own sister had suffered a severe C4 injury when she dove into Lake Serene in high school and her head hit a submerged log. It was tough getting her down from the mountains, as there was no place for a copter to land for about two miles. Some suspected that during the carry out, by the mountain rescue team, over logs and rocks, her spine was damaged. But they did their best with what they had.

Her sister lived for over twenty years, as a quadriplegic who needed ventilator assistance at times, before—like Erika—succumbing to sepsis. Those life events propelled her into nursing and neurosurgery as a career. Being sixty-four, she had given up hope of seeing a cure in her lifetime and was ready to retire—until she heard about Dr. Eisner's work.

With Clay on Bryan's left, a surgical technician, Ahmed, was on his right. Ahmed was an expert on the complex array of instruments, which were on the trays beside him. He could anticipate the next instrument needed and have it ready before even being asked. He handled the suction machine and the electric cauterizing tools. He had made himself an expert on the operation of the top-of-the-line Leica operating microscope. Ahmed even knew how to adjust, to perfection, the lights and anything else in the room including the temperature. He did his work with great passion. He came to America as a refugee from Syria. There he worked with the White Helmets, rescuing victims from bombed-out buildings. That experience had sealed his desire to learn more skills, to one day take back to Syria. A sponsoring church helped pay for his vocational training. Now he aspired to go on to college and eventually follow in Bryan's footsteps and become a neurosurgical PA.

Sitting comfortably at the foot end of the table were the two electronic technicians, a woman and a man. They were collectively called the "Geeks" by the rest of the team, although they had real names of Traci and Christopher. They were responsible for producing and setting up—with great precision—the bridge matrix that would fit between the two ends of the spinal cord.

The Geeks were also experts in positioning the CDWs using tiny magnetic dots to create X, Y, Z axis reference points. The surgeon would cement the dots to the vertebra bone above and below the wound with UV activated glue. The dots had to be

197

removed at the end, or they could greatly interfere with post-op MRIs.

Traci and Chris were also responsible for setting up the software that coordinated what was seen in the microscope with what was imaged by the patient's MRI and stored digitally as a 3-D model. This image was being projected on an eighty-inch, high-definition screen, which showed in real time the position of the surgeons' hands in relationship to the patient's spinal cord. With a click of a mouse, it would hold the image being captured by the microscope and, if needed, project that simultaneously over the MRI image. Once they had captured a perfect image of the cross section of the spinal cord with the CDW, the pair would then transfer that image into the 3-D printer computer controller. The printer would start to grow—or print, in other words—the bridge matrix. Before bringing the bridge couple out to the patient, the technicians would infiltrate it with the neuron growth solution by submerging it in a bath of the suspension. Curtis had found that, upon briefly exposing the bath to ultrasonic waves, the mixture would penetrate the tubular matrix much better. Last, the Geeks would inspect the bridge coupler under a microscope and present it at the appropriate time to the surgeons for implantation.

Curtis and Bryan had worked together in New York in several hundred cases, both human and animal. They could just glance at one another's eyes and know what the other was thinking. Curtis looked at Bryan and spoke, although Bryan had said or done nothing. "Not just yet, I feel like I need to say a few words."

198

Curtis looked around the table and said to the group, his voice being muffled by his paper, surgical mask, "People, I'm not sure if you can grasp the historical significance of this moment in time. From the prehistoric years, when someone had been trampled by a mammoth or short-faced bear and their spine was severed, people have felt helpless to do anything about it. I think of the thousands alive now whose lives were changed in an instant without hope of recovery. Today is the culmination of eight years of hard work and patience and lots and lots of money." He chuckled lightly. "From this point forward, everything changes. I dedicate this moment to Erika and her sacrifice that put us on the trail of curing this god-awful injury."

Curtis looked at Ahmed and asked for the mini, power bone saw. Then he nodded at Bryan. Bryan held his left hand on the patient's back, which had been covered in a layer of a transparent sterile membrane.

Bryan pressed down on the fleshy back to stabilize both the patient and himself, his right hand meanwhile holding the scalpel. There was a big purple H on the transparent membrane covering the patient's back, which Bryan had drawn with a surgical marker. He carefully cut through the dermis and subcutaneous fat following the lines carefully. Brenda quickly suctioned away any blood and loose material.

Clay was about to speak when Curtis interrupted him, "Clay, as I explained before, Bryan and I came up with the idea of the H-figure opening wound for this unique procedure. This will allow us to roll back the superficial layers and stabilize them with clips, leaving a wide space in which to set up our coordinates and to work. We need a much wider operating window than other spinal surgeries. Now watch as Bryan makes small, vertical cuts in the paraspinous muscles, separating the bundles, so that we can lengthen then retract them out of the way. We try to limit our horizonal muscle incisions, avoiding removing all the paraspinous muscles from the spine. That was my idea and a bit unorthodox. But, this saves valuable recovery time."

Bryan continued to work, methodically cutting small lines down the muscles that support the spinal column. Curtis used a retractor to gently pull back the layers and then anchor them out of the way using his special clips, which he had modified for this purpose. With all the soft tissue out of the way, Curtis took his small bone saw, which looked more like a Dremel tool than anything else. Before him was now a large, square depression that kept trying to fill with blood. Clay was cauterizing small vessels to end the bleeding while Brenda gently suctioned the bloody exudate. The tips of the white spinous processes rose above the pink and red pool, on which small pieces of subcutaneous fat floated. Rather than a spinning blade, Curtis's bone saw had a single tongue of serrated titanium that vibrated side to side by a couple of millimeters, a thousand times per second. He paused to look at the group. "We'll need to remove the bone and then have a full view of the entire spinal cord. After that, we will need to attach our magnetic dot markers to the vertebra, for later positioning the CDW accurately."

Curtis looked up at Clay, thinking that he might be disappointed that he, a board-certified neurosurgeon, wasn't doing more and may be finding the H incision as odd. He spoke to him with a preemptive intent, "I know you've already done a lot of spinal surgery and that you are very good at what you do. This technique is what works for me. Bryan and I have worked through a very steep learning curve to get to this point. If you can learn our way first, then find a way to work efficiently through a single linear incision, then do it. Maybe we can learn from you, too. But I had to create a new way, and Bryan is doing the incisions correctly."

Clay remained silent as Bryan, with a silence of great focus, continued to work to clear the way to the vertebrae. Once exposed, there was an obvious deformity in the fourth thoracic vertebra as much of it was missing and a piece of metallic hardware helped to bridge the space.

Over the next thirty minutes, Curtis, working like a sculptor, first removed the metal, which didn't come out easily. Then he cut away bone in a precise and highly controlled use of the saw. Clay pitched in by removing debris and the larger bone fragments for later re-grafting. The larger pieces of bone were placed in glass containers that contained a chilled, oxygenated solution of autologous (the patient's own) red blood cells and glucose. This was another one of Curtis's innovations. The team began to work together as a single unit with only an occasional, trivial misstep.

Despite a state-of-the-art ventilation system, the air was quickly filled with the miscellaneous smells of blood, burning tissue, and antiseptic cleanser.

Although Curtis had been in and out of ORs for over ten years, the smell of blood always brought back a vivid memory of visiting the butcher shop with his mother in Jonesborough. He didn't like putting the two settings together, but that's the memory journey his amygdala and hippocampus would take him on once the smell had penetrated his olfactory center.

The butcher shop was owned by the local farm cooperative. In one end of the facility, steers and lambs would walk in. In the other end, customers would buy beautifully wrapped lamb chops and roasts. The building was set up to provide the customers with a psychologically sanitized experience. The customers couldn't see the animals walk in or hear their cries. But the thick smell of blood hung in the air throughout the building.

With the back sections of the patient's thoracic vertebrae, numbers 2, 3, and 4 (also known as T2, T3, and T4), were removed, fully exposing the milky white membrane of the dura mater (the tough membrane that holds the spinal fluid). Curtis paused to look around the group. "Is everyone ready?" He looked at Brenda, "Ready with suction?"

She nodded her head.

"Remember, be careful," Curtis said, "and do not make contact with the spinal cord."

Clay and Brenda both nodded from each side of the table, indicating they were ready. Then he took an electrical probe and created a tiny arc of electricity that cut through the membrane, coming down from T2 to T4. A perfectly clear fluid began to flow from the linear cut, and it was quickly suctioned up by Brenda, with a flawless touch, holding the suction tip with both hands. Curtis arched his own back to relieve a spasm. "That my friends, is the water of life—the true waters of Bimini."

He carefully cauterized a few small bleeding vessels around the edge of the wound as he continued talking. "Yes, Ponce de Leon was searching for the legendary waters of Bimini that would sustain life forever, but he never knew the waters were right inside his body all the time." He paused to look closely through the surgical microscope at the edges of the wound and then adjusted it to start studying the cord itself. He pulled his head away from the eyepieces and looked around the table. "There was an idea in the nineteenth century that we evolved from the little blue fish, which swim in the sea. That alone isn't shocking. However, the idea also stated that we started our lives as humans, looking like tadpoles, and changed into small fish-like creatures, swimming within the amniotic fluids. But the theory went on to say that we are still fish, just that we don't swim in the sea or even amniotic fluid anymore." He placed his eyes back on the big microscope and continued talking. "We brought the sea with us, as the amniotic saline was wrapped up and sealed within our spinal cords and cranium." He looked up again and continued, "The story goes on that the real us—meaning the brain—still spends its life as a fish swimming in this salty sea of spinal fluid. What we know as our bodies is just the outside, mechanical application of what the fish wants and needs. The fish is like a little man inside a giant robotic suit or exoskeleton."

Bryan, chuckling through his mask, commented, "Reminds me of something I saw in *Men in Black*."

While the injury to the spinal cord was clearly in view to the unaided eye, Curtis could see the intricacies of the wound though his binocular scope. Most of the fractured vertebra had been removed by surgery at the time of the injury. Curtis commented, "In the future, if we can get to the patients first, this part will be much easier. We would still have all the bone to work with, but this time, it looks like we may have to take a graft from her iliac crest to create a stable bone medium around our repaired area." He paused for a moment and then continued, "Hey, Bryan, move down and prepare her hip for the bone graft extraction. I will need a piece that is one centimeter by... hmm... let's say five. Clay, move across from me and help me. The last thing I want is to give someone the gift of walk only to have it taken away again later by an unstable cord. I am very anal about creating a good boney protection around the wound."

Brenda, who was busy with retractors and using the suction on Curtis's side of the table, spoke for the first time, "Her?" The people around the table just looked at Brenda, so she continued, "You said 'her' so this is a woman?"

Curtis shook his head. "I'm really sorry, folks. I usually give the introduction to the patient before we begin, but in my nervousness, I seemed to have forgotten. This young lady is Kayla. She suffered a T4 injury while playing freshman—freshman high school—soccer. It was a freak accident when she fell forward over the ball and the defensive player pursuing her fell on top of her. This force caused a hyperflexion injury of her upper back and an SCI. The vertebra itself fractured, and the ends severed her spinal cord. The injury happened four years ago. Maddie and Chris, her parents, are nice folks… both Microsoft executives. I think, between their own funds and the settlement from the suit against the soccer association, they found the money to pay for this procedure. I suspect that her parents are sitting above us right now."

Curtis looked up to the surgical balcony for the first time. It was dimly lit, so he couldn't see who was inside, but he could tell that someone was. He even saw a quick flash behind the dark glass as if from a camera. The observers couldn't see his face behind the mask, but he tried to smile with his eyes and give them a nod of reassurance.

Six hours later, after the debridement and mapping, the bridge matrix was carefully put in place and secured with four fine carbon fiber suture threads on each end. Additionally, the bridge was secured with a UV-activated adhesive. The tiny electrical wire power source was attached to the inside wall of the dura, and the ends of the Y-shaped gold wires were attached to each end of the bridge with electro-conductive UV-activated glue. Curtis was finally ready to, as he would say, "work our way back out." They closed the dura, and then Curtis placed a needle through it to infuse his proprietary mixture of liquids, saline, and a little autologous serum, devoid of most of its proteins, which was intended to help replace the volume of spinal fluid lost.

Next, he withdrew the needle and painted the dura wound site with some of the same autologous red blood cells that he used to soak the bone grafts, except this part had not been hepatized, thus it was thickly coagulated. Curtis called it his preemptive blood patch, which would prevent leakage of spinal fluid and help in the healing process. He painted it on, as a paste, with a sterilized artist's bristle brush. He purchased high-quality brushes from Italy that was guaranteed to never lose a bristle. The two neurosurgeons worked, bridging the vertebra with the bony graft, which Bryan had harvested from her iliac crest. Before they had closed the skin, they had carefully punctured it with titanium alloy screws and screwed them deep within the vertebrae above and below the wound to add stability. On the outside of the patient's body, they were connected to long braces like Tinker Toys in a process called "external fixation." In cervical cases, it was typical, to use a "halo" cast, with metal screws in the skull and the rest of the cast resting on the patient's shoulders. Curtis used the external fixations on all his spinal anastomosis procedures, even those in the neck. He had borrowed the idea from a Cuban orthopedic surgeon he had trained with in his first year in New York. When all of this had been done, the wound site was carefully closed.

For the first three weeks, they had only one case on the schedule each day. By the fourth week, Dr. Emerson was ready for his own cases. He had his own "right-hand man," but in this case a talented woman, Tiana. She was a surgical PA who had trained at the University of Washington. They scheduled both surgeons to be operating at the same time in case there was a problem. They could communicate by speaker and, if necessary, Dr. Eisner, or Bryan, could change his gown and move into Suite 2 to assist. If Dr. Eisner had to leave, he felt quite comfortable leaving Bryan to close the case.

By their third month, they were, collectively, doing three cases a day on a routine schedule. They rarely had complications. The first patients, including Kayla, were reaching the point of near full motor movement. It was extremely rewarding for Curtis, and he felt the best he had in years.

His work schedule, now that they were operating, shifted. The pace was certainly still hectic, but it was the type of busyness that neurosurgeons expect. The team would round on the pre-op patients in the morning, then spend six to ten hours in the OR. If they had an easier case, a lower and fresh injury, they could combine it with a more typical case; in that way, one surgeon could do two in

207

one, ten-hour day. At the end of the day, they would round on the post-op patients. Sometimes, in the middle of the night, he would get called. They had a few complications and setbacks. A couple of patients required another trip to the surgical theater, both to drain hematomas that were forming around the surgical sites. However, because Curtis was so methodical and had planned things out in advance, things went quite smoothly. In contrast, his personal life was complete mayhem and was to get worse before it got better.

There were a few moments now and then that Becky's ice seemed to thaw a bit, and she would talk to him, but even in that conversation she was illusive. She was moving along in her PhD program in biochemistry, specifically plant biochemistry, at the University of Washington. She also, to Curtis's surprise, started to attend an alcoholic recovery group on Wednesday nights. He knew that she had been consuming a lot of wine, but a pure addiction to alcohol, while not surprising, wasn't something he had seriously considered. She made it clear that she didn't want his help or pity, just that she "needed to be left alone."

Curtis devoted himself to his work, as always. But this time the patient interactions helped him to manage his days. He looked forward to the early morning rounds when he would meet with the patients and their families. Even though there was no need for a surgeon in the NLAU, Curtis insisted that he be there to watch them take their first step. He would always whisper, "This step is for Erika." Those in earshot often thought it was praise for the procedure, but to Curtis it was in memory of the girl.

Those who walked were very grateful. He got his share of hugs and kisses from moms, dads, patients, and patients' husbands, wives, sisters, brothers, and/or children. This gave him only a brief feeling that it was worth it. Then he would return to his office in the basement at the end of the day, and there would be the mail. Always more mail. The mail room tried to sort it the best it could, but some of the hate mail got through. "Greedy pig!" was a name that Curtis heard more than once. He tried to put himself in the writer's shoes. He tried to imagine having a spinal cord injury and a cure was available but was off-limits because the patient couldn't afford it. He tried to feel their pain.

One day, Curtis was in his chair, leaning back, still in his teal scrubs, including his surgical cap. His eyes were closed while an open letter sat on his desk. He heard someone walk into his office and he peaked between his eyelids to see it was Jennifer. She began to tiptoe back out of the office, obviously thinking he was napping. He opened his eyes and said, "I'm awake. Do you need something?" He sat up and looked at her and explained he was attempting to "lie in the pain" of the family, whose letter he had just read. "I just want to put myself in their shoes and try to understand why they were using such hateful words."

She immediately shouted, "Stop it! This self-flagellation must stop! This isn't a healthy way to read letters." Then she grabbed the letter off his desk, threw it into the post office container box, and carried them all away, forgetting why she came into his office to start with.

While surrounded by people at work, Curtis's condo was quiet, dark, and very isolated. It seemed that Becky was always gone. He assumed she was at the university library or her lab. When she did come home, usually late, she would go directly to the guest room and close the door. It was probably that loneliness that prompted him to start a search for his father. The only lead was his aunt's name and the general area in which she lived. He had to purchase an online subscription for a people search service. He came up with four women, all named Elizabeth Carter, the name of his aunt. He started to call them, one by one. All of them denied knowing his father, but he left his number with each one in case they knew someone who knew him. He was thinking that, if one of them was lying to him, and really was his father's sister, maybe she would come to her senses and call him later. That is precisely what happened.

One day, he received a voicemail for one of the Elizabeth Carters. "Hi, Curtis. This is Libby Carter in Kingsport, Tennessee. I think I know more information if you want to call me."

He wavered for three weeks before he called. She quickly apologized for lying to him and admitted that she was, indeed, his aunt. She tried to explain that when his father, her brother, "turned queer" and left with "that young man," it was a profound embarrassment to the entire Eisner family. They weren't mad at Curtis or his mom, but they just couldn't face them again. It was as if their entire family had been shamed. However, regarding the whereabouts of his father, she didn't know.

Libby added that her own father, Curtis's grandfather, strongly rejected his dad. "Your father saw us once after he announced that he was in love with that young man. He came by the house to meet with all of us. Dad sat in the living room on his easy chair watching *Perry Mason* and pretended not to see him. It was bizarre, like he was pretending that Wayne was invisible. Finally, your dad began to cry and say, 'Dad, I love you, please look at me!' He got down on his knees beside Dad's La-Z-Boy. It was sad, sad and pathetic at the same time. Your grandfather finally stood up in rage, shaking his fist, and shouted at Wayne, 'I don't know you! I don't love you! I wish you had died in Vietnam rather than come home and bring disgrace on this family and that sweet family of yours!'"

She added after a brief pause, "Wayne stumbled out of the house. The young man was in the car waiting for him, and we never saw either of them again. I think it was Wayne's intention that, once he 'broke the ice,' he would bring the young man in to introduce him to the family. We never met him. Your grandfather died later the next year. The only thing I heard was that Wayne and Bobby, I think that's his name, moved to San Francisco, where homosexuality was more accepted in the early 1970s."

Curtis decided to wait before he restarted his search, this time in Bay area.

CHAPTER ELEVEN: SUCCESS

In the coming months, the complex procedures found passage into the routine. Clay moved out into theater #2 and became quite independent, managing his own surgical team. He even adopted Curtis's H incision form as his own, not finding a better way to create a broad-enough field for the mapping. Word started getting out about their successes. Their first patient, Kayla, was now up and walking without assistance and quickly won the attention of Seattle's Channel 5 news. It didn't hurt that her parents were well-known socialites of Bellevue. After airing a segment on her road to recover, their parent network, NBC, had her and her family on *The Today Show*.

If anything, it was a little surprising how long it did take before the Erika Procedure collected the fame it deserved. Curtis had the hunch that some nebulous force was already lurking in the dark to discredit their work. Or had Raymond made him paranoid?

Previously, attention had been given to the hope that wearable battery packs and computers with exoskeletons fixed to the lower extremities would help people to walk again. Others have approached the problem with brain implants that communicate, electronically, with stimulators distally to the injury site, thus bypassing the spinal cord injury. But to say that Erika was a game changer was a gross understatement. These other techniques had far inferior outcomes and more opportunities for technical breakdowns over time. But the world was not, yet, being rocked by the breakthrough the way that Mack had imagined.

A pivotal point came when *Time* magazine, picking up on *The Today Show* story, became intrigued with the procedure but wanted to focus on the genius behind Erika rather than the patients. They flew in a group to interview the Neurogenics team and take many photos.

While Curtis had some media attention for his work during the early days in New York, it faded during the long delays of boring paperwork and battles with bureaucracy. It didn't help matters that Curtis didn't associate with patient groups (which he later realized was a mistake). He became so consumed with the work before his nose that he stopped writing papers or attending professional meetings. So, neither the patient nor professional communities were as informed about their work as one would imagine until the news broke in the public domain.

Six months from the day they finished their first case, their work was the lead story in the "Medicine" section of *Time's* July 2021 issue. To Curtis's disbelief, his photo, holding the hands of a patient taking their first step, was the cover with the heading, "The Gift of Walk."

It was the highlight of his mother's life. When the pharmacy tech at her Walgreens showed her the magazine and asked, "Isn't that your son?" She put her hand over her mouth and impetuously said, "Oh, shit!"

At that juncture, things at Neurogenics exploded. Curtis, in some ways, wasn't as busy as he was during the lead up to the first case.

Yet, it was a different kind of distraction. He started to know what it was like to be a rock star. Their phones were ringing all day. Thomas set a hefty price for personal interviews with his staff or patients, yet the requests for Curtis's attention only escalated. Journalists from Dubai, Tokyo, Moscow, and even Ulaanbaatar were knocking on their doors, sometimes literally. It was insane to step out of the shadows of constant frustration and what felt like disrespect into stardom, and no one loved it as much as Thomas... except for maybe Mack.

Requests from paying customers were starting to come in from the whole world. Curtis had a strict protocol for the type of patient his team would operate on. For one, he wanted the easiest cases to begin with, those with injuries less than three years old and clean spinal lacerations. Large crush injuries would be more difficult and would have to come later... if at all. Curtis also wanted mentally stable patients. He never wanted to repeat his experience with the man who sued them.

Thomas had an additional criterion, simply that they could pay. Besides the up-front deposit of one hundred grand, he did a credit check on each potential patient to make sure he or she was worth as much money as they claimed.

Curtis persuaded Becky to join him for one night out for dinner. After a wonderful meal of Blanquette de Veau for him and a Cassoulet for her, they sipped sparkling waters (to avoid tempting

214

her with alcohol) and sat back in their chairs in the dimly lit bistro overlooking Salmon Bay. He had her full attention for the first time in six months, and they could talk. He tried his best to convince her that he could really see the light at the end of the tunnel, and this time it was for real.

He tried to force her hand by asking her to decide to stay with him and try to redeem their marriage, or to let him know if she was leaving him. Still, she was somewhat immobilized by hurt and just couldn't shake it. Her malignant ambivalence, once again, seemed unsurmountable. "But Curtis," she said. "I've heard this all before about the light and the tunnel stuff. I don't believe it anymore. You are now a celebrity for goodness' sake. Now the women will be throwing themselves at you." She leaned further in his direction, "Do you realize that you could have any woman on the planet."

Without hesitation, Curtis said, with a big smile, "That's fantastic… I'll choose you!"

Becky paused, looking down at the dessert menu the waiter had just placed before them. She looked back up with a sad look. "Here's the problem. I don't know if I love you anymore. I'm really confused."

His confident echo was, "I still love you, always have and always will. How can I take away your hurt? How many times do I need to say I'm sorry? A million? How many months or years will you need to sort this out?"

Becky chuckled. She then leaned over the table again and put her face in front of his and said sternly, with an animated face flanked by active hands in the air, "Curtis, I followed you here to Seattle where I knew no one. You took off the next day after we arrived. You took off to your lab and disappeared. I never saw our old New York Shark friends in the lab because they were as busy as you were. You saw them every day. I held up in our condo for months not speaking to one person. I was so lonely that, on some days, I thought of taking a bottle of pills just to escape. I couldn't stand it. For that I am so disappointed that I don't know if I can ever forgive you or trust you again." She sat back in her chair... no tears on her face, but her eyes were becoming sodden.

This time Curtis leaned forward, but without the hand gestures. "Becky, I've said a hundred times that I'm sorry for that. I think we've had this conversation over and over, but you knew that I would be busy; I was just busier and for longer than I had anticipated. But it was for a good cause—a damn good cause. I know men who spend this much time out of the house just to go fishing or lift weights in the gym." They both sat in silence for a few minutes. Curtis sat back in his seat creating a distance between them. Finally, he spoke again, "When I asked you to marry me, you knew my dream, and you wanted to be part of it. I still have dreams. I want to pay off my debt with Thomas and get out of my contract. Then I want to go and work for a public institution where we can treat all people. I want to create a training center where I can share my secrets to the world and wipe paraplegia and quadriplegia off the

216

face of the earth. Those are my dreams, and I can actually see them coming true for the first time."

Becky fumed and shouted, while pointing at her chest, "What about my dreams!" She said it so loud that it got the attention of everyone on the outside dining deck.

"What are your dreams? Share with me your dreams and let's…" Curtis made a big circle above his head with both hands, "sew them together like some damn celestial dreamcatcher web." He punctuated the comment with a boyish smile.

She had the look as if she couldn't tell if he was being serious or just being sarcastic and felt no wit in the matter. "Curtis, you knew that I was in graduate school when I met you. I had ambitions, too. I wanted to work to find ways to feed the world in a new, warmer climate. Those were my dreams. What's more important, feeding the millions of people who are and will be starving or helping 300,000 to walk again?"

Curtis looked up and noticed that the waiter was standing beside them. He first thought he had come over to ask them to be quieter, but the waiter just said, "Did you make a decision about dessert?"

Curtis answered, "Just some coffee for me… uh, cappuccino." The waiter smiled and then looked at Becky. She responded with a sweet, but false smile, "I want the dessert with the largest number of calories."

The waiter seemed speechless at her request but then smiled back and answered, "O … kay. That would be a large bowl of our famous crème brûlée… and I can add a couple of scoops of our vanilla bean ice cream if you like and whipped cream, real whipped cream, to top it off." She gave him an affirmative nod. He smiled and walked away.

Curtis leaned over the table and whispered, "What was that all about?"

"Oh, it doesn't matter anymore. I don't think you noticed that I lost over forty pounds last year."

"Of course, I did."

"You never said anything about it!"

"I didn't know I was supposed to! I didn't want you to feel that it mattered to me. I love you if you are fat or skinny. I don't care!"

Moments later, the waiter returned with their order. They both sat in silence, Curtis drinking his coffee, Becky eating her creamy-saccharine desert. She leaned over and said, this time in a whisper, "Have you noticed everyone staring at us?"

"I guess we were pretty loud," Curtis whispered back.

"That's not why, Curtis. Don't you get it? They recognize you. You're famous. They are taking photos with their phones. Curtis, you've done it. You are successful! You must be really happy now."

"I am miserable without you. I'm not happy about my work, either. I'm not successful until everyone with a spinal cord injury walks again. I won't be happy until I can find a way to make you love me again. Those are my two dreams. So, maybe I can fix a few broken spinal cords, but I can't seem to fix broken hearts." It was soon after that night that Becky stopped coming home.

One night, Curtis came home early after they had to cancel their afternoon case. It was a problem of payment. The Pakistani government had set up an appointment for the son of an army general. Through an oversight, the young man had been admitted and scheduled, but then they found out that the funds for the deposit had never arrived. It was complicated, but the young man had to be discharged after having his hopes—profoundly—dashed. The father was very angry and kept promising the money would come. Curtis felt terrible about that and pleaded with Thomas to make him their first charity case. But Thomas wanted their first charity case to come after a year of paying patients and insisted that case be a photogenic American. Someone they can use for their public relations propaganda. He added, "Someone like Kayla, our first patient. She was a beautiful blonde, all-American, and grabbed the attention of the press."

When Curtis arrived home at four in the afternoon, the first time he had been home this early in years, Becky wasn't only gone, but she'd left a message taped to the refrigerator, "I'm moving out, Curtis. I need to be closer to school. Talk to you later."

"Are you kidding me?" he said out loud when he read her note. He wadded it up and threw it toward the trash can… but missed. It rolled across the linoleum and Racer jumped down. He started to pat it around with his paw. Curtis poured himself a Chardonnay, one he kept in his Jeep and away from Becky. He then grabbed the only cheese he could find—Kraft Singles.

For the first time since his father had left him at age twelve, Curtis cried. He lay in his bed, in his condo alone, and cried. He ate all twenty-four slices of the cheese, leaving a pile of clear, thin wrappers beside his bed, looking like cellophane ghosts. He rolled over, buried his head in his pillow, and cried more. The tears belonged to Becky, of course, but also to the years of mental exhaustion and disappointment. He cried until he was too dehydrated to cry anymore. He wrapped himself in the old, lime-green bedspread, as if its loose ends were Becky's arms, holding him. He had not been held in over two years, by anyone. He had said to Becky many times how she needed to throw that bedspread, that relic of the 1970s, away. This night he was glad she hadn't.

Before the evening was over, the sadness completely engulfed his soul, and, from his vantage point, there seemed to be no way out. Would she come back if he abandoned his whole dream? Maybe. In this emotional moment, it seemed worth it to him. But in other moments, he felt that the hope he could bring others was so much bigger than his own life and that personal sacrifices had to be made. He felt so torn, seeing the eyes of Erika and her mom haunting him day and night. He made a promise to them, a promise that he had never fulfilled, yet it was finally within reach for other Erikas. Could he abandon them?

In the following weeks, once again Curtis turned his thoughts around and totally devoted his attention to his work. They were now up to three or four cases per day, one or two for each surgical team. They were working hard, reducing their time to four or five hours per case if there were no complications. He told Thomas that was stretching both teams to their limit; something had to give, or his staff would eventually burn out. A twelve-hour day had become the norm.

On many days, he was working on perfecting techniques for rejoining lesser nerves. They had already received requests to treat old war injuries from Iraq and Afghanistan. He hesitated at first because, as much as he wanted to help those folks, their injuries weren't only old but had resulted from blast injuries.

Blast injuries were different from lacerations, including lacerations from fractured vertebra fragments. Lacerations left relatively clean, although serrated, wounds. But blast injuries caused a multitude of forces on the nerve, cutting, tearing, shearing, and crushing. It was hard to tell, even with electrical feedback from the nerve and microscopic examination, where the injuries ended, and good nerve material started. The age of the wounds, some over a decade old, would likewise be a challenge.

Because violence had now broken out between the Reds and Blues in American politics--some were even predicting the coming of a second great American Civil War–Curtis wanted to be prepared for all possibilities. So, he had to start thinking of treating the injuries of violence, as senseless at that all seemed.

The first non-spinal-injury patient that Curtis chose to treat was a young man who was on a support mission in Syria in 2017. A large shell exploded near his unit's station, and the blast wave fractured his Kevlar helmet, turning one fragment into a sharp blade. The sliver of Kevlar severed his right facial nerve just in front of his ear. The man had a facial droop that left him disfigured and unable to open or close his eye on that side. To keep the eye moist, his plastic surgeon chose to suture the lid almost closed, leaving only a tiny peephole.

While Curtis had experience with connecting cranial nerves during his experimental years in New York, it was a brand-new procedure to his Seattle team, except for Bryan. They did have to adjust the operating theater with a different table, lights, and even a new setup for the anesthesiologist because the patient's face would be inside their field of operation. His friends at MIT were kind enough to take the time to create three CDWs, to cover all sizes of cranial nerves, costing the company $300,000 each.

Thomas wanted his team to do a few practice-runs in their original theaters before he invested in creating operating theater # 3 for cranial nerves. They expected to create at least one more theater, theater # 4, for more spinal injuries, and then another, theater # 5.

Neurogenics was sponsoring two neurosurgical fellows each year. The fellows had finished their neurosurgical residencies and had applied for the funded one-year training program to become skilled surgeons in the Erika procedure. Thomas required them each to sign contracts that said they would give Neurogenics a three-year payback of service and would be prohibited from performing the procedure anywhere else, or it would be a patent infringement. His hope was to force them to work for Neurogenics. Curtis placed emphasis on searching the country for good female neurosurgeons, a male-dominated field. He did find one excellent candidate in Alisha Smithers, as well as another man, Alan Bloom.

To everyone's surprise, Mack sent two neurosurgeons, one from Thailand and one from India, to be fellows. He did it without talking to Thomas or Curtis. Because the original two slots had been filled with signed contracts, they had no choice but to create two additional fellow positions, which strained all the staff even more. Curtis, Clay, and Bryan had to take turns supervising surgeons, sometimes two at the same time. A few applicants were bewildered by the concept of being supervised by a PA. However, Dr. Eisner was very clear, in his program, the letters after your name did not carry as much clout as what you know, what you don't know, and the discernment to know the difference. Curtis often cited his early days, as a resident, when a scrub nurse took him under her wing for weeks, until he could get on his feet in the OR.

Over the following twelve months, the program moved forward. By the end of the year, they had completed the procedure on 422 individuals. Thomas had a meeting with Curtis to celebrate their first year in business. Raymond joined them for breakfast at the same downtown restaurant where Curtis had met Thomas a year and a half earlier.

Thomas with a big smile announced to Curtis, "Dr. Eisner, you did good work. We just had an over half billion-dollar year." He lifted his orange juice, and the three men tapped their glasses in a toast.

Curtis asked with a bit of sarcasm, "So we're rich?"

"Well," injected Raymond. "I would just say we are financially healthy. We have a waiting list of about 4,000 people, so we should be in good shape by this time next year. But running an operation like this is expensive. We've paid out over $25 million in salaries and benefits. We've purchased over $35 million in new equipment this year, including our new higher-resolution MRI machine that you asked for. We have made a twenty million dollar—first payment— to Mack." He paused to sip his juice and continued, "And, I think Thomas has some good news for you."

Thomas spoke up, "Curtis, you *are* the goose that has laid the golden egg. It is time that we start to reward you for your hard work. I am going to increase your salary going forward from the $350,000 per year you're making now, to paying you at a partner level. That will be one million dollars per year. It's time you move out of that damn rathole condo and into a real house here in Seattle. You need to be Bill Gate's neighbor, and it's time you bought your own Desmond Merrion suits."

Curtis looked at Thomas and Raymond and said, "Partner level. Does this mean that *you* have already been paying yourselves at this rate?"

Raymond responded, "We earn on par with other corporation's CEOs and CFOs."

Curtis chuckled, "So you do. But, what do you do? I mean, we are busting our butts every day for twelve hours in the OR and taking care of patients, and you two are up in your offices playing with spreadsheets and looking at photos of furniture while you eat caviar and drink good wine? I know that your positions in thriving hospitals can be demanding, but we have been in the buildup phase most of the time under your watch." He paused for a minute and then added, "Oh, yeah, and I hear that you play a lot of ping pong."

Thomas had a frown—a contagious frown. "It's table tennis, and Curtis, if you don't want the raise, we can retain you at your current salary." His frown morphed into a smile with those last words. "You should also know, we do some of our most creative thinking during those games. Raymond is rather good," he added, implying that Curtis should be surprised due to the man's physique.

The smile that came to Curtis's face wasn't the idea of a new luxury home or fancy clothes with the increase. He felt comfortable in his Macy's wardrobe. However, now he could buy out his contract much sooner than he thought, maybe within seven years. "No, I'm not complaining, and I'll accept the raise with gratitude, but my Dockers will suffice for me. But knowing that we are doing so well

will also permit us the opportunity to do some charity cases...
right?"

Raymond was shaking his head while taking a bite of his hash browns with Tabasco. When his throat cleared, he spoke, "That's right. We'll start with one this year. But we must do this very carefully. I've seen other hospitals start a charity program, and it creates a lot of hard feelings. Think of the hundreds or thousands of patients who we'll have to turn away. I know about the hate mail that you receive. Well, you haven't seen anything yet if you start to do more and more charity cases, meaning that you are turning away more and more people for their life-changing treatments. So, keep that in mind. For each patient you bring a miracle to in that program, there will be thousands who apply, and we must reject. You will become their nemesis... and they will hate you. So, if you can let the love of one family override the hate of a couple of thousand, then we will go for it."

Thomas leaned across the table and said in a low, intentional voice, "But Curtis, remember, people are only animals in clothes. Even those charitable cases, like the guy in New York who sued you, may not be as grateful as you assume."

Curtis looked puzzled and said back, "But gratitude wasn't my purpose."

Another six months passed, and Neurogenics had five trained neurosurgeons, not including the four fellows—who had become quite independent—working on their backlog of cases. Curtis

226

opened the new suite devoted to cranial and other nerves, as those procedures hadn't been perfected yet.

One early October morning, about 2 a.m., Curtis's phone rang. He was thinking it was a call from the post-op recovery area. He quickly remembered that Bryan was on call for their patients, and Bryan would only be calling if they needed to go back to the OR. He could handle everything else. Curtis knew that Bryan could even do the emergent surgical intervention by himself, but it would be a problem of appearance and license limitations.

Curtis turned, set his feet on the floor, and reached for the phone. The screen on the phone showed that the number of the incoming call was long, as if it were an international number. His next thought was that Mack was calling from some exotic harbor. He would likely be drunk, with women on his lap kissing him while he talked, and he wanting to talk business. It had happened before. The ringing stopped before he could answer it, and he laid the phone back down. As soon as his head hit the pillow, the ringing started again. "Damnit, Mack!" He shouted and sat back up, grabbing the phone. He said in a sour voice, "Hey."

"Dr. Curtis Eisner?" came the accented voice.

"Yeah?" responded Curtis, with a voice soaked in annoyance.

"Dr. Eisner, this is Viktor Sorensen of the Nobel Assembly at Karolinska Institutet."

Curtis, now thinking it was just a gag call, said in a more hateful voice, "The what?"

The man continued, "We are the nominating and selection committee for the Nobel Prize in Physiology or Medicine."

Curtis sat quietly on the edge of the bed, thinking to himself. Was it possible that their work had been nominated for a Nobel Prize? Or did they just want his advice on another nominee, maybe for Dr. Richter at Mayo?

"We are happy to announce that you have won the 2021 Nobel Prize in Physiology or Medicine."

Curtis felt dumbfounded and asked, for clarification, "You mean we're nominated?"

"No sir. I mean you, you alone… well, have won. We will be announcing this decision to the public in two hours in Stockholm."

"Are you serious!" shouted Curtis.

"Yes, we are quite serious. Please be available to be in Stockholm on the tenth of December for our prize banquet and award ceremony. Congratulations on your great work!"

"But it was a team effort. What about Dr. Jacobs, Bryan Rogers, and the others?"

"No sir. The committee is clear; this award belongs to you and you alone. We recognize that others may have been invaluable to your efforts, but the results would have been the same if all those people were replaced, but they would not have happened without you. So, we will be mailing you more information in the coming weeks. I do warn you that the media will be seeking you out for the next few weeks. It happens to all our winners. And, as I said, the media will know in two hours."

Curtis, with great wisdom, immediately turned his cellphone off. He dozed off and on and was startled when his landline started to ring at 4:20 in the morning. He just rolled over in bed. It never stopped ringing, so he decided to get up and dress for work.

He had a full day of cases, so he knew that he would have to be razor-focused despite what chaos might be playing out around him.

Even though the announcement was made to the public at noon Stockholm time, that was six in the morning New York time and three in Seattle. Within minutes, the announcement was shared on all the national TV news outlets, NBC, CBS, ABC, and CNN. Quickly their affiliates in Seattle were abuzz with the news, and it was the first item when they went on the air at five. It was the top story that a local man had won the Nobel Prize. Next, the news outlets in NE Tennessee figured out from the published bio that he was a "local boy." The news passed over his mother, being unobserved.

By the time that Curtis got to work, there were no less than four TV news satellite trucks parked in front of the Neurogenics building. He drove past them and parked at a public street parking lot a block away. He pulled his collar around his face, as if anyone would know what he looks like anyway and made a bee line toward the nearest door that he had a key to. As soon as he was inside, unnoticed, he turned on his cellphone. It started to ring even before it was finished booting up. He had missed fifty-six calls and his voicemail storage had reached its limit. He scanned them for any he recognized. There was one from the pre-op area. It was a routine call that he got every morning, updating his schedule. He played it, "Dr. Eisner. Your first case is scheduled at 7 a.m. in ST-3 (Surgical Theater # 3). It is with Henry Carson, with a severed left ulnar and radical nerves. And by the way, boss, congratulations! We are so proud of you!"

Curtis had to hang up the phone quickly. For reasons that he couldn't understand, he felt like crying, and crying hard he did. It was like Becky's leaving him unplugged the—figurative—tear ducts and now weeping came too easily about too many things. He had cried every time a patient took his or her first step, making him feel like a fool. But this morning it was a torrent lurking at the doors of his eyes. He darted into the stairwell, which went to the basement. In the cold, darkened well, which smelled of concrete with a hint of urine, he squatted down where he felt no one could find him. He began to sob. Despite his struggle, he was feeling that maybe, just maybe… it was all worth it after all. It was an overwhelming feeling of euphoria and happiness that he had not felt in a very long time. Yet, he felt guilt for savoring in the self-glory.

When he finally regathered his composure, he looked at his phone again. He had several calls from Thomas and two from Mack. He looked at the time: 6:30 already. His scrub-in ritual, including scan review, usually took an hour, and now he only had thirty minutes. The fact that it wasn't a spinal case made it somewhat easier, at least for the scan review. He called Bryan.

"Hey, Bryan?"

"Yep."

"Are you upstairs?"

"Absolutely. What do you need, boss?"

"Hey, I'm running a little late. Can you go over the checklist with the team before I get there?" The checklist was a ritual where they went over each step of the surgery, making sure the equipment was working correctly and that they had everything they needed in place.

"Absolutely. And don't worry, boss, the Carson family saw the news this morning. They are delighted to have a Nobel laureate operating on their family member, so they will understand your delay."

"Thanks, man. You're a gem." Tears started to stream down his face again. He felt more guilt, as if the tears were gloating tears, and he wanted to return his mind to focus on the patient. The tears had to stop before he reached the tenth-floor operating area.

To his surprise, his attempts at self-composure were in vain. He opened the door from the stairwell on the tenth floor. A crowd of no less than twenty people were facing the elevators. Employees, staff from the lab, and patient families stood in anticipation of his arrival. Bryan nodded and shouted, "There he is!" They all turned and started to sing, with Bryan in the lead, "For he's a jolly good fella, for he's a jolly good fella," and soon the non-alcoholic champagne began to fly.

The tears began to flow again, and Curtis raised his hand to quiet the crowd. "Thank you. Thank you so much. I'm so grateful; however, this has been a team effort. I want to thank everyone for your help in seeing this dream come true… and most of all," he started to sob again… "I want to thank Erika Ledbetter for her sacrifice in helping the rest of us see… what a horrible thing a spinal cord injury can be. I want to thank the families for their hope and determination to support their family members. I wish I could say more, but we need to get to the OR."

Bryan appeared from the crowd. "Hey, boss, take your time. We have worked together to move all the cases back an hour, and Dr. Simons [one of the new post-fellow surgeons on staff] will be taking your last case, so you can go home to celebrate with your family."

With the word "family," Curtis felt a poignant absence. Then again, maybe this would be an excuse for Becky to dine with him once more. More likely he would dine alone with a sandwich, cold Alaskan amber, and "Seinfeld" reruns.

The following weeks were more chaotic than Curtis ever thought they could be. The media hounded him for interviews. Yet, at the same time, he had to forge ahead, as many patients were depending on him to give them their lives back. Probably the happiest were

Thomas and Mack. Thomas could veil his economic interests behind a "we are proud of you" attitude. However, Mack was clear, "Damnit, son, you have given us a hundred million dollars' worth of PR… and for free. Good work, you son of a bitch! I envy you and what I would give to walk in your shoes. You must be the happiest man on the planet."

Even after his big raise, Curtis continued his lean lifestyle. He stayed in his condo, drove his ten-year-old Jeep, and had no social life. He created a budget for himself of $55,000 a year, and he put the rest into an investment account, saving to buy-out his contract.

Within Curtis's head dwelled a self-generated voice of his father. He imagined that voice saying now, "Son, you are a success. I am very proud of you. I wish I had stayed with you and your mom and helped you navigate life." That also hurt because he didn't know if his dad knew, would ever know, or was even still alive. If he did know, would he be proud or not? Likely, he wouldn't care one way of the other.

His mother could not understand what all the fuss was about. She could not be there for him mentally as her memory seemed to be drastically fading as she was getting older. Even to Curtis himself, success—once the novelty of it started to wear off—left him feeling empty. He would much rather be walking down a hospital corridor full of poor people, from India, Africa, Asia, and America, whose loved ones had been cured, than walking into a grand hall receiving a Nobel Prize.

Becky did come, reluctantly, with him to Stockholm and seemed to enjoy the banquet but avoided the ancillary parties. They stayed in separate rooms, and her coldness waivered only slightly. Her excuse, this time, was her own research paper, for which she was trying to meet a publisher's deadline. She stayed in her room, her devotion lost into her MacBook's screen, as she worked on her paper. Curtis toured the beautiful city and attended meetings alone. At the awards banquet, she smiled at him once and kissed him after he returned to their table. That was the extent of the affection.

She agreed to accompany him the following evening to a private dinner, just for the two of them, at the Stallmästaregården Wärdshuset. They sat by a large window, looking out on the Brunnsviken Bay. There were daffodils on the table—a full yellow bloom in the dead of winter. Curtis made a great effort to only look upon her. His tunnel vision overtook his senses, by design. He thought of five questions to ask her about her life and her work. He wrote them on the palm of his hand, so he would not forget them. He started by asking about her work. She reported that her paper was based on a research project, which she had totally devoted her first year of graduate school to. She was working with a post-doc to create a drought-resistant strain of millet that has no GMOs in it. As scientists, they knew that inserting a gene from a desert grass into the millet would cut years off their research and yield a safe product in the end. However, the political climate was changing with a worldwide opposition to GMOs, at least in the first world. Curtis certainly agreed with her on that point, as it came up at his own IRB meetings in New York. Curtis asked her, "How then do you do this?" Then he sat in a tripod-stance, his back arched forward, his elbows on the table, and his fists supporting his chin. He awaited her answer.

Becky explained their research project. "At the University of Washington, they had a group of greenhouses and warehouses, where they could reproduce almost any soil, climate, and season that you could imagine."

He looked at the daffodils and back at her, "And any season?"

"Sure," she said. "They simply planted a crop of millet and programed the artificial climate control to reproduce a situation that was so harsh that only fifteen to twenty percent of the crops survived. The light and dark cycles determined the season, along with the ambient temperature. The computer would even send rain, from sprinklers in the ceiling, on a programed basis. Then they took the survivors' seeds and planted a new crop, then nudged up the conditions to a slightly harsher environment and waited until only fifteen to twenty percent survived. They repeated the cycle over and over. They could only do three cycles in a year, so it could take five years to end up with a strain that would equal the same strain they could have in six months by using the desert grass gene as a genetically modified organism (GMO)."

"That's fascinating," said Curtis, exhibiting a sincere curiosity.

Curtis felt that he had gained a little ground in his relationship by trying to focus on Becky, while at the same time, juxtaposed to that, the whole world was focusing on him and his accomplishments. His time with Becky in Sweden, once again, left him disappointed. He wasn't sure why. But he started to realize that it was the notion that he had given the relationship his best shot, and yet there was still no evidence of Becky changing. He still came up wanting. Once they were back in Seattle, she didn't call him again or return his text messages.

Curtis's greatest satisfaction from the trip was having an additional $700,000, the after-taxes total from the Nobel Prize money, to put into his savings account. He now had almost two million dollars and needed about seven and a quarter million more for his emancipation.

CHAPTER TWELVE: SANDRA

Curtis's mother's memory was continuing to decline rather rapidly, and he had been too busy with work and the prize to focus on her. Her muddled mind couldn't appreciate this moment of fame for her beloved son. "Mom," Curtis said with pride, "did you hear on the news that I won a Nobel Prize?" She seemed excited again but then forgot all about it by the next time he called. He wanted to keep reminding her, so that she could bask in the glory of her son's accomplishments… for her sake, not his. If there was a bright side to a failing memory, it is reliving a glorious moment over and over. She would, however, forget his phone calls from the week or even day before.

He had taken a trip to Tennessee in October to check on her. He noticed right away that there had been a decline in her cognition and that she certainly had some type of dementia, beyond simple aging. It took several calls for him to set her up with a neurologist. She was taken for her first appointment in late November with the help of a neighbor. Curtis was preparing for his trip to Sweden and couldn't make another trip to Tennessee at that time. He was determined to accompany her on a follow-up appointment with the neurologist in January. Despite how busy things were, the intense surgery schedule, the media hype being at its peak, he knew that he would have to go be with his mom.

On that visit, the neurologist was confident that she had Lewy Body Dementia, which would not only take her memory but also give her a body of a Parkinson sufferer. Curtis felt devastated and knew that her future would be methodically unravelling like an old sweater. He started to search for a memory care center to admit her if she progressed. He looked in Seattle, but there was a long waiting list, and he knew that, in Seattle, his mother would be separated from the few friends that she did have.

Curtis left the chaos once again and flew back to Tennessee in March. Somehow his trip was leaked to the media this time, and the local Tennessee news channel asked him for an interview during his visit. He spoke to the Johnson City TV station in a meeting room at the airport but declined a more in-depth interview, at least during this trip.

He drove his mother to Dr. Kimber's—the neurologist—office two days later. He walked in from the car, inter-locking his arm with hers. Her walking had declined, and she had some shuffle in her steps. Once inside, he sat his mother down in a waiting room chair and walked up to the window to check her in. He returned to his seat. He noticed one of the nurses looking at him. He had noticed the same nurse looking at him during the previous visit in January, but they never exchanged more than glances. He was startled when he looked up from a waiting-room Southern Living magazine, and the nurse was standing right beside him. She spoke to him in that conversant, East Tennessee enunciation, "Curtis, I don't think you remember me, do you, hon?"

At that second, looking into her robin-egg blue eyes, he suddenly recognized her. But the eyes didn't fit. But her voice and the general shape of her face were clearly recognizable. He could tell that she had gone through many physical changes, more than just the normal aging process. It was not just the blue scleral contacts over her original brown eyes, either. He laid down his magazine and stood up. Fortunately, her name finally found him. "Oh my, Sandra, is that you?" They spontaneously embraced.

She sat down in the seat beside him, and he slowly sat, too. "It is me. I knew you were in town as I just saw you on TV the other night. I couldn't believe it. You were nominated for a Nobel Prize or something like that, right?"

He nodded.

"You're the most famous graduate from Jonesborough High School. I thought it was you sitting out here, and then I looked at the schedule to see your mom's name. I think I had met her before but didn't recognize her."

"Well, I doubt if I'm the most famous graduate," not mentioning that he had won the prize. "There was Bundy, who played in the NBA. His little sister was in our class. I think he would get that title."

"I wouldn't know, as he was before our time."

Sandra asked Curtis how long he was in town, and he told her five more days. After the appointment, as they were scheduling his mother for her next visit, Sandra came back out to the check-out window. She asked if they could go out to dinner or get coffee. He agreed to meet her the next afternoon at a local coffee shop.

On the way home from Dr. Kimber's office, Curtis was deep in thought about her. She had never crossed his mind since they parted ways at graduation. He wasn't going to say anything, but his mother spoke up with a surprising comment. "That nurse, that's Patsy Smith's daughter, isn't it?"

Curtis, being surprised at the detail of her memory about old things, chuckled, "It is, Mom. Her name is Sandra, and she had a brother named Tim and another brother, Mark, who was a Marine killed in Lebanon, in the early 1980s."

"Oh, I remember that. It was horrible about her brother. But wasn't Sandra your girlfriend?"

Curtis was a shy boy in high school but did date a few girls briefly, all of whom had taken the initiative. "Yeah, Mom. Well, I wouldn't call her my girlfriend. We were friends, and we dated for a few weeks, maybe, at most. I did take her to the senior prom. But then I went off to college and lost touch."

"Are you going out on a date with her now? What would Becky think?"

He laughed out loud, "Mom, how can you remember some things so well and other things you can't? No, we aren't going on a date—we're just having coffee."

"Well, that's how these bad things start, you know. A married man goes out with another woman for coffee, and then bam, it's adultery."

240

Curtis burst out laughing. "Oh, good grief, Mom. It's just coffee." Curtis pondered in his mind if he should let his mother know that he and Becky weren't living together. It occurred to him that it probably wouldn't matter, as she wouldn't remember the conversation the following day. "Mom, Becky and I are separated."

She turned and looked at him with her mouth agape. "Now why's that?"

"I haven't a clue. I mean, I know she got mad at me and that was because of neglect. I was so consumed with my work. But now I don't know why. I'm not as busy as I was a couple of years ago. I have apologized to her many times… but, Mom, she can't seem to get past that. She went with me to Amsterdam when I got my Nobel Prize, but I haven't seen her once since then."

"Well, then I guess it's okay if you date that nurse."

"Mom, I'm not going on a date with Sandra! We're old friends, and we've a lot to talk about. I think she's married anyway."

"She wasn't wearing no ring on her finger."

He laughed again. "Mom, you noticed and remember that? I didn't even notice. Of course, I wasn't looking. You didn't remember I was at your house this morning, and I've been there for three days. I think your memory is selective." Then he chuckled out loud again… but his mother didn't see any humor in that comment.

The following morning, Curtis took his mother to visit a memory care center. He could tell that this made her angry, and she barely spoke to him for the rest of the day. Then he met Sandra at the Franklin Coffee Shoppe on East Main.

When he lived in Jonesborough as a kid, the location for the coffee shop was a ramshackle, old red-brick storefront, with large plate-glass windows. Now, the antebellum building had been renovated into a wonderful space. The glass was clean with the name of the coffee shop stenciled on the glass in large, white Canterbury lettering. Behind it ran the glistening, Little Limestone Creek.

The hour with Sandra turned into two, and then three. They talked about old high school friends and what happened to each one. Sandra was much more in touch with them than Curtis. She also described how she and Rusty Painter, her high school boyfriend whom she started to date after Curtis, were married, but then he became hooked on amphetamines. He was a long-haul truck driver and used stimulates to stay awake, which led to snorting speed and then smoking meth. He became totally hooked. He lost his job when he had an accident, and his blood draw was positive for drugs. She left him at that point, and he continued a downward spiral until he overdosed on heroin a year later. She had remained single for twenty years.

She also told the sad story of her parents. Two years after her divorce from Rusty, there was another personal tragedy when her father was killed backing out of their driveway. As if losing her big brother to a stupid truck bomb on a hopeless mission in the Middle East and her ex to a drug overdose wasn't enough misfortune for one person.

242

She explained that her mother had become what they all called a "new-ager." This was in late 1980s, after losing Mark in the bombing. Maybe it was her way of coping with the loss. She was into Shirley MacLaine spirituality after someone—with good intentions—gave her Shirley's book *Out on a Limb*. She planted "healing plants" all around their house and had giant quartz crystals everywhere. It was a strange turn of events when Sandra's mother planted a row of lavender bushes down the driveway to "escort good feelings" to their house. She wanted the bad feelings of grief to leave after a prolonged period of incapacitating bereavement. She planted them in a funnel shape, one row on each side of the driveway. The wide end of the funnel was at the road and near the house they closed in to the very edge of the driveway.

But her father hated the bushes and all the "spiritual crap," as he called it. Then one ironic twist came when he was backing out of the driveway in his mid-life-crisis 1968 Mustang convertible, which he had restored with a great passion. He was going to the hardware store on a sunny, Saturday afternoon. He couldn't see traffic above the lavender bushes, which were then quite high, while in his low-sitting car. This was especially true where the rows mushroomed out near the road. He backed right in front of a brown delivery truck. It struck his car at the gas tank and it immediately exploded into flames killing her father.

He had spent hours working on that old car and only drove it around town on sunny days with the top down. The seatbelts were old and hard to release. That day he was trapped." So, Sandra concluded, "Mom's healing plants murdered my father." Then she—peculiarly—burst into laughter.

Curtis looked at her curiously, "You have some morbid sense of humor. Are you joking about all of this?

"No," she answered. "This really did happen. I know, it's bizarre. The other sad thing is that after Mom watched Dad burn to death in the driveway, him yelling and not being able to get out of his seat, she went completely nuts. Mom was watering her lavender bushes up near the house when this all happened. All she could do was point the hose on the car. But soon the car erupted into a ball of fire that even a fire truck had a hard time putting out later. So, it was no match for her little garden hose."

Curtis sat, spellbound to the horrors inhumed within the story.

Sandra continued, riding on Curtis's heightened interest, "On the surface, she seemed to take it well. She kept saying that fire was Dad's destiny, and he had already come back. She believed that he had been reincarnated into a cockroach, which she saw scurrying up the driveway from the rock retaining wall that was baking in the fire's heat. She collected that cockroach and put it in a matchbox beside her bed. The bug died, but she kept insisting that it was just sleeping in the little box. She really believed that the little bug would wake up one day and go dancing with her, like Dad did when they were dating in 1960." Sandra sipped her latte, reached out, and put her hand on Curtis's arm, and continued, "Can you imagine, Mom

244

and the cockroach doing the twist?" Sandra had such a burst of laughter that her coffee dripped from her nose.

Curtis was staring at her with an intense perplexity wiped across his face as if this whole story was some type of bizarre embellishment.

Sandra added, "Mom was getting nutty before, but after watching Dad burn to death, and realizing that it was—in a way—her fault, she went off the deep end. I mean, completely off the deep end. She was admitted to Eastern State Mental Hospital with a psychotic break a few months later. She eventually returned to her house but has been a zombie since. I don't know if it's from the five psych meds she's on, the electrical shock therapy, or if being a zombie in her natural form. I kept thinking that she would just die and end her suffering, but she's still alive, in body at least."

"Were you at home when this happened—I mean, when your dad died?"

"Fortunately, no. I had just started nursing school at East Tennessee State. I was living back home after my marriage was over, but I wasn't there that day. No, I got the terrible call while I was on clinicals at the hospital." Finally, a passing show of grief came to her face and watery eyes. She wiped them with her napkin and flashed a big smile. "I'm fine."

Curtis had been studying her face as she was talking. With just a tad of squinting of his eyes, Sandra appeared to him as she did the last time he had seen her, on high school graduation day, save her blonder hair. He remembered giving her a hug as she was leaving with several of the football players, heading to Gatlinburg for an overnight graduation party. Curtis, of course, wasn't invited but went home to eat a special green bean casserole with his mother and his aunt. They drank alcohol-free champagne to celebrate. But when he looked closely at Sandra, his eyes—trained for identifying anatomical subtleties—could see the layers of work that she apparently had done. Her real hair was more auburn than blond, but he wouldn't be surprised if it had a touch of gray now that she was around forty-three or forty-four. Her real, brown, eyes were well hidden beneath their blue facades. Her face looked as tight and smooth as it did in high school, if not middle school. He first thought it could be the effects of Botox, but he could see the edge of the skin as it joined the turkey-neck, which she—like most people in their forties—had. It indeed had a mask-like appearance up close. Lastly, it was clear her breasts had been augmented. He couldn't remember anything about her breasts in high school, so surely, they were not as prominent of a feature then as they were now.

Curtis thought about her choices to make these so-called improvements on her physique. She was a beautiful girl in her teens and if the hopes of keeping that beauty were her purpose, then—in his eyes at least—they had failed. Sure, maybe a man, whom she had never met before, might be more attracted to her in her present state than in an au naturel version of her. However, to Curtis, there was no comparison.

246

After Sandra had finished her personal story, it gave Curtis license, in his mind at least, to candidly share about his own struggles, including those with Becky. He described how they had an affable trip to Sweden together in December, with real conversations, yet when they got back to Seattle, Becky never returned a single call. Sandra listened carefully but her only comment was, "That sucks." She also assumed that the trip was a simple vacation, not connecting the dots with the Nobel Prize or realizing the prize was a Swedish institution.

It was four in the afternoon and, after another half-hour of talking, Sandra looked at Curtis and said, "This has been fun. Why don't you come over to my cabin on the lake and I make you dinner?"

Curtis, smiling, responded, "I don't know. Mom's probably worried to death already. I better get back to her place."

They said their goodbyes, and Curtis gave Sandra a big hug, somewhat like the last hug twenty-six years ago. He put on his jacket, left the coffee shop, and drove home to his mom's house. He couldn't find her anywhere inside, and it was getting dark outside. As he walked around the yard, he heard moaning in the garden area. There was his mother lying, face down, on the ground between her rose bushes. Her mouth was covered in muddy red clay and her old, galvanized watering can was on the ground in front of her. He stooped beside her and in a fleeting panic asked, "Mom… are you okay?"

"Oh!" She screamed. "Oh, God help me!"

"Mom… what is it?"

"Oh, my God!" she moaned in a slightly quieter voice.

Curtis looked down at her legs and noticed her right leg was turned outward. He pressed into her groin, and she screamed, "Oh, shit! Don't do that!"

Curtis pulled his cellphone from his pocket to call 9-1-1. He didn't realize that it had been in airplane mode since his flight. Maybe he had left it that way in a subconscious attempt to escape the stress back in Seattle. As he turned the cellular service back on, immediately voicemail after voicemail began to download. He called the medics, who were quickly on their way.

While waiting for the ambulance to arrive, he tried to console his mom. He ran back into the house and got a wet wash cloth to clean up her face. He had always felt bad for not cleaning off Erika's face, while they were waiting for her CT scan. Her dad was certainly upset about that.

The medics pulled a stretcher out of the aid car, jerked it, and the wheels dropped down to the driveway asphalt. They rolled up into the yard, following an old brick path, which the crab grass had subverted under its roots and stolons. They rolled up beside her and released the wheels, letting the stretcher collapse to the ground. The two medics, caringly, loaded her up, and they were off to the Johnson City Memorial Hospital. Curtis locked the doors and stuck the keys in his mom's purse, something he would later regret.

He was sure that his Mom's hip was broken... and it was. While he waited alone in the ED, he started to listen to his voicemails. He had a total of thirty-eight in the three days he had been in Tennessee. Thomas had called several times and left messages stating that Mack had flown in from his new place in Thailand's Similan Islands. He showed up—unannounced—in Seattle, hoping to meet with Curtis, Thomas, and the whole executive team. Of course, Curtis wasn't there. He deleted each message, one by one, and turned his phone back to airplane mode. He reasoned that he could excuse his missed calls by "accidentally" leaving his phone offline. He was known to be absent minded, and he used that image to his advantage when he could.

The orthopedic surgeon came out and spoke to Curtis. He was a tall, slender man with short gray hair held up in front by a somber face. He said in a raspy voice, "Yes, she does have a broken hip," which didn't surprise Curtis at all. However, the surgeon added, "This isn't your typical broken hip. I looked at her bone density tests from last summer, and they were very good for her age."

"Yes, I know," said Curtis. "She was just diagnosed with dementia, Lewy Body to be precise, by Dr. Kimber, the neurologist. I'm sure that is why she fell... you know, with the changes in her gait. She seems to suddenly be aging quickly."

"I see," said the surgeon. "Well, her femoral head (not realizing that Curtis himself was a surgeon and explaining in very simple terms) is the bone that connects the hip to the leg. It's broken. However, it looks like it'd been weakened by a bony tumor. That's what I see on the CT. I don't know what kind of tumor it is. I think the best thing is to take her to the OR, and we can look at the mass and take a biopsy. If it looks benign, I can cut it out and try to create a new hip for her. If we get a real-time biopsy report back, and it is cancerous, we must make a new plan."

Curtis's mother was admitted to the hospital that night. They wanted to run some tests, including taking a couple of scans looking for a primary tumor source that may have spread to her bones. "It would be a huge mistake to take her to the OR," the orthopedist said, "and then find a lung filled with cancer."

The surgery was planned on Thursday, two days away, and that was the day that Curtis was supposed to be flying back to Seattle.

Curtis felt an intensification of his grief for his mom. Dementia was plenty to deal with. Then the changes in her movements from the Lewy Body disease were yet another blow. Now, a—possibly cancerous—tumor was the worst of it all. He felt like he should be calling someone. He was afraid to call anyone at Neurogenics, or they would know his phone was on. He was sure that Becky wouldn't even answer his calls.

He did call Jennifer. The phone rang a couple of times and her lively voice answered, "Hi, boss. How's it going down there?"

"Well, there are some complications. Mom broke her hip, and now I need to see this through. So, I will be here at least for a week."

"Okay, but Thomas is about to go out of his mind. Mack is here and wants you here ASAP. He's about to drive everyone crazy. Mack has been down here to ask me where you were several times."

"Mack? Down there? In the lab? That's strange. Can't I even get away once a year? Okay, explain to Thomas about my mother and that my cellphone was turned off. I want to get one night's rest, and then I'll make sure my phone is working tomorrow morning. I'll talk to him myself."

For reasons that Curtis wasn't sure about, he then dialed Sandra's number. He thought it was because he had a good feeling after talking to her over coffee. She was a sounding board for his thoughts and feelings, something he hadn't experienced in quite a while. He tried hard to avoid talking about his personal life at work. There would be many days when he would look back and have remorse about that call, but at the time it seemed the right thing to do.

"Hello," came her familiar voice with the southern drawl.

"Hi, Sandra, it's me."

"Well, hi, Curtis, hon. How's your mom?"

"It's funny that you should ask. There're complications."

"I'm so sorry to hear that. I hope she's okay."

"Well, to make a long story short, she broke her hip. I found her when I got home last night. I thought it was a simple fall due to her problems walking. Now it seems she has a tumor in her leg and it probably broke first. She's going to surgery on Thursday."

"Oh, Curtis, I am sorry to hear that. It's sad that she's diagnosed with dementia and then breaks her hip and has a tumor. Poor thing. You must be exhausted."

"I am. Plus my boss is in a frenzy looking for me."

A few seconds passed, and she asked him, "Curtis, they won't need you at the hospital tonight. Come on over to my lake cabin and let me cook for you. It is quite lovely here… and peaceful."

He thought about it for a few minutes. "Sure… why not? I don't think I can do much here at the hospital."

"God no. I was a floor nurse for almost ten years, and we couldn't wait for the families to leave. With people in the room it made our work twice as hard. I bet your mom is sleeping anyway with the pain meds."

Sandra gave Curtis clear directions, and, at six in the evening, he kissed his mom on the forehead. She awakened briefly. "Mom, I'm going to step out for a few hours. I'll be back later and stay with you tonight."

She smiled. "Just go back to the house and I will see you tomorrow. I hope I can go home tomorrow."

"Mom, like I said, you'll be here for a few days, as you need surgery for your leg."

"My leg is feeling fine now. I think they'll let me go tomorrow." Then she seemed to doze off again.

Curtis made his way to Sandra's house. It was on a high bank overlooking the lake and, while smallish, was quite a beautiful setting. The bank was steep and covered with young maples, pines, and bushes, leaving no real beach to access. Her home was a log home, looking like it was built in the 1970s or '80s from a kit with logs uniformly milled to about the diameter of a teacup saucer. Curtis also noticed right away that the stones around the foundation and fireplace were fake, probably concrete, or what they call cultured "river rocks." When Curtis commented on her cabin as "cute," she responded that she thought it was built by some of Daniel Boone's family when they lived in the area in the 1700s. Curtis thought of correcting her, but he just let it go. However, he was surprised about how unobservant she was about the world around her. Obviously to Sandra, at least on this night, the structure's history made little difference.

Sandra had welcomed him at the door with a wooden spoon in her hand. She was wearing cut off jean shorts and a button up blouse tied in a knot at the bottom, looking like she was auditioning for the old show *Hee Haw*. Her shorts seemed out of place for a dinner date and the seasonally cool evening. She was just finishing setting up the table with fried chicken and some type of sausage and spinach-noodle lasagna. It was a reminder to Curtis that southerners often prepare two main courses with dinner. Curtis helped make a salad. She paused in the kitchen to drink from a wine glass.

253

"What can I get you to drink, Curtis?"

"Oh, wine would be fine with me. A red wine like yours would be delightful."

She handed him a new bottle and asked, "Can you uncork this one? I am afraid that I finished off my bottle."

"I hope you didn't start it tonight."

Sandra laughed. "No, it just had one drink left in it."

They sat at the table and Sandra reached out and held his hand, giving it a squeeze, and said, "It is so good to see you again, Curtis. I can't believe it. And you've hardly changed in twenty years. Now, let's pray." Sandra led him in a brief prayer of thanksgiving.

He responded to her statement after the prayer was done, "Except for gaining about twenty-five pounds and thinning hair. But you look remarkable." Curtis was telling just a white lie. Sandra did look remarkably well for a forty-four-year-old woman—but with help.

"Well, I bet I could still fit in my prom dress... which is in Mom's closet. You do remember that dress, don't you?"

"Uh... sure," while his mind raced looking for the image and came up with nothing.

As the dinner progressed, they once again found themselves talking about their families and the changes they had seen in their lives since high school. They talked about the profession of medicine and how it had evolved. Everything had become more complicated now, where most of your time was documenting for, or fighting with, insurance companies for payment.

After dinner, Sandra fixed up strawberry short cakes, and the two of them took a seat in the living room. Sandra turned on her gas fireplace and turned down the lights. She pushed some buttons on her sound system and Michael Bublé's voice came on softly, surrounding the room. This was the line of demarcation in Curtis's mind, where a dinner between friends was taking a romantic flavor, whether he liked it or not… and frankly, he was unsure. Would Sandra become Becky's surrogate in that lonely place in his soul? Could she be the one to pull him from his private desolation?

Sandra seemed to be totally engrossed in his story of Neurogenics and his great trials and frustrations. However, she changed the subject any time that he spoke of Becky except to say things like, "That must've been hard for you" or "You deserved better than that."

Sandra kept the wine flowing and Curtis lost count. Was it his third glass or forth? He could feel the effects with weak legs and a sense of humor with a hair trigger. Sandra got sillier and sillier as the night went on. Then she opened the wooden trunk, which served as a coffee table, and pulled out an old cedar cigar box. He watched her with great curiosity. She flipped the lid and pulled out a small, glass, smoke-stained bong and a zip-locked bag of what appeared to be cannabis. She started to work stuffing a small cluster of dried buds into one end, finally pausing to look back at Curtis.

"Do you smoke?" she asked him.

"Believe it or not… never have. Not even in high school or college. It just never interested me, you know, trying to alter my brain with chemicals."

She lit it up and puffed through the glass stem until the smoke was thick, and in a stream, looking like a genie was about to appear. She savored the smoke in her lungs and slowly released it through her nostrils. "But pot is natural," she said as the lingering smoke puffed from her lips behind each word. She handed it to Curtis with a melted smile on her face.

He added, "Chemicals are chemicals… no matter where they come from. But I'll try it." He took one puff and started to cough and choke. Not absorbing enough THC through his nose and mouth to have an effect, he handed it back to Sandra while still coughing. She took one more draw and then put it out. "I guess pot isn't your thing?"

"Nope," he said in an awkward way. "Sorry."

"That's fine," said Sandra. "Rusty taught me how to smoke. He introduced me to it in high school the same night I lost my virginity. I think that was his plan. He got me so high, I couldn't hardly move, not knowing where reality ended… and fantasies began."

She moved close to Curtis and kissed him on the lips. Still, sitting very close, she asked him, "How did you lose yours?"

Curtis pulled back and shook his head, "I'd rather not talk about this." It wasn't just because of embarrassment that Becky had been his only one, but the topic also seemed inappropriate to him.

She poured him another full glass of wine, and they drank together. After finishing if off, she looked back at him and giggled, "Curtis, you're in no shape to drive home, young man. You can stay here… on my couch." Even a simple comment like that drew loud chuckles from both. Then they stared into the fire in silence. Curtis wasn't sure what she was thinking, but he had a spectrum of thoughts and emotions that even four (or was it five?) glasses of wine could not subdue. They both slid down and sat on the floor in front of the couch, pushing the coffee table away from them. She leaned against him, the shine of her eyes dancing with the flickering blue and orange light of the flaming ceramic logs. Curiously, Curtis found himself putting his arms around her, with her back resting on his chest. It felt surreal. Finally, Sandra spoke, "What happened to us?"

Curtis was thinking of the big picture of how they each had changed over time but then she was more specific. "I mean, why didn't we become a pair? If I hadn't fallen for that loser, who knows, maybe I would be the wife of a brilliant and famous neurosurgeon living it up in Seattle now."

Curtis chuckled. "I don't know. I mean, I never had the sense that you liked me."

She turned her head and looked at him, "Curtis, every girl in the school liked you. I mean, you were, and still are, the spitting image of a young Omar Sharif—you know, the Doctor Zhivago guy—but with lovely blue eyes. The only problem was... you were square."

Curtis looked at her with some confusion on his face and laughed. "That movie was well before my time." He paused for a moment and then added, with an inflection of wonder in his voice, "Square? What is that supposed to mean? Oh, and my eyes are green, at least the last time I checked."

"Curtis Eisner, you were a nerd before nerds were invented. You were awkward around us girls. I remember the night of the prom. You brought me home and kissed me on the lips at my parents' doorstep and went away. I loved that kiss, but you didn't try for anything more. I honestly felt sorry for you. Now, you're a few levels above me. I'm just a small-town nurse, and you're out there changing the whole fucking world."

Her compliments left a vacant awkwardness, which Curtis felt obliged to fill, "Look who's talking. You were one of the prettiest girls in our class. I guess I never asked you out again because I thought you were *above me*. You proved it when you started to date the quarterback."

Sandra rolled her eyes. "I guess that was my curse and my destiny. Yes, I could get the quarterback with my so-called good looks, but Rusty was a loser even then." She paused, and her eyes were drawn back into the fire. She yawned and leaned her head back against Curtis's. She said softly, "It didn't take me long to figure out that he wasn't just a 'party boy' but a full-fledged alcoholic, even in high

258

school. Then, when he didn't get a chance to play college ball, his dad gave him a job with his trucking company. He couldn't drink and drive, so he thought, but he reasoned that uppers and eventually speed would enhance his driving… which it didn't. I only married him because I was pregnant. Then I miscarried, and that marriage was for nothing. Absolutely nothing! A complete sham. My life was ruined, and I've never left this town."

They both sat and stared into the fire as they looked for conversation. Curtis was savoring the statement that all the girls in high school found him attractive, which he would never have guessed. With Becky's coldness, he felt like a real loser in the relationship department. All those letters from the public telling him that he was a loser confirmed that. He was sick of hearing that he was cold-hearted, cruel, money-hungry, and just plain evil. His mind had a way of being dismissive of the huge amount of acclaim that came with the Nobel Prize. The negative was weightier.

Sandra interrupted his thoughts when she asked, "Did you ever roleplay?"

He glanced down at the side of her hair against his face, "Do you mean as a kid?"

She turned her head toward him and rolled her eyes. She took another long, hard drink of wine and sat her empty glass on the floor. "No, goofball, I mean, did you and Becky every roleplay in the bedroom?"

Curtis felt a wave of awkwardness despite the disinhibition from the alcohol. "No… that wasn't something we ever considered."

Sandra looked at him and moved even closer, laying her ear against his chest. She listened to his heartbeat for a minute, counting each thud out loud. Then she added, "Well, it's never too late." Then she sat up and kissed him on the lips again. She turned and straddled his lap, her face in front of his and her arms on his shoulders. He kissed her, with a bit of passion. Eros was starting to prod him with the tip of his arrow.

She leaned back, still facing him, sitting on his lap, his belly between her thighs. Then she leaned forward again, looking at him eye to eye, with their noses touching. She whispered, "I think it would be a lot of fun to relive that prom night… but then you break out of the shy Curtis mold and put some pressure on me. Let me push you away, but you be persistent. Be like that Biff guy in *Back to the Future*. You just might be surprised what you can get." She just stared at him for a minute. Then her eyes lit back up, "Hey, I could run to Mom's house and get my prom dress and be back in twenty minutes… then we could see if you could rip if off me."

Curtis never remembered giving her an answer except that she didn't need to go get her prom dress as things became a blur. He just remembered them kissing and finally him starting to really like it. He remembered her pushing him back onto the floor and even slapping him once, as she burst into laughter, which in turn caused him to get the giggles. He remembered her biting his lip, hard, until it bled. He screamed, "Ouch!" and then they both laughed again.

Then she started to lick his neck… licking it like a cat. His sober mind thought it was weird, but his drunk mind could only laugh, plus it tickled. She eventually looked up and whispered, "I love the taste of a man's salt. It's an aphrodisiac for me."

Before long they were in her bed making love. He hadn't had sex, except once, in two years. That time was very strange, as he and Becky seemed to need each other physically, even though she wasn't talking to him. It was like two androids recharging some primal urge without an emotional intersection. It felt like a one-night-stand, although it was with his wife of six years.

Curtis awakened in the middle of the night feeling sick and empty. The hole in his soul was still there… maybe stretched out bigger. The sickness was real, a consequence of a bottle of wine… or more. He leaned over and vomited into the trash can beside the bed. He looked around the bedroom feeling dizzy. The curtains were all open, and he could see the moonlight reflecting over Boone Lake down below. It would've been romantic in any other circumstance. It was strange, but he thought of Becky and how he wished it was her in the bed with him. Curtis wasn't feeling any romance toward Sandra, just nausea and disappointment… in himself. Shame was seeping in, and it wasn't even morning yet.

"That stinks," mumbled Sandra without opening her eyes, referring to the vomit in the trash can.

"Sorry," was the only response he could give. He felt too sick to get up and try to clean things up. He was hoping that he would feel better by daylight. He laid his pounding head back on the pillow. As he was trying to go back to sleep—to sleep off the nausea—suddenly there was a knocking, then a pounding, not inside his head this time, but on the cabin door.

Sandra suddenly sat up in bed, "Who the hell's that?"

Boom, boom, boom, came that agitated knock. Sandra rubbed her face and rotated, putting her feet on the floor. She turned on the lamp on her bed stand. Curtis put his pillow over his face to block the light, leaving a peephole through which he could gaze on her nakedness in the light.

Boom, boom, boom, came the knock and then a man's voice yelling, "Sandra! Sandra! Open this damn door!"

"Oh, shit," she said softly.

Curtis, still peering from beneath his pillow, "Who's that?"

She stood up and walked toward the en suite, where her bathrobe hung. She put it on and shuffled back into the bedroom. "That's Robert… he's my boyfriend."

With the word "boyfriend," Curtis suddenly felt a wave of fear overcoming him, enough fear to subdue the nausea a bit. Taking the pillow off his face he looked at her, "Boyfriend? Are you kidding me! You didn't tell me you had a boyfriend."

She sat on the edge of the bed to regain her balance as the banging and screaming at the door got louder. "Well… it's complicated." She paused to shake her head as if to clear her thoughts. "It's an on-again, off-again type of relationship. I guess tonight… Robert seems to think it's on." Then she looked at him and added, with a frown, "I don't know why you're so surprised… *you* have a wife."

Curtis felt that he didn't need to be reminded of that. "What should I do?" he asked. He was feeling that he would rather be anywhere in the world right now than in Sandra's bedroom dizzy and nauseated with her angry boyfriend beating the door down. He would fight for Becky, but the relationship with Sandra wasn't worth fighting for. Honestly, he didn't want to ever see her again after this night. He felt like a foolish rabbit in a snare.

"Nothing. There's no back door, or I would say go for it. Robert is quite hot-tempered. Let me see if I can calm him down." As she was struggling to stand again, she added in a low voice, "My god, I hope he didn't bring his gun. He can be so silly sometimes." Then she exited the bedroom.

Curtis hastily turned on his bedside lamp and started to look around the room for his clothes. "Gun" and "silly" were not two words he would normally associate with each other. "Gun" and "serious" seemed to work much better in his mind. He saw a shirt on the floor but not his shirt… and no pants. He figured that he must have left all his clothes in the living room, just inside the front door where the madman was knocking. Could he make a dash for them and get back? He didn't think so.

He quickly stood up and donned the shirt. He opened Sandra's drawers looking for something he could put on, but the choices were limited. He did find a pair of flannel pajama bottoms, but he couldn't get them over his thighs. He felt ridiculous and just laid back in the bed.

About this time, he could see through the door, which was still ajar, Sandra slowly walking (obviously with a hangover as well) to just inside the outside door and shouting through it, "Rob, now calm down. It's four in the morning; why are you here?"

"Let me in, damnit! Sandra, who the hell's in there with you?"

Curtis felt a panic when she unlatched the door and whispered audibly, "Oh no, don't let him in… are you crazy?"

Apparently, she cracked it open to where the security chain became engaged. Shouting through the door wasn't working for her. "Rob, listen to me," she said without shouting, "There's an old high school friend here. He had no place to stay so I gave him my bed, and I was sleeping on the couch. Nothing happened here last night."

This Robert guy could see through the door crack and looked around the room. "You're lying to me, bitch! I see the wine bottles, and the couch doesn't look like it was used as a bed."

Then he started kicking the door. "Stop it, asshole!" Sandra shouted again while wincing at her headache, "You're going to break my damn door. Just calm down, and I will open it."

With those words, Curtis's anxiety quickly morphed into a pure panic attack. He felt like he was in a nightmare, the kind where you are swimming to get away from a hungry alligator, but instead of water, you are swimming in honey… while the gator was right behind you—making no metaphysical sense—swimming in water. The fatigue, the alcohol-induced vertigo, all made it hard for his reflexes. He stood up and stumbled to the window. He opened it and took out the bug screen. It slipped out of his hands, falling into the dark void. With the light coming off the lake through the trees, he was blinded by the shadows to what was below the window. However bad it may have been, this route offered him the only escape.

He walked over to the en suite, turning on the lights and closing the door in front of him. He thought that would stand as a decoy for his escape. He caught his reflection in the mirror over the sink, just before the door closed. He felt ridiculous wearing nothing but a silky shirt, only now realizing it was Sandra's pink blouse. If she hadn't been a busty woman, it would not have fit his chest.

About that time, loud arguing broke out in the living room. Curtis walked over to close the bedroom door and lock it. A locked door, so he figured, would provide a temporary obstacle for the deranged man. He peeked through the crack, wanting to get a look to size him up… and to see if he was carrying a weapon. To his disbelief, he quickly recognized the man as none other than Dr. Kimber, wearing gray dress pants and an untucked white oxford shirt. There was a rapid flashback in Curtis's mind, to when he was sitting with his mom in Dr. Kimber's office. He saw the large photo on his desk of him, a lady, and two boys. It appeared to be a family photo, and the lady certainly wasn't Sandra. Now he was mystified.

He saw the man look in his direction. Sandra was pushing him away from the bedroom, but she had no chance of stopping him. Kimber was a big man. Curtis shut the bedroom door and locked it.

Curtis ran to the window and stuck both legs out, one at a time. He sat on the sill looking back over his shoulder and once again into the darkness below him. He inched further through the window as he heard Kimber pushing his way toward the bedroom door. Up to his waist and looking down… Curtis saw nothing but darkness below. Even the moon was flirting with the clouds, obscuring its humble light now and then. He quickly rolled over on to his belly and tried to gently let himself down, far enough at least until he could find something to stand on with his foot. There was nothing… nothing but air. There came a huge crash at the door, like a hard kick. Then another. Robert. Kimber shouted, "Open the door, you sorry son of a bitch. Open the damn door, or I will beat you unconscious with it, asshole!" There was a short pause and a peculiar change in the man's tone, "Okay, man, let me in, I just want to talk to you."

In the background, Curtis could still hear Sandra saying, "Rob, go home! We can talk about this tomorrow."

Then came another loud kick, and Curtis thought he heard the door crack. He dropped feet-first out the window. He had no idea that the lake bank was over fifteen feet below, followed by a steep landing on brush and rocks, and then several more feet down to the water's edge. On the way down from the window, he felt a sharp stab in his abdomen when he caught something… maybe a nail or a metal flashing. The object must have been protruding out of the side of the house. Then his feet hit hard, and he began to tumble and roll in the direction of the lake, being poked with sharp branches and pounded with rocks as he rolled over them through nature's gauntlet. It seemed like minutes, but was only seconds, before he came to rest with one leg in the cold lake water. He had never felt so horrible—bodily—in his life. He vomited again. After the heaving was over, he had a very sharp pain in his abdomen and felt it with his hand. It was wet and sticky, so he knew he was bleeding.

Curtis looked up and saw the lights on in the bedroom far above him. Robert Kimber's head was sticking out the window as he continued to shout, "Hey, you coward! Come up here and fight me like a real man. No one screws my woman and lives to tell about it, you damn asshole! I'm coming down there to beat the living shit out of you… and now I know who the hell you are!"

Curtis laid his head down in the slimy mud and held his hand over his abdomen. Was he dying? Did he disembowel himself on the way down? He fingered his wounds carefully in the dark. His muddy finger-tips caused a hard sting when they touched the open flesh. He felt no deep, penetrating spaces, but he could tell that the cut was well into his fatty layer, cut cleanly as with a fillet knife. While not feeling any penetrating wounds in his gut, he was cut well enough to cause him to bleed to death. He washed the mud off the cut with dirty lake water. He held his wound edges together with his fingers as best as he could while trying to apply pressure at the same time. Was this his destiny to die in the mud outside his lover's—not a lover but a mixed-up woman's—bedroom? He prayed for the first time in a long time, except for the strange pretend prayer at dinner the previous night. But this time he was sincere. "God, please help me!" If only the moon was a little brighter, he might see how severe the wound had been.

He heard a scuffle at the top of the bank on the left side of the cabin. It was Kimber, now outside with a flashlight, trying to climb down the seventy-five-degree embankment. Sandra was yelling at him, "You idiot! You are going to break your neck. That's a thirty-foot drop to the lake." Oddly, Curtis felt some hurt as she seemed to have no regard for his own well-being.

The man, in an unhindered passion of purpose, continued climbing down, thrashing and moaning, and then the flashlight appeared to fall out of his hand or his mouth or wherever he was carrying it. The flashlight bounced between trees on the way down, casting its light like a disco ball in all directions as it tumbled, landing a few feet from Curtis.

"You're a dead man!" came another shout through the dark brush. Curtis had a real fear for his life. Was this how it would all end? What a stupid waste of everything.

CHAPTER THIRTEEN: TRANSFIGURATION

Kimber had now slid three quarters of the way down to the lake. From the left side of the cabin, he slid through the mud, rocks, and brush… while Curtis started to climb up on the right side. With Kimber now deafened by the noise of his own scrambling, impeded by branches rubbing across his clothes as he tumbled through the brush, and blind from the loss of his flashlight, it seemed an opportune time for Curtis to try and make his escape.

Curtis reached up with his right hand and grabbed a small tree. As he pulled himself up, he tried not to dislodge it completely out of the ground, which would result in him falling back to his starting point, or even into the lake. He was entangled in vines and had to tear his way through them via brute force. He reached again until he felt another small plant with his left hand. Back and forth he worked his way up the bank, digging his toes into the soft, wet clay, while Kimber was battering around twenty-five feet away screaming, "Where are you… you sorry son of a bitch? I'm going to beat the hell out of you! I'm gonna drown your sorry hide in the damn lake."

Curtis could hear the man slipping downward and above him came Sandra. She was sliding in the dirt in her house coat, which seemed to be coming off as it was getting hung up on the bushes. He could barely see her in the remnant of the—now unclouded—moonlight. The weak light barely penetrated the edge of the thick undergrowth. Finally, he reached the top of the bank, and he grabbed onto a big rock and pulled himself into a standing position. He looked back down, and there was Kimber at the lakeshore, crawling around in the mud looking for his flashlight, which had lost its light from either being submerged in water or being switched off from the tumble. Curtis took the opportunity to run for his car. He found the car door locked. He remembered that the keys were in his jacket. He wasn't sure where his jacket was but assumed it was somewhere in the living room. "Shiiiiiit!" he quietly screamed.

Fortunately, Kimber, in his haste, left the front cabin door standing wide open. Curtis ran in and looked around. He saw his jacket over the back of a rocking chair. He grabbed it and the weight of the left side confirmed to him that the keys were in the pocket. He was about to run out the door when he paused and ran back, grabbing his pants off the floor, and then made a run for it.

When he started his little red, rental Civic, only then did Kimber realize that the man—his prey—had escaped.

Through the sunroof—that he apparently had left open—Curtis could hear Kimber screaming at Sandra, "Stop that bastard!"

Curtis hit the gas and backed out, clipping off the passenger mirror of Dr. Kimber's black BMW as he swerved around it. He backed into the street, threw it into drive, and the front-wheel drive spun out on the asphalt. He finally got traction and was down the short street in a few seconds. He turned right, heading toward the main highway.

When Curtis hit the main highway, he also hit the gas. The little car had a hard time keeping up with Curtis's intention. However, he had only gone three miles when he went around a sharp elbow in the highway and then flashing blue lights were behind him.

"Shiiiiiiiiiitt!" screamed Curtis to himself again, but this time in a loud voice. "I can't believe it, a damn cop!"

A thousand thoughts crossed his mind in a second. Should he try to outrun the officer? Not in this Civic. What will he say to him? He couldn't come up with any believable story… except the truth.

Curtis slowed down and pulled over to the shoulder of the road and the police car pulled up behind him. He looked over at his wadded-up pants in the floor of the passenger side. He thought about trying to reach for them and putting them on, but that hasty movement could be interpreted by the cop as a hostile action… and Curtis feared he could be shot. However, at this juncture he wasn't sure that would be a bad thing. He had never—in his entire life—been afraid of being shot before. This night he had faced such a possibility twice and by two different men… in the span of ten minutes.

The cop sat in his car for what seemed like an eternity. Curtis sat frozen with his hands on the wheel. Finally, the cop opened his door and slowly walked up to the car with a flashlight in his hand and a radar gun hanging from his belt. He came up to the window and asked, "May I see your driver's license and car registration?"

"Sure," answered Curtis. Then he opened the glovebox and pulled out the rental papers, which included the registration. Then he leaned over to grab his pants and the cop seemed alarm, "What're you doing?"

He sat back up. "Uh, sir, my billfold is in my pants, and my pants are on the floor."

The cop, who had been shining his big Maglite in his face, then worked the light downward on Curtis's body, first to his muddy, exposed chest, then down to the gash in his abdomen that was caked with gooey blood and dirt. Then the light shone farther down to his groin, where his pubic hair was all matted with coagulated blood. He then worked the flashlight back up to study the pink, unbuttoned, blouse he was wearing. Then he spoke, appearing to be unshaken or even surprised, "Okay, get your billfold."

While Curtis was reaching for his pants, the cop spoke again, "Sir, do you need an ambulance?"

He sat back up in the driver's seat. "Uh, no sir, I'm fine." He handed the officer his open billfold.

As he took it out of Curtis's hand, he remarked, "You look like hell. I think you need to see a doctor."

Without thinking, Curtis said, "I'm fine. Besides, I am a doctor."

The cop looked at him and mumbled, "A doctor? What kind of doctor?"

"Uh… a brain surgeon, sir," he replied, using the term he reserved for laypeople to avoid having to explain what a neurosurgeon was.

272

As the cop studied the driver's license he looked back at Curtis, "A brain surgeon, you say?"

Curtis thought that if he had added, "A Nobel Prize-winning brain surgeon" for sure the cop would think he was high, or delusional.

The officer walked back to his cruiser and sat down. Curtis was shaking because he felt so nervous and cold. Being in the cool spring air, wet from the lake… and wearing nothing, his body core temperature started to plummet. The fear of being chased by a madman and now being caught by a cop speeding while naked and dirty was the substance of nightmares. Now he was shivering and facing hypothermia. He was afraid to start the engine to turn on the heat. The cop would think he was going to make a run for it. Could this all just be a bad dream? A very, very bad dream? He only hoped so, but the pain he felt from limb to limb assured him that this was no reverie.

The cop returned. He had something in his hand. "Sir, I'm going to ask you to take a deep breath and to blow through this straw."

Oh shit, Curtis thought, remembering the bottle of wine he had consumed the previous night. As a scientist, he was trying to quickly calculate if the alcohol could be out of his system by now through vomiting and respiration and hepatic processing. He had no clue what time of day it was, but he could see some light in the sky to the east, so sunrise couldn't be too far off. He quickly calculated that it had been four or five hours since his last drink.

He followed the policeman's command and blew into the straw. The officer studied the reading and then he replaced the straw with a new one. "Okay, let's get one more reading for good measure."

Curtis blew into the new straw and the cop studied it again.

"Son, you just missed a DUI by a point. Now, do you want to tell me your story? You were driving fifteen miles per hour over the limit, and I can just give you a warning for that, or I can give you a ticket. You just missed the DUI. There is no law against driving naked or driving wounded. I would like to hear your story, so I can decide if I need to take you in for more questioning. I would like to know how you got cut."

Curtis rubbed his face and then said, "I'm sorry for all of this. I mean, I'm a respectable professional. I rarely drink alcohol."

The cop seemed, at least to Curtis, to be rolling his eyes as he had already heard every excuse possible.

Curtis continued, "But a friend invited me to her cabin. She got me drunk. Then we slept together. Next thing I know, her boyfriend showed up threatening me."

The cop seemed alarmed. "So, he did this to you? He beat you up and cut your belly?"

"Oh, no. He never touched me. I fell out of the cabin window, trying to get away. I caught my belly on something. Something sharp, like a nail. Maybe I caught it on a piece of metal flashing on the way down. It could have been the bug screen, which I had tossed out earlier. I tumbled down a steep hill and got all scratched up."

"Really?" asked the cop.

Curtis, feeling like he wasn't being believed, added, "The man was mad at me. Very mad. He was also after me… but he never touched me."

"So, what happened to him? Why isn't he after you now?"

Curtis thought about Robert Kimber for the first time in a few minutes. "Uh… I guess he's still at the cabin. But again, I wouldn't be surprised if he was still coming for me."

The words were barely out of Curtis's mouth when a black BMW came flying around the sharp corner behind them with the wheels squealing. The cop quickly turned and pointed his radar gun at the approaching car with a steady head like a gunslinger in an old western.

As the BMW passed, it was like a slow-motion or stop-frame film. Curtis and Kimber locked their eyes, one on the other. Curtis could even see the broken passenger-side mirror dangling by a cable. He saw mud on Kimber's face and his teeth clenched. Once Kimber had passed, his bright brake lights were lighting up the highway in reflective cerise. Then the red went off and the engine roared to pick up speed.

The cop looked at the radar in his hand. "My Doppler clocked his speed at eighty-five miles per hour when he came around the curve. Is that the guy who's after you?"

"That's him," said Curtis confidently.

"Man, that guy is pissed! Okay," said the officer, "I've gotta go. Get home safely and get yourself to a doctor… a real doctor."

The police officer jumped back into his cruiser, which was still idling, and took off in a big hurry after Dr. Kimber. Curtis decided to take an alternative route to his mother's house. He certainly didn't want to play a game of leapfrog with Kimber, where he would pass the man beside the road after being pulled over by the same cop.

When Curtis arrived at his mother's house, it was still quite early… maybe 5:30 at the latest. He slipped on his pants in the car before he made a run for the house. Only when he got to the door did he remember that his mother had her keys in her purse at the hospital. He had a way to monitor and deactivate the alarm system and even to unlock the doors with his cellphone, but he felt his pants pocket and his phone wasn't there. He realized that it must be somewhere on Sandra's floor—that's if Kimber didn't get it.

"Damnit!" he shouted as he slapped the door with his open hand. He stood in the darkness contemplating his next move. Should he try to go to the hospital to get the keys? What would they think with him wearing a muddy and bloody pink blouse that wouldn't button? How would they take him being barefoot and hemorrhaging from this belly? They would call the cops for sure. Maybe if it were Halloween night, he could pass it off as *moulage*. Then he thought about the present date. It was the first of April… April Fools' Day. He felt like the fool.

"I doubt if Kimber knows where I'm staying," Curtis whispered out loud. Then a thought came to him. Kimber said he knew who he was. As a physician, the neurologist surely had access to the electronic health records, even remotely. It would only take him a few clicks to figure out his mother's address. He felt a sudden state of panic again, realizing that Kimber might pull up at any moment. He preferred to be inside the house, rather than standing in the driveway without cover.

Curtis walked around and pulled a garbage can up beneath the bathroom window. He climbed up on top of the can and then tried to open the window. This was the window he used to crawl into when he came home past his curfew. If he came in late, it wasn't because he was out partying, it was because he was at a friend's house watching an episode of *Nova* or *Nature*, which ended at eleven. Now, the window was painted shut and wouldn't budge. Then he, out of frustration, kicked the glass window with his bare foot. It broke alright, but not without leaving a small gash on the bottom of his sole. "Shit!" he screamed in pain as blood started to drip.

He reached in and unlatched the window. Then he pounded it open, hitting the frame from the inside with his fist, trying hard not to cut his wrist on the remaining glass. He took one of the pieces of pane

277

and used it like a knife to scrape some of the paint off the edge. Finally, it budged. He opened it and climbed in. He sat down to look at his cut foot. It was a deep cut. Now he had two medically significant wounds needing a cleansing and closure. He had to do it himself, as he wasn't about to go to the ED and suffer even more humiliation.

He stumbled into his old bedroom and picked some clothes out of his suitcase and his running shoes. He hobbled back into the bathroom to shower. The room was small with brown plastic walls of faux tiles. It had a tub with a shower head and a curtain to keep the water inside. He looked in the mirror. He had scratches, mud, and dried blood all over his face that he had not noticed before. He had a brief flashback to three months earlier, standing in his room at the Radisson Blu in Stockholm in his tux, looking in the mirror, trying to figure out how to tie his bowtie. On that day, he felt like a little boy playing James Bond. Now he felt like an old and addlepated version of himself or even a homeless crack-head living the lowlife.

He said to his reflection, "Curtis, man, you look like shit!" The anger suddenly built in him. He screamed at the man behind the glass, "You stupid fool! What's wrong with you!" as he pounded the mirror with soft sides of both fists. He was in tears.

He turned the bathtub water on as hot as he could stand and stepped in, switching the water to come out the showerhead. He gently soaped and washed the wound on his abdomen. He wanted to make sure that the cut had not penetrated his abdominal wall into his gut. With close inspection in light, he found that it had not. But the probing with his fingers stirred up the pain, which his adrenaline rush had subdued until that point. He next turned his attention to his lacerated foot. While the noise of the water was drowning out all the background noise, suddenly he was shocked when a bright light came in through the broken window and—simultaneously—a pounding came from the front door. His heart fluttered within his chest and then took off at an amazing rate. He immediately assumed it was Kimber at the window with his flashlight and maybe Sandra at the door. In a reflex, he fell to the bottom of the tub in the fetal position, as if to hide. But with the water running, he knew that he would soon be discovered.

Then came a shout through the window. "Come out of the house… and keep your hands where I can see them!" The voice wasn't Kimber's.

Oh, shit… the police… again, thought Curtis to himself.

"Okay, I'm coming! Let me get a robe on!" Curtis shouted back.

He turned the water off and dried off his face. He padded his abdominal wound, which was starting to seep blood again after the washing and cleaning. He reached over to the wall and found his mother's lime-green housecoat with fishnet edging. It was hideous. He made a quick decision that it would be better to don the bathrobe than to take the time to put on his underwear, pants, shirt, socks, and shoes. Hoping to resolve this issue quickly, he grabbed the robe, put it on, and tied it snug. He held the towel, firmly, against his abdomen for a minute, trying to dam the flow of blood and restart the coagulation.

He limped to the front door wrapped in the gaudy garb. He dripped blood along the way as the wound on his foot was reopened with the walking. He unbolted the door. There stood two officers, a woman and a man. The woman had a can of pepper spray pointed at him. He then looked at the male officer and he had his gun drawn. "Hey, please put the gun down. I'm unarmed."

Neither officer put their weapons away. The woman officer asked him, "What are you doing breaking into this house?"

"This is my mother's house. She's in the hospital. I came home and had forgotten the keys and had to break in."

There were just stares from the two cops.

"Really," Curtis added.

The male police officer asked, "Why didn't you just go back to the hospital and get the keys?"

"I don't know. I just thought I could fix the window today."

The woman officer asked, "Do you have a form of ID?" The thought quickly came to Curtis's mind that he had never felt the presence of his billfold when he had put on his pants to run to the house. Surely, he had left it in the car from when he showed it to the previous officer.

"I'm thinking about that. It has been a long night at the hospital, and I think I left my billfold in the car. Can I get it?"

The police, seeming to fear that he had a weapon in his car or that he would make a run for it, denied his request.

"Is there some other form of ID I can use?" he asked and waited for a response with raised eyebrows.

The officers said nothing as the question seemed circular.

"Come into the house, and I will show you my photos on the wall with Mom."

The officers, with hesitation, did follow him into the house. They saw the photos of Curtis and his mother on the wall, but that didn't solve the issue for them. Their silence suggested that they were in as much of a quandary as Curtis was. Curtis then suggested that they call the hospital to confirm that his mother was there and that he was the one who brought her there. The male officer went out to his squad car to make the call; when he returned, the woman officer walked out to the car to look for his billfold. She returned with it. Curtis noticed that when she came back into the house she was staring at his feet. He looked down to see a pink-tinged water dripping down from under the bathrobe.

"Sir," said the officer. "Can you open your robe?"

"Uh, well it's my mother's robe." The officer said nothing but continued staring at him. He opened it. She had a grimace on her face. "Oh, my God! What happened to you?"

Curtis rolled his eyes thinking, here we go again. "Mam, I cut my abdomen crawling out of a window."

The male officer spoke up, "I thought you crawled *in* through the window?"

"It's a long story, and I've already told it to another officer this morning." He could tell they weren't backing down, so he continued, "Okay, I was with my girlfriend last night and her ex-boyfriend came home, and I crawled out the window in the dark and cut my belly. I came back home to Mom's house to clean up and go back to the hospital to check on her."

The officers stood in silence trying to decide if they believed his, expanded, version of his story. Curtis added, "The officer that pulled me over was on Old Boones Creek Road and his last name on his badge was Cole. Yes, Officer Cole. I remember his name because I went to school with some Coles." Curtis started to feel that he had already said too much.

It took another thirty minutes before the police were satisfied enough to leave. Fortunately, they knew Officer Cole, and a quick call on the car radio seemed to substantiate Curtis's story. The male officer's last words to him were, "You should go to the ER and see a doctor when you go back to the hospital." Rather than announcing that he was a doctor this time, Curtis just smiled and said that he would.

Curtis felt exhausted. He figured that he had only had about three hours sleep before all the commotion had started, and he had a full-blown hangover. He took care of the wounds on his belly and his foot with what he had available to him in his mom's house. Duct tape and a few drops of superglue was all he had to work with. He tried to put a stitch or two in, with his mother's sewing kit, but the pain of the dull sewing needle made it too difficult to pierce his flesh. He got fully dressed and decided to head to the hospital.

He walked into his mother's room from a hallway with a hint of fresh fecal smell. She was sleeping quietly as the IV dripped and the infusion pump rapidly flashed a white light in a musical 3/8 time. Without awakening her, he kissed her on the forehead. He walked over and sat in the recliner beside her bed, with a sigh of exhaustion. He was just drifting off to sleep when the door swung open. In walked a tall, thin man with gray hair wearing surgical scrubs. It was the same orthopedic surgeon he had met in the ED when his mother had fallen. Curtis sat up. The man was accompanied by a nurse, and he had an electronic tablet in his hand.

At first the pair didn't seem to notice Curtis, but then the tall man looked at him and reached out his hand to shake Curtis's as he stood up. "Hello, I'm Doctor Ambrose, and I will be doing your mother's hip surgery."

"Oh, hi. I'm her son, Curtis. I think we met in the emergency department, but I didn't catch your name before."

The surgeon smiled and looked back at his mother.

The nurse spoke into his mother's ear, trying to wake her. "Mrs. Eisner! Hello, Mrs. Eisner, the doctor's here to see you."

283

Her eyes shot open, and she looked around the room with a startled, wide-eyed look. Curtis reached for her hand. "Hi, Mom."

"Mrs. Eisner, my name is Dr. Ambrose, and I'm the surgeon that will be operating on your hip in a couple of days."

"A couple?" asked Curtis.

"Yes," said Dr. Ambrose. "We will be operating on her Friday morning. We were going to do it tomorrow, but there were some more tests that we think need to be done. It would be too late to work her into tomorrow's schedule, so we need to put it off a day."

"What kind of tests?"

"I have been looking at the CT scan, and, as you know, there's a tumor growing in her leg. I also read her notes about her recent cognitive changes. The thing I would like to sort out is if the two are related or just a coincidence."

Curtis knew instantly that the only relationship between the two could be a metastatic bone tumor that had spread to her brain. He looked at his mom, and she was already back to sleep. He looked at Dr. Ambrose again, "Really?"

"It's possible, and it could change the course of our plan. I mean, if she had other parts of her body affected—lungs, liver, or brain— then we may not choose to operate at all."

"Okay. I am a surgeon myself. You can be candid with me."

"General?"

"Uh... no, neuro."

"Oh, then you know exactly what I'm talking about. I think I could've asked you which tests we should order, but I already have asked her neurologist, Dr. Kimber, to stop by this morning to see her. I wanted him to rule out a brain metastasis before we move forward."

With the mention of Dr. Kimber's name, Curtis felt the breath knocked out of him... so much that he sat—more like fell—back into his chair.

"Are you okay?" asked the nurse.

Curtis looked at her and answered, "Sure, I'm just overcome by the possibilities that lay ahead." He paused for a moment thinking about the change in plans. "She did have a brain MRI in November when she was first diagnosed with dementia."

Dr. Ambrose smiled at him. "Yeah, that's been a few months, so I wanted Dr. Kimber to decide if we need to reimage her now."

Soon Dr. Ambrose and the nurse left the room, and Curtis sat back in his chair with a wave of extreme apprehension. Would Robert Kimber really show up, or was he at home nursing his own hangover and beat-up body from the tumble down the hill? Maybe the man was in jail for a DUI? But what if he came in? Curtis needed a nap badly, but for now... there was no way he could sleep. He was afraid that Kimber would walk through the door at any minute, and there would be a nasty confrontation right in his mother's room, maybe even a fist fight… something he had never done in his entire life. Should he go and try to sleep in his rental car?

He was startled about half an hour later when Sandra, unexpectedly, came through the door. She looked totally different than the last time he had seen her. She was now in her professional clothes, wearing a bold striped shirt, tan skirt, and coffee jacket. She was, inconspicuously, carrying a brown paper bag at her right side, the large kind that they use in grocery stores. Curtis felt a medley of emotions ranging from bewilderment to right out anger. Nowhere did he feel affection.

"Hi, Curtis. Are you okay?"

"Yeah," he said with hesitation in his voice.

"Hey, I'm sorry about last night. I never expected him to come to the cabin. He'd been drinking and must've come to check on me."

"You think? Yeah, he'd been drinking, and I thought he was going to kill me. Now, he's coming to round on my mom in a few minutes."

"So, you figured out who he is?"

"Yeah, I saw him through the crack in the door. It makes no sense to me."

"Are you leaving?" Sandra asked.

I feel like I should be here for her, but I would hate it if a scene broke out here in her hospital room. I have already had two run-ins

286

with the police since last night--the first and second in my life. My only hope is that *he's* in jail for a DUI, or at least home sleeping off a hangover."

"I'm sorry, I really am." Sandra looked at his mom, who was sound asleep, and then sat on the foot of her bed and looked back at Curtis, "He'll be here. But, there's not going to be a scene, I guarantee you that. Robert has a way to compartmentalize his life."

"How do you know he's coming?"

"He's as elusive as a cat. I don't know how he does it, but I've already heard the cop didn't catch him last night. His car is fast, and he knows how to pull into a driveway with his lights off. When he has been caught, and last night's drinking and speeding wasn't his first time in such state, he talks himself out of a ticket or an arrest by saying he is on his way to the hospital to save a patient's life. Then he gets a police escort… not an arrest." She quietly chuckles.

"Do you think he really knows it was me?"

"Of course, he does. He probably knew I was with you from the start. I mentioned that you were an old high school friend after he saw your mom in the office. But understand, he's very professional. I will be shocked if he said a word about it. He will just pretend that nothing happened between the two of you last night."

Curtis looked at the floor and shook his head. Sandra added, "Cheer up, Curtis. It was fun while it lasted."

"It wasn't *fun*, Sandra!" He said snappishly. "That was the worst night of my life. I should say 'day' as well, because I almost got arrested for speeding and a DUI. Then I almost got arrested an hour later for breaking and entering Mom's house."

Sandra started to giggle.

"Sandra—really—this isn't funny!" said Curtis in a loud voice.

"Curtis, lighten up. Robert will come in here and take good care of your mom and treat you with the same respect that he would any family member. He's a great neurologist. Think about this, he's happily married with two sons. He's the deacon at the big Jonesborough Baptist Church. He goes on medical mission trips for his church and the whole nine yards. As I said, the man knows how to compartmentalize his life, and I mean pigeonhole, with big, thick dividers between each section."

"And he sleeps with you… and his wife doesn't know?"

"Well, he has slept with me and about every girl in our clinic, that's every girl under forty-five. I think he's slept with a bunch of his patients, too. Do you realize how vulnerable a woman can be when she is thirty-five and diagnosed with MS? And you ask, doesn't his wife know? Oh, hell, she knows. She walked in on us once after hours in his office in what I would call a very compromised position. But she niches her life in boxes even more than he does. If she brought his debauchery up to him, she knows she would have a lot to lose."

Curtis, looking serious, asked, "The man would hurt his wife?"

"No. He's a bully alright, a black belt in martial arts and all mouth, but he wouldn't hurt a fly, or you. What I mean about Annie, is that she would lose her reputation as the great doctor's wife, the matriarch of the perfect Christian family, her husband's $300,000 a year income, the huge colonial up on the hill overlooking the valley, and—worst of all—a happy, peaceful family life for her sons. Yeah, it's much easier to just pretend you don't see it and just gracefully close your eyes. I could make love with her husband on her dining room table, in the middle of dinner, and she would pretend not to notice."

Curtis looked down at the floor, then shook his head back and forth. He looked back at her, "I don't get it, Sandra. You guys live in a world that I don't understand. Don't you realize that you're nothing to him?"

Sandra laughing out loud, said, "Curtis, my dear Curtis... of course I'm nothing to him, and he's nothing to me. We are all nothing, just big pieces of talking meat taking up space and air."

Curtis, shaking his head and frowning, said, "What a cynical way to see the world. Is life just a game to all of you? Do you not have any values... any external reference point of morality? Any kind of code? Any hope?"

Sandra just smiled at him in silence.

Curtis added, "You know, for a moment last night I thought I was starting to feel something for you."

She cringed like a chill was going up her spine and immediately answered, "Oh, God no. Don't feel. Feel nothing at all. Hell, yeah, it's a game. Losing a brother when I was only eight and living with a meth head taught me to take nothing seriously. Having a wacko mother and a father burned to death in the driveway taught me the best way through this life is to pretend it's a game. This so-called life that we live is nothing but a sick comedy."

Curtis was shaking his head again, and this time he sat in silence. Finally, Sandra spoke again, "I think Mark Twain said that all of life is a stage. That's all I'm saying. We each have a different role to play on different stages, and some of those stages are for satire."

Curtis sat back in his chair with his head tilted back and closed his eyes, almost like he was sleeping, but of course he wasn't.

Sandra broke the silence again by adding, "Okay, Curt. I've some stuff of yours. I have your belt, shirt, and your cellphone. I had to turn it on to see whose it was. I would hate to give Kimber your phone or you his. I had to quickly turn the damn thing off because it wouldn't stop ringing." She handed him the bag, and he leaned forward looking at the floor. Finally, she set it on the floor in front of him.

She turned toward the door and looked back, "Goodbye, my dear Curtis. If you ever need me, you know where to find me. I will be your friend forever." She gave him a flirtatious wave and exited.

Curtis gave her a half-cocked smile and said, "Shakespeare."

"Shakespeare who? Hmm? What are you talking about?"

"The one who said life was a stage… it was William Shakespeare, not Twain." He then looked down and opened the bag and peeked inside. His shoes weren't in the bag, so he had no idea where they ended up. He took out the phone and saw it had maxed out at thirty-seven new voicemails. He sighed. He then put the phone to his ear and hit the first voicemail, which he could tell was from Thomas, "Hey, Curtis, where the hell are you, man? We can't find you, and we need you here ASAP. Call me, buddy. Mack is here, and he is driving me crazy wanting me to locate you in a hurry." As he was listening, Sandra's presence faded from the doorway like a lost thought.

Curtis dialed Thomas's number. Immediately he picked up and answered, "Hey, man, where've you been? Lying on a damn hammock down there while we're working our asses off?"

"No," said Curtis in a serene voice. "Uh, it's been busy… I've been helping my mom. She's here in the hospital. What's up?"

"Sorry to hear that about your mom. Now, can you get away today?"

Curtis sat up in his chair. "Today? Get away to where?"

"Here," said Thomas. "Where else?"

"There's no way. My mom is having hip surgery on Friday. She may have cancer."

"Oh, dude. I'm sorry to hear that, too." There was a long pause on the phone. Then he added, "But I think there's a way we can get you here and back before then."

"To Seattle? I don't think so. Even if I could get a flight that was leaving in ten minutes."

"Well," said Thomas. "I think we can arrange something like that. Mack has a 'door to door' air taxi service contract, and he has already called them and has a plane ready for you at Tri Cities Airport. It's been sitting all day."

"Are you freaking kidding me? He did all of this without asking me?"

"Hey, the man is made of money and $3,500 an hour for a plane to wait on you is nothing. But we need you for a big powwow and getting you here and back is somewhat of an emergency."

"Can you give me more than that?"

"Hey, man, I don't even know." Thomas paused for a few seconds and then asked, "What time's your mom's surgery?"

"It's Friday morning at seven." Curtis heard a noise and looked over and was shocked. There stood Robert Kimber at his mom's bedside looking at an electronic tablet. Out of instinct, Curtis walked to the outside window and turned to look out to the parking lot with the phone covering half of his face and his back toward the neurologist. He was trying his best to refocus his mind to the conversation with Thomas. His voice started to whisper into the phone, "Uh… what? Oh, yeah, Friday morning at seven."

Thomas said, "Well, that's about forty hours from now. If we got you to the airport in one hour, then took off immediately, you could be in Seattle in about six hours. I could have someone pick you up at Boeing Field and bring you here. So, all that will take about eight hours. We could meet for about three hours. Now we are looking at eleven hours. Then get you back to the plane, and back to Tri Cities in about eighteen hours total. Let's say, twenty hours at the most."

"Thomas, I'm really exhausted. I've had very little sleep," Curtis then guarded his words carefully as he knew that Kimber was still within earshot.

Thomas responded, "These are luxury jets, and I've flown in one. You'll have no problem getting a good nap and good food, too. Just tell me anything you want, and it will be in the plane for you."

"Okay… I guess, if I have to." Curtis would have said no, but the thoughts of flying away, far from Kimber and Sandra, seemed like a godsend. He was afraid the man would come after him again, even though he seemed quiet and professional as he was examining his mom.

Thomas gave him the instructions for finding the plane. He didn't want to put down his phone and to face Kimber in real time, but Thomas hung up first and he felt silly trying to air-talk. When he did put down his phone, Dr. Kimber spoke to him in the same manner as he would any family member of one of his patients and as if nothing had happened between the two of them. He was scheduling a brain MRI with contrast. If that was negative, he was still interested in doing a spinal tap to look for cancer cells. Curtis started to doubt if this was the same maniac that was trying to kill him in the woods seven hours earlier. It was an unreal moment. Kimber seemed sober and alert now, although his face was scratched to hell, as he had endured the same gauntlet of brush, thorns, and rocks as Curtis had.

Curtis had a passing thought that the spinal tap was a little extreme. Was it just to punish him by punishing his mom in a subliminal or even subconscious attack? He spoke to Dr. Kimber, "Really, a spinal tap? Do you think that's necessary? Mom's in a lot of pain with her hip and doing a tap will be difficult."

Kimber stared at him and smiled with a creepy half-smile. Then he said slowly and softly, "She won't feel a thing." There was a long pause where the two men just stared at one another across a room filled with ice. Then Kimber spoke again, suddenly appearing more animated, "I'll have the anesthesiologist do it after he puts her under for the surgery. He will probably do an epidural anyway... you know, so he can go light on the general. He'll get some fluid then." Kimber looked back down at the electronic tablet where he was writing orders and then back up at Curtis. "That's right, you're a neurosurgeon, aren't you? So, you understand that I'm trying to rule out a leptomeningeal metastasis that, theoretically, could be involved with your mom's mental decline. I think it's unlikely, but a necessary rule-out."

CHAPTER FOURTEEN: EMERALD LANDING

The jet reached a cruising altitude above the parallel ranges of small mountains that rolled out westward toward Kentucky, like a crumpled, green bedspread. Inside the plane, Curtis felt great comfort. It was like an isolation booth or womb above the clouds where no one could bother him. Finally, he had solitude. There was a bench seat covered in rich burgundy leather that opened into a bed. Mack had already arranged to have sheets and a blanket on the plane as well as a basket of tasty treats with a theme of Spanish tapas. There was also a bottle of a French pinot noir. He pushed the bottle away from him. He didn't even want to be tempted. He did partake of the food. Soon, he was lured into a dream world by the soft purr of the Lear's engines.

He awakened once and was surprised that they were sitting on the ground. He looked outside and saw a couple of feet of old, muddy snow pushed up beside the tarmac under the bright airport lights. He knew it couldn't be Seattle. The copilot was sitting in the cockpit looking at a laptop. "Is everything okay?" Curtis raised his head and asked in a loud voice.

The copilot looked back, "Oh, sure. We are at Salt Lake refueling. A routine stop."

Curtis nodded and pulled his blanket back up over his face. He wavered in and out of a hypnagogic state as he heard the door close and felt them take off again. When he was sleeping deeply, he started to feel itchy, very itchy. He woke up scratching his legs, his

296

arms, his neck, and his back. He rolled over and fell asleep again, only to be awoken by even more attacks of extreme itchiness. When he did sleep, fire ants intruded upon his dreams, biting him up and down his arms and legs. He would awaken to brush them off to find there were no bugs. He was in want of sleep, and now the crazy itch was cheating him of it. He sat up and looked at his excoriated arms and legs and even places where his scratching was of such intensity as to bring blood. He rubbed his eyes. The first thing that came to his mind was that he was allergic to something in the plane… or maybe the multimillion dollar jet was infested with bedbugs. He remembered reading once that Sir Richard Branson's Caribbean mansion was infested with bedbugs, so it wouldn't be unreasonable to think the same thing could happen in a luxury jet. But then, in the moonlight coming through the oval windows, he could see little lines of raised red bumps, some with blisters.

Curtis lay back down and sighed with frustration. "Damnit!" he said with a whisper. He knew what it was. He remembered the infirmity well from his boyhood. His tumble through the bushes was also, apparently, a tumble through poison ivy. Since the plant wasn't indigenous to Seattle, or even New York or Ann Arbor, as far as he knew, it had been decades since he'd partaken of the little vine's allergens. He had forgotten how awful it was. He continued to doze off and on, as he dug into his skin with his fingernails, being driven crazy by an insatiable itch. Each scratch dug deeper and deeper. He was starting to fantasize about a wire brush connected to a drill or angle grinder to tear his flesh apart and stop the insatiable itch buried within.

Eventually, exhaustion overtook the pruritus to the point he could sleep—and sleep soundly he did. In his dreams, the army ants would return to devour him, and he fought them off… with karate. The next thing that Curtis knew was the copilot standing over him and shaking him saying, "Hey, chief. We'll be landing in about fifteen minutes. Did you want to freshen up? We have a lavatory, you know."

Curtis sat up and stretched but felt the sharp pain in his belly, like he had torn his wound open once again. He waited for blood to start seeping through his white shirt, but none did. The layer of impermeable duct tape was doing its job. He went into the little WC, relieved himself, and washed his face. He looked into the small mirror. His hair was a mess. He put some water on it to flatten it. He felt the plane bank hard and grabbed the handhold to keep from falling over. He looked down at his belly and unbuttoned his shirt. He peeled back enough of the tape to see the top of his wound. It looked nasty. He knew as a surgeon that it wouldn't be superfluous to have a few stitches. With the new pain, he thought that it might be a good idea to have Bryan look at it when he got to the office. With his abdominal wound, his foot wound, and his new extremely itchy blisters that covered him from head to toe, he felt no inferiority to Job himself, and he looked no better, either.

The wheels hit the runway with a screech and a bounce. He smelled burning rubber. The plane, methodically, taxied across the wet runways, pulling up to the small passenger terminal at Boeing Field. He had always flown in and out of SeaTac and didn't know his way around this smaller airport. It was dark out and raining hard, giving the typical Seattle early spring's night a coating of a glossy black lacquer. Or was it morning? Curtis was clueless. He turned on his phone and waited for it to boot up. Finally, the time came on, and he saw it was only 7 p.m. That would make sense, as it was 10 p.m. back in Tennessee.

He stepped down the three-step ladder to the tarmac and walked, with an obvious limp, through the automatic glass doors. There stood Jennifer wearing a bright bumble-bee-yellow raincoat. Her black hair was wet around the edges. She looked like a little girl who had been playing in mud puddles. A big smile came to Curtis's scratched up face.

"Hi, Nef, I can't believe they sent you to fetch me."

"I volunteered," she replied with a big, wet smile.

"That's so kind of you." He gave her a little hug. "So, which way?"

"Uh, do you have bags?"

"Nope, just a toothbrush in my jacket pocket," Curtis said.

Jennifer pointed to the left, and they walked in that direction. She looked at him, "I hate to say this, boss, but you don't look so well. What's with all the scratches on your face and what's with the limp? Did your leg fall asleep on the plane?"

Curtis shook his head and frowned, "That's a long story, but it's been one messed-up trip to say the least." He knew that would not satisfy her curiosity, so he added, "In summary, I fell out a window then off a small cliff through a poison ivy patch and then into a lake."

"Really?" she asked. "Or… are you joking?"

"Really," he said.

Jennifer let that comment go, resisting the temptation to ask for more details, so she just chuckled and added, "Poor thing."

They made it out to her seagrass-green Prius, Jennifer skipping to avoid the rain. Curtis tried to keep up, but his sore foot wouldn't allow it. She unlocked the doors and they both climbed in. The car smelled new. She looked at him after closing her door. She threw her head back so that the rain hood fell off her hair and onto the headrest. She sat in silence while still carrying a big, contented smile. Then she morphed the smile into a pout, "How's your mom?"

"Not well… she may have cancer."

Jennifer remarked, "I'm so sorry, that must be rough." Curtis didn't reply but flashed a sad kind of smile, where the lips curve up, but beneath clearly frowning eyes. Then she turned to look behind the car, before they backed out and then pulled away in an unfamiliar quietness.

They left the airport, heading north toward downtown. Once on the freeway, Curtis started to drill her for more information about this important meeting. However, she had no idea what this meeting was all about. She said that Thomas had asked her at least thirty times if she knew where Curtis was and how to reach him. She told him, once again, that even Mack was hanging around the lab talking to her, trying to find out more about his whereabouts, and, asking her very personal questions. He made her feel uncomfortable at times. Yet, no one had made her privy to the reason for the urgency.

After ruminating over her statements for a moment, Curtis turned and looked at her, tilting his head, and asked, "How did Mack make you feel uncomfortable? What did he say?"

She hesitated at first, fiddling with the defrost controls as her windshield was starting to fog. She leaned onto her steering wheel, with a focus on the wet, shiny highway—giving a glance toward Curtis now and then—and said, "It was odd." She paused for another minute to gather her thoughts. "Out of the blue, Mr. Pendleton remarked that he has an Asian girlfriend, I guess he was considering me as sort of 'Asian.' But then he said that she, his Asian girlfriend, favored silk panties rather than cotton. He added that his American girlfriend, speaking of both girlfriends in present tense, favored cotton. So, since I was a 'half-breed Asian,' his words not mine, he was curious which I preferred."

"Creep," said Curtis abruptly. "He really called you 'half-breed?'"

"Yeah." They both paused in silence as she navigated the traffic. Then she added in a passive tone, "So *that's* the part that bothers you the most?"

301

Curtis answered, "Oh no," but thinking he did not want to enter a dialog with Jennifer about her panties, "I mean yes, but all of it bothered me. I hope you ignored him."

Jennifer turned and looked at him, flashed a big smile and answered, "I did."

Arriving at the Neurogenics building, Jennifer mumbled, "I'll go up with you," driving passed the entrance and into the parking garage. They walked together toward the building's door. She gave him updates on the lab, the surgeries, and, of course, the boxes and boxes of mail. She rode up the elevator with him to the 23rd floor. Then she walked with him toward Thomas's office. The door was open, and they could see people inside. She paused just outside, "Hey, boss, I'll give you a ride back to Boeing, just text me. Do you need to run by your place?"

"Actually, I do. I need to pick up some shoes and check my mail. Somehow I lost my shoes in Tennessee."

"Really?" She said with a puzzled look. When Curtis, again, made no attempts to explain, she continued, "Okay."

She started to walk away but turned and, with hesitation written in her voice, asked, "Is Becky back? I mean, is she living there now?"

Curtis shrugged his shoulders, "Maybe? I also wouldn't be surprised if she has served me divorce papers." He frowned. Then quickly added as Jennifer was turning to walk back to the elevators, "Oh, also, could you have Bryan meet me at the surgery suite later? If you

302

could call him, and if it's okay, he could text me, that is if he can do it. I will text him back when I'm done with my meeting."

"Sure," she nodded. "Why?"

"Uh, well, it's a personal matter."

Jennifer frowned when the thought quickly passed through her head that Curtis had secrets for which Bryan had privilege, but not her. She turned again and walked down the hall and pushed the button to the elevator. Her yellow raincoat was dripping, leaving a puddle where she stood. She had a little girl's grin of discomfiture when she saw the puddle around her. Then she shrugged her shoulders, smiled at Curtis, and turned her palms up to indicate, "Sorry, I can't help it." Curtis, stood, and just watched her smiling until she got on the elevator.

Curtis's concentration was rudely interrupted when Mack stepped out the door from Thomas's office and spoke, in a whispered voice, into his right ear, "She's a real cutie."

Curtis looked back at him, "Hi, Mack."

"So, who's the chick? I talked to her in the lab, but who is she? Don't tell me she's your niece."

"No, that's Jennifer. She's like my personal assistant and lab manager."

"Jennifer who? What's her last name?"

"Baker." Curtis looked at him as if to ask, "Why's it your business?"

"She's gorgeous. I mean, like I'm talking supermodel material."

Curtis dismissed the comment with a brief, "I hadn't noticed." He turned and looked fully at Mack. He was standing just like the last time he had seen him, with a glass of amber liquid and a couple of ice cubes. Jack Daniels, Curtis assumed. "So, what's so important that you wanted me back in Seattle?"

Mack turned to look Curtis in the face; he was about to say something but then paused and frowned. He looked Curtis up and down. Finally, he spoke, "Curtis, son, what in the Sam Hill happened to you? You look like a piece of shit."

Curtis shrugged and answered with reluctance, "It's been a rough week at Mom's. I had a fall and got into some poison ivy. I'd rather not talk about it right now."

"What, does your mom wrestle alligators?" Mack chuckled.

Curtis looked at him with a smirk on his face for a few seconds. "No, she works on carburetors. Dad, he's the one who wrestles alligators."

Mack gave Curtis a confused look.

Curtis added, "Mom... her name's Virginia. You should meet her."

Mack's confused look didn't abate, so Curtis added, "Never mind... it's a joke."

Mack chuckled, although you could tell he didn't know what was supposed to be funny. He put his hand on Curtis's elbow. "Hey, let's go inside and get started, and you will find out why I needed you here so badly."

As they went toward the door, Mack asked, "How did you like that ride from Tennessee?"

"Oh, the jet? It was great. Much easier than taking a commercial over to Charlotte and then here. I don't remember much, as I slept the whole way, or at least the times I wasn't scratching."

"Did you ever get poison ivy on your dick?"

"No," said Curtis ardently, wanting to change the subject before Mack headed down some convoluted path about his sexual exploits as a teenager in Arkansas. He had heard them all before, the virgin cheerleaders and the beauty queens, all part of his litany of conquests. And there was even the story about the incredibly beautiful forty-four-year-old mother of Mack's best friend, whom he "seduced" and had sex with in her garden shed, when he was just fifteen, or was it fourteen? The story kept changing, except for the most disconcerting part, about him holding her down, cutting off her black-laced brassiere with pruning shears. Curtis remembered Thomas asking Mack—in a pandering tone—if he obtained his manhood that day. Mack sneered and responded no but… it was the morning that Mrs. Wilkinson became a *real* woman. Curtis then reflected on Mack's disturbing conversation with Nef, which she had shared in the car, and he felt nothing but disgust for the— whiskey breathed—social slob.

305

The two men entered the office suite, and already seated were Thomas, Raymond, and—to Curtis's great surprise—two of the neurosurgeons that Curtis had trained during the Neurogenics fellowship, Dr. Thanchanok Bidaya from Thailand and Dr. Vihaan Kaur from India. Curtis looked directly at the doctors with a smile and a perplexing facial expression. "Hey, gentlemen, what brings you to town?"

Mack interrupted, "Curtis, sit down and let me tell the whole story; it is an exciting story of the next phase of Neurogenics." Mack looked at Curtis up and down, and then he tried to explain to the group, "My man Curtis is looking a little rough. I think he got into one of those cockfights down in Tennessee?" Then he laughed out loud.

This time, Curtis was the one clueless to the humor.

Mack went on to deliver a presentation with some multimedia support that Thomas had supplied. Mack just held his drink and yelled out orders such as, "Show that damn video now!" or "Next set of slides!"

The presentation showed a beautiful tropical island and a lot of construction. Mack explained that he had purchased a two-hundred-acre island in Thailand's Andaman Sea, northeast of Ko Payang Island, and was building a new center for spinal anastomosis. He had named the island in honor of himself, Ko Pendle. He explained—seeing Curtis's bewilderment—that the buildings were completed, and they had started doing preliminary cases six weeks earlier. He had set up Drs. Bidaya and Kaur as the medical directors of this new facility.

Curtis spoke up and tried to explain, even though he thought the surgeons were well-trained, that he just couldn't imagine that they could establish the infrastructure needed to carry out a successful program. It took them over two years to get all the parts in place in Seattle, and that was with a lot of expertise and years of preparation and research.

Mack laughed and explained, "Curtis, most of your problem in America was the damn red tape. I bet if you had started your work in a place like Thailand, you would've been up and running five years ago. You completely wasted that time at Apple Health and all those studies, IRBs, applications for approval, and all that crap." When he observed Curtis's hesitation, he finally said, "Curt, I thought you would be our number one cheerleader in this endeavor. Wasn't it you who wanted to take your cure for spinal cord injuries around the damn world? That's exactly what we're doing, son."

Curtis never trusted Mack, not from the day he first met him. He was trying to think of a way to channel that distrust into honest, intellectual questions for the man. They needed to be questions that wouldn't push Mack into a defensive stance of only giving sarcastic responses with no definitive information. "So, who'll be your patients? I mean, you're setting up shop on a remote exotic island that requires a long flight just to get there. I don't see you catering to the poor of Calcutta."

"We will leave that up to Mother Theresa's people," remarked Mack with a big condescending smile and a wink. "We'll have paying customers at first. We will have a hell of a lot from the OPEC countries, China, and SE Asia. There's a hell of a lot of money in Russia these days. We have a tremendous amount of interest already. Once we take care of them, we can start to see some of the charity cases." Then he winked at the other doctors.

The wink was lacking in comfort for Curtis. He spoke back to Mack, "First, Saint Theresa's people don't have a way of healing spinal cord injuries, and we do. And why on a tropical island? Why not in a major city where the injured would have better access? Why not downtown Bangkok?"

"Have you ever been in downtown Bangkok? It's nasty, A real shithole," said Mack while lifting his eyebrows like two gray caterpillars rising on their heels.

Mack, without yielding a serious answer to Curtis's questions, had them put up a few more slides to show artists' conceptions of the facility. "This place will be a six-star resort that these poor sufferers deserve. We have rehab facilities. We have started another project on a different island that will be a world-class medical spa for families of the injured or for people who just want to restore their bodies through rest, exercise, and a good diet. That island has a gorgeous beach."

Curtis knew that Mack was trying to talk in terms that would make him feel better, but they didn't. His feeble elucidations made him feel even more suspicious. Curtis had never imagined that his work on spinal anastomosis and "spa" would be associated in the same breath. He had to ask, "Who is paying for all this luxury?" No one answered him, so he asked different questions, "Why did you feel the need to tell me about this? What does this have to do with me, if you got this all worked out all by yourselves? Why spend $80,000 on a jet to haul me here?"

Mack smiled, finished off his drink, and put one of the ice cubes in his mouth to suck on while he continued to talk. "Curtis, your good man Thomas here has agreed to loan you out for three months to see this get off the ground. Also, your reputation precedes you, even in Asia, especially now that you are a Nobel laureate. It is like having Magic Johnson come and help us set up a basketball camp. The camp doesn't need him, but they need his name. We must do this right, even from the start, or our brand will be worthless. We need your experience and expertise now, not to mention your notoriety." He sucked on another ice cube and looked back at Curtis, "And I'll fly you in on a damn SpaceX rocket next time for ten million bucks if I want to."

Curtis sat back in his chair. He looked over at Thomas, whose face carried a sheepish grin. He looked back at Mack, shaking his head. "I don't know. I can't get away right now, not for three months." He paused for a few more seconds and added, "My mom's sick… maybe with cancer. I can't see me leaving the country now. The timing is terrible."

Mack spit his ice cube back in the glass and remarked, "Do you have a choice?" Then he chuckled, before adding, "I'll hire someone to take care of your damn mother. Like Jesus said, 'let the dead bury the dead.' So, we can put Virginia in some good hands while you're with us."

Curtis was somewhat taken aback and had to bite his tongue to keep from yelling at Mack. He stood up and walked over to the window to allow the anger to dissipate. He looked down on a dark and rainy downtown Seattle. The tops of all the buildings, including theirs, were now penetrating the dipping clouds. He could still see through the fog enough to make out the streets and the rhomboid intersections.

Meanwhile, at the table, Thomas looked at Mack with a bit of confusion, asking, "Who's Virginia?"

Mack looked back at Thomas, "His damn mother... who the hell do you think I was talking about?"

Thomas gave his head a quick shake to clear his thoughts. He then whispered to Mack, "Never mind... I just thought his mother's name was Helen."

Curtis eventually walked back over and took a seat. "So, when do I have to leave?"

Mack smiled and added. "We need you in Thailand in about six weeks. I've already asked Thomas to clear your schedule here. Dr.

Emerson, from what I understand, can manage here without you. Doesn't he have a new intern to help him?"

"He has a new fellow, not an 'intern.' An intern is a trainee before they are a physician, and a fellow is after they are a full-fledged neurosurgeon. Yes, he has one, but it will be months before Dr. Smithers is up and running on her own. But Mack, I don't think you realize how complicated it is to set up such a brand-new program. We are barely keeping up here and now you want to double our work?"

"Of course, I understand, son. I wouldn't be a billionaire if I didn't know what I was doing."

Curtis looked baffled. "We'll need to get a Jones-Fahlner device designed and produced just for your facility. We need to get the 3-D nanotube printers set up. We need to get the complex lab set up to create our, what you called 'pixie dust,' neuro growth factor soup. All of this must be done before you could ever even consider starting your first case. I have a whole team here working on these things, and I couldn't just fly to Asia by myself and start up a new program overnight."

Mack leaned over the table and looked Curtis directly in the eye and spoke softly, in a condescending tone, "Now calm down, son. We have these things under control. The nice Drs. Jones and Fahlner from MIT have been out and set up both the CCWs for us and a 3-D nanotube printer, and I paid them handsomely. We have folks trained in the mapping and production of the neuro-bridging

311

matrix. They've already practiced on dogs and baboons. Son, I'm telling you that we have one hell of a team already in place. As I said, my fine surgeons have been doing routine spinal cord work cases, in preparation. They are ready to start their first full case next week. We don't need you! So, don't get your panties in a bundle. I just want to err on the safe side, and I want you there to supervise. I, uh... what I mean is... I also want you to make sure the standards are high enough to associate the place with your name. We'll only need you until our first five or ten cases are done and are sent home. Oh, and your pixie dust? We have a supply from your lab here... and I, also, have some very smart biochemists from China who are reverse-engineering your work to create our own line of neuro-growth factor on site."

Mack looked over at Drs. Bidaya and Kaur, who had been sitting quietly and respectfully as their culture would dictate in such a circumstance. "Doctors tell Curtis about your work."

The two Asian neurosurgeons went into detail about the work they had done setting up the program. They had already operated on several spinal injury patients, fresh injuries that needed stabilization. So besides repairing the acute injuries to their necks or backs, they also carried out debridement in preparation for an eventual anastomosis procedure. They were set up to do their first case as soon as they got back.

Curtis looked back and forth between Thomas and Mack and added, "I'm sorry but I feel a bit betrayed. It had to be deliberate. I mean, if you are involving Jones and Fahlner, you had to purposely hide it from me. Did you order them not to talk to me? I haven't heard a word from them about this. I even talked to Jones before I went to Tennessee, and he never mentioned Thailand."

Thomas squirmed in his seat a bit and answered, "Curtis… it wasn't a conspiracy. It was more like a surprise for you. I know how busy you've been, and we just didn't want to bother you until it was the right time. If it would help, I would approve sending Bryan with you."

"No, I need Bryan here! He's the one anchor when I'm gone. He knows more about what's going on here than anyone, except myself."

Mack interrupted Curtis, "I don't know what your problem is, Curt. When I first met you two years ago, you were like a wide-eyed young boy who wanted to bring this cure to the world. Now I'm trying to do exactly that. Yet, rather than being excited about it and thanking me, you are stressing out about it and—do you know what? I think it's your damn ego. We got this far without your help—thank you—and I think that pisses you off."

Before Curtis even had a chance to answer, Mack continued, "Thomas is partially right that we kept this from you because you were so busy, but the other reason is because I was afraid you'd get a damn burr under your saddle just as you are right now." Without breaking stride, he looked over at Thomas. "I need another drink, bro." Then he continued speaking to Curtis. "Now, you only know

313

the half of it and I will fill you in on the rest… as soon as I get my drink."

Mack sat back in his chair in silence except for motioning to Thomas to switch the PowerPoint to the next presentation. Once his drink was served, he continued, "Curtis, I want to show you what we have in the ground now. The major hospital is complete. It has two wings. One wing is for nerve anastomosis, and the other is our transplant unit."

Curtis looked puzzled; with a furrowed brow, he leaned forward, turning his palms up in the air. "Transplant unit? Transplanting what?"

Mack looked at him and said softly with a pompous tone, "I am getting to that." He continued, "Many transplants, such as hands, legs, faces, and others are limited by the nerves, right?"

Curtis thought for a moment and then nodded and added, "And rejection."

Mack continued, "So, with our expertise in nerve regeneration and anastomosis, it was a perfect fit to create a transplant unit. I recruited Osaka, that's Dr. Osaka Takahashi, from Tokyo. Do you know who he is?"

Curtis shook his head in the negative.

"Well, you've heard of face transplants, haven't you?"

"Sure," answered Curtis confidently.

"Well, Dr. Takahashi did the world's first full face transplant in Spain in 2010. He then went back to his native Japan and created a face transplant program there. He was limited by the fact that the facial nerves don't grow back well, and it often leaves the patient with the inability to show expressions. Some are left with what is known as a 'rubber face.' When I met with him and reviewed your work with repairing the facial and trigeminal nerves, he was thrilled. He had already heard about your work, but not the gory details. Then, when I offered him a luxury surgery suite, not to mention a hell of a lot of yen, he signed a three-year contract."

"So, you're going to do face transplants there, too?"

"Yes, and more."

"And for cash, I assume," responded Curtis.

"Absolutely! They don't have health insurance in many parts of the world, and if they did, it wouldn't pay for anything we do... just like here in good-ol' U.S. of A."

They continued their discussion about the transplantation program for another half hour. Curtis felt some unease about it, mostly because he felt that it would take away vital resources from the Erika program. He emphasized with Mack that he wouldn't have anything to do with transplantations. Mack kept stressing that the two parts would be intimately related. He showed Curtis more PowerPoint slides of the transplant facility, which was even ahead of their own anastomosis side.

Mack was trying to bring his argument to a close when he said, "Curt, you are obviously not a business man, and I respect that. A good business man—which I happen to be a hell of one—is always looking ahead to the future. All the dinosaurs of the business world failed to do that. My late friend David McAllen was a futurist and a genius, and that's why he made so much dough in the warehouse retail stores. So, for us to survive, we must diversify. You told me that in the entire world there is a potential of only 300,000 customers… or patients, in other words. Of those, maybe we can help less than 20,000 due to financial barriers. But moving into this area of limb and face transplantation, that would more than double our market."

Curtis answered, "That's 300,000 new cases per year, not a total of 300,000! I'm doubtful about that, that face transplants will double our market. I mean, the need for face transplants must be a much smaller group than spinal cord injuries."

Mack looked at him and grinned. "My people have estimated that at least .7% of the people in the world have a facial deformity of some level. That would mean about 450 million people. Of those, there's at least ten million who would qualify, due to the severity of their disfigurement, for a transplant today. But it isn't just for disfiguring burns and injuries. There're others."

"Others? Like who?" asked Curtis.

"Now, son, I want you to take me seriously. I have had long talks with Dr. Takahashi, and he and I see things eye to eye, at least more than you and I do. Besides the disfiguring injuries, there's a hell of a lot of people who are just born—to put it bluntly—shit-faced ugly."

Curtis sat motionless, other than stealthily scratching and digging into the poison ivy vesicles on his arms and legs beneath the table. He sat up. Looking into Mack's eyes with a bit of annoyance, he asked, "Are you kidding me? Now our work is going to become an aesthetic clinic?"

"Curtis, remember that Dr. Takahashi was a plastic surgeon first, trained in aesthetics. Fixing a patient who was disfigured from a burn or trauma is no different than fixing a human being who was born a freak of nature. And Curt, not that it's important to you, but in America alone, over $15 billion were spent last year alone on aesthetics. This is a tremendous market, son."

Curtis looked over at Thomas. "Are you on board with this new direction?"

Thomas, clumsily answered, "Well, I guess I am. I mean, Mack has some logic to what he's saying." He paused and then quickly added, "But, Curtis, you will just be helping us with the nerve anastomosis part. You won't be involved with the other side… not that much."

Curtis looked back at Mack. "And where in the hell are you going to find all the donors?"

"Son," Mack said, "do you realize that we bury in the dirt 30,000 pretty faces every day? That's our best estimate. We just need to get our hands on a few donors. They can still give their corneas to others, which we don't need. They can still give their hearts, livers, and kidneys… we just want the one inch of skin on their faces."

Curtis sat in a state of disbelief. While he was quietly thinking, Mack spoke again. "So, Curt, my man, my golden goose, while you are processing this thought, I wanted to bring up the next concept."

Curtis's eyebrows raised again, and he looked back at Mack with the expression of "what else could there be?"

Mack stood up and walked around the room and then, leaning his shoulder against the window, looked out over Seattle, beneath the lifting fog. With his back toward the others, he spoke as if he were talking to the entire city, if not the world. "Let me ask you—as a surgeon—a hypothetical question."

"Okay," answered Curtis from across the room.

"Imagine that there was a young, healthy man, and some bastard— maybe his lover's jealous husband—blew his damn brains out and killed him. Say, he shot him in the back of the head, not in his pretty face. Then you have a patient with kidney, liver, lung, and heart failure. What would be the easiest way to donate all his organs to the poor, suffering man with the tools that you have now?" Mack meandered back to his chair and sat back down, resting his chin on his fists, staring at Curtis and waiting on an answer.

Curtis knew instantly what Mack was alluding to, so he didn't need time to figure that out. But he did need time to watch several thoughts trudge through his mind. The first, primal thought was the empathy he felt for the man shot in the head by a jealous husband. Less than twenty-four hours earlier, he was being chased through the dark brush, like an animal, by a jealous man, whom he thought was going to blow his own brains out. But then he thought of Erika, the girl. He felt so far removed from her… and his promise. He felt like he was standing on some strange threshold into the "Brave New World," where there was a complete loss of universal reference points, at least in the areas of morality and decency. It was like his whole life's mission was being commandeered and directed into some murky place… and all for money. He looked over at Mack, "Of course, with our present spinal and cranial nerve anastomosis abilities, doing a head transplant, or what would be better called a 'body transplant,' would be the easiest course. But that would be the most complex surgery ever done in history. It would take a big team over twelve hours for one case. Don't tell me, for God's sake, that's on your agenda too! If it is, we will have now officially gone back to the nineteenth century and the days of Mary Shelley and her monsters."

Mack smiled. "Son, I am a futurist and not a historian, and I'm not even sure who Mary Shelley was. Yes, the world will be shocked at the first case, just as they were with Dr. Takahashi's first face transplant back in 2010, but now, several hundred cases later, it's accepted as normal and the moral thing to do. Did you know that the first time they implanted pigs' heart valves in humans, there was a moral outcry? Mixing animals and humans was considered by many as a sacrilege? The same moral outcry appeared with the first kidney transplant, and of course, the first heart transplant. Did you know that many argued that the soul was in the heart and it would violate some religious principle to replace it? But now we know better. We know the soul resides in the brain and not in the body. There's a continuum of change and development, and I can see the future where ugly people pay for new faces, and people with failing bodies will pay—and pay handsomely—for new bodies. I can see setting the price for a new body in the tens of millions of dollars, and I'll be their damn broker."

Curtis abruptly stood up. "I think I'm done here." He looked at Thomas. "Did you need me for anything else?"

Thomas smiled and said, "Let me walk out with you."

Curtis walked over and stood beside the two surgeons; they stood up, bowed, and shook their hands. "I guess I will see you in Thailand in a few weeks."

He nodded goodbye toward Mack.

Thomas and Curtis walked into the hall as Curtis pulled out his phone and looked at the texts. He had one from Bryan saying that he would be happy to meet him in the surgery suite. He was already in the building reviewing his charting. Curtis texted him back that he was on his way there now. Another one was from Jennifer: "Let me know boss when to pick you up." Curtis looked at the time on the phone: 10:20 in the evening. He texted her back, "In an hour." Then he added, "Is that too late for you? I can take a taxi."

"No problem," came her text in return.

Thomas stood in silence watching him. Curtis looked back at him and said, "Oh, I almost forgot, I need my ride back to Tennessee."

"Sure," said Thomas. "What time will you be at Boeing?"

"Hmm. I need to run by my place on the way. Let's say midnight."

"I'll get word to the pilots. I think they had to get a fresh pair." As Curtis walked down the hall toward the elevators, Thomas walked beside him and put his hand on his shoulder. He gave him one last bit of advice, "Hey, Curtis, just focus on what you do best and stay out of Mack's other ambitions."

"Sure," he said despondently as he pulled away and stepped onto the elevator. The doors slid closed. Thomas's presence lost immediate relevance.

He stopped by his office, briefly, to grab his sport coat because he was chilled from the dampness. He kept it in the office for official meetings, when a lab coat would not suffice. Curtis went up to the surgery suite. He climbed up into the observation balcony to look things over in the operating theater without having to don his sterile gear. It seemed quiet now, except for the night cleaning team working down in the post-op room. He leaned over, placing his crossed arms on the railing and his chin on his arms. He looked down through the windows and did a quick survey. All things seemed in order. It felt to him, on that night, like a holy place—an inner sanctum of peace. It was a special space for miracles, where people were born again or given a second chance on life.

About the time his mind was starting to journey further into that place of mystical contemplation, he heard the automatic door open below him in the pre-op area. Curtis climbed back down the corkscrew stainless-steel stairs, favoring his left foot. He walked through the set of sliding doors that entered the pre-op area. "Hey, Bryan. I'm here." The two men shook hands and then hugged.

"So, what's up, boss?"

"Bryan, I need a personal favor. I got injured at my mom's and then had to fly here, so I didn't have time to go to the hospital. I think I need some sutures."

Bryan had a surprised look on his face. "I had noticed that you were looking a little rough. What happened to you?"

Curtis didn't answer that question at first but started to slowly remove his jacket. "It's here on my belly."

"Okay, let me see."

Curtis paused before unbuttoning and taking off his shirt. He took a deep breath. He slowly started to pull it loose from the dried blood and duct tape. Inch by inch he freed his tender skin from the cotton material. Then he pulled his arms out of the sleeves.

Curtis methodically pulled the duct tape off the wound, exposing the ragged edges and chunks of dried blood. Bryan gasped, "Oh, my lord… what the hell happened?"

He knew that he didn't want to get into the details. Not that he would have any problem with Bryan knowing about his private life, but he just didn't have the energy to explain. So, he told him the abridged edition. "Well, I left Mom at the hospital, I don't know if you heard that she broke her hip?"

Bryan shook his head, "No, I didn't. Sorry about that."

"Well, she did, and I took her to the hospital yesterday… or was it the day before? Anyway, she was admitted. Then I went back to her house, but I forgot the key. I had to kick the window in. That's how I cut my foot. Then I slid through the window and caught my stomach on something that cut me." Of course, that was a lie, but Curtis had no intention of trying to explain the convoluted, but honest, version.

"Okay, that explains part of it, but what happened to your face?"

It seemed to Curtis that Bryan was catching on to him. He let the silence hang in the air for a moment, then added, "I also fell through some bushes and got into poison ivy." He paused and added, "Bryan, it's a long story, and I'll tell you about it when I'm back."

Bryan was taken aback by the abrupt answer and secrecy from his close friend. However, his instinct told him to let it go, and he did.

He had Curtis lay back on the stretcher. He went into the supply room and came back with a bag of saline IV fluid. He punctured the bag with a large needle and sprayed a jet of sterile saline fluid over the wound. He placed gauze pads over the wet scabs to soften them; then he went into the scrub area for a couple of Betadine-infused brushes. Beneath the clump of hair matted in dried blood were the remains of a few strips of duct tape. The superglue had completely failed, and the wound was wide open.

As Bryan worked gently with the brush to clean up the old injury, he impulsively asked, "Geez, boss, were you trying to disembowel yourself?" There was no response other than Curtis's moans from the pain.

After Bryan did his preliminary wound cleaning, he injected lidocaine around its edges so that he could clean more aggressively, and to prepare for suturing. He closed the gaping laceration using two layers. At one spot, the cut had penetrated through the fatty layer and into the top layer of the muscle. This required a couple of deeper stitches. Then he used a fine, absorbable suture, hidden just beneath the surface, to close the final layer with a good cosmetic result.

"I am concerned," voiced Bryan, "with an old wound like this, that there could be an infection starting." He ran down to their pharmacy and came back with a tetanus booster syringe. He gave Curtis the shot in his right arm and sent in an electronic prescription for an antibiotic from his laptop.

324

"Can I look at that foot?"

Curtis, lying on his back on the pre-op stretcher, reached down, pulled off his sock, and flipped over to lie face down, being careful not to put pressure on his abdominal wound dressing. Bryan began to work on cleaning up his right foot. "Hey, boss, I think you could use a couple of sutures here, too. Fortunately, most of it is superficial." Then Bryan injected lidocaine around the deepest hole and paused to let it take effect.

While Curtis was lying on the table and they had a moment, Bryan said something that Curtis wasn't sure how to respond to.

"I've asked Jennifer to go out with me several times, but she won't... not even for coffee. When I pressed her, she first said that she just didn't want to date right now. Then someone in the lab said that she's in love with someone else, but they wouldn't say with whom." He focused on setting up his second suture tray: an array of gauge sponges, needles, a syringe, surgical scissors, sutures, and a tweezer-like instrument called "pick-ups." Then he said, almost in a mumble as he put the first stitch in, "I have the hunch... that someone else... is, well, you."

"Me!" shouted Curtis as he rose up, briefly, from the stretcher. Then he started to laugh. "You're crazy. Don't get me wrong, I love Jennifer to pieces... as a daughter. I know she looks up to me, but I don't think she looks at me that way. Good heavens, I'll be forty-five this summer, and what is she now, twenty-four?"

"I think she's turning twenty-six pretty soon."

325

Curtis didn't say another word about that. He changed the subject to asking Bryan how Dr. Emerson had been doing in the OR. Bryan reassured him that he was doing good work. Bryan thought with each passing week, Dr. Emerson was becoming more confident.

Then, as Curtis was lying face-down on the table, he raised his head back up, supporting his weight with his elbows rather than his abdomen, to look at Bryan and asked a rather philosophical question: "Hey, Bryan, do you believe in a code of life? I mean, a universal reference point for morality, or purpose for that matter? I remember that philosophy was one of your majors and must be an area you are interested in. You see, I keep hearing from people that I'm too idealistic. That life's a game or, even worse, it's all about the money. Would you agree with that?"

Bryan paused in his suturing and looked up. "I don't know, Curtis, that's a difficult question." He went back to work on the foot, putting another stitch in and then tying it off and cutting it. He started to clean up the wound to see how it was lining up. He looked back at his patient. "Yeah, I think I believe in a higher calling to life, a common principle that we should live by. It isn't just about money. I think you're an idealist, but not too idealistic… but an idealist in a positive way. I mean, I followed you here to Washington because I saw you as the kind of person who gives us hope. You're the kind of man who believes in something more than himself. I've certainly worked with plenty of self-centered, asshole doctors, but you're different." He paused to focus on dressing the foot, so walking wouldn't cause it to re-open.

326

Then Bryan added, "Game? No, life isn't just a game."

Curtis swung around and sat on the side of the table and picked up his sock. He paused to scratch at the skin on his arms and legs a few more times, which he had tried to restrain from while Bryan was suturing his wounds. As he was slipping his foot into his shoe, Bryan asked him, "Do you believe in a god or a higher authority?"

Curtis chuckled. "Now *that's* a loaded question. Like so many people, I don't think about it a lot."

"Well, you live like you believe in God," said Bryan.

Curtis seemed puzzled by that statement and flashed a crooked smile. "I'm not sure what you mean by that. I don't go to a church or a synagogue. I did go to Sunday school as a little boy, but we— my mom and I—stopped going after Dad left us. I sense something is there, but I haven't invested much energy in trying to figure out what it is. But I do think that there's some reference point and meaning to life that's bigger than just 'living in the moment.'"

They walked out of the pre-op area and Bryan turned out the lights behind them. The cleaning crew had finished and left several minutes prior.

As they were walking down the hall, Bryan added, "Well, I'm definitely a theist. I say this with confidence because I was an atheist my whole life and became a theist by a deliberate choice. My mom was a professor of anthropology at Columbia, and she made sure she raised me as an atheist. But the more I thought about it, the more nonsense it seemed to me. To live faithfully as an atheist, you must be a nihilist. Mom was a hypocritical atheist her whole life... and I say that in a kind way. I love my mom dearly. She is a wonderful woman, very kind to others and involved with many humanitarian issues."

They stopped in front of the elevator and Bryan pushed the down button. It lit up. He continued, "She led a big campaign in Manhattan for decent low-income housing. She was also a big supporter for the arts. So, she was a terrible atheist. That's why I see you as a practical theist. You believe in saving humanity and relieving some of the suffering, like there is more to life than a string of moments or self-fulfillment. If there is nothing out there, on the other side of the grave, then there can't be anything on this side, save a grand illusion of meaning."

Bryan paused when the door opened. He observed Curtis as he walked on his newly dressed foot, entered the elevator, leaned against the wall, and pushed the ground floor button.

Bryan entered the elevator and, as the door closed behind him, looked over at Curtis and added, "Boss, you're my hero because you see people as worth saving. I see God in you, even if you don't know who he is."

Curtis turned to watch the digital numbers change as they dropped toward the ground. He looked over at Bryan and was starting to choke up. He whispered, while looking Bryan in the eyes, "That's kind of you."

At that moment in time, after the experience with Sandra, he didn't feel like anyone's hero. He looked down at the floor and then back up. "Bryan, I really screwed up when I was at Mom's house. I did something terrible and was almost killed for it. So, I wouldn't be such a great hero if you knew the real me."

Bryan gave him a shocked expression framed by a soft smile. "Really? You?"

Curtis just nodded his head. "Yeah, I will just say it involved another woman, too much wine, and a jealous lover." He raised his eyebrows and asked, "Do I need to say more?"

"Well, I'm shocked… a bit disappointed… but at the same time… I don't really care *what* you did in Tennessee. I'm just glad you're okay."

They both watched the digital numbers as they closed in on "1."

Bryan looked over at him with a scowled face as the door was opening, "So, someone did this to you?"

"No, answered Curtis. "I did it by accident falling out of this woman's window."

Bryan shrugged his shoulders. "Really?" he mumbled as his facial expressions seemed to imply he was trying to sort this all out.

They reached the juncture where Curtis was going to take the steps down to his office to wait on Jennifer. Bryan was going out the door to his car. He asked Curtis, "You don't want me to give you a ride?"

"No, Jennifer's on her way. You could ride with us?" He winked.

Bryan smiled. "I think you're trying to set me up."

Curtis flashed him a kind smile. They shook hands as they were preparing to part ways. Bryan added, "I have the freedom to decide who my heroes are, and you're still on my list. Yeah, definitely."

Then Curtis responded with a startling statement, "Yeah, and you're mine."

Bryan was shaking his head as if to unscramble the confusion. A grateful smile erupted from Curtis's face and turned into words of explanation, "Bryan, I'm no smarter or kinder than you are. I just happen to have 'MD' after my name and lucky enough to have been around some great mentors like Lennard Jacobs. I think many other people, including yourself, may have done a much better job with it. For one, I've somehow gotten myself deeply entangled in patent problems and a chronic lack of funding. Others could have navigated this legal process much better than I have. You could have done this better."

About that time, before Bryan had a chance to respond, Curtis's phone buzzed. It was Jennifer texting that she was almost there. Curtis turned and followed Bryan outside, where he stood on the curb waiting for a sight of the Prius. Curtis turned to him and added, "One more word of advice, Bryan ..." then he paused.

"Yeah?" asked Bryan.

He pointed at him with a stern smile, "Don't ever tell anyone that you can save them … and certainly don't tell them that you promise you will." Bryan smiled and about that time the car pulled up. He waved goodbye to Curtis and leaned over to wave hello to Jennifer in the driver's seat as Curtis jumped in and they pulled away.

They drove north toward Ballard. He directed her to his condo. "Nice," she said as she turned into the driveway. Curtis knew that she was just being polite.

He looked at her. "Not bad. It's small, but we do have a view of the canal. That's the greatest value here."

He jumped out of her car and walked up the three steps to the front door of his condo. He searched around a group of rhododendron bushes, flipped over a flat stone, and picked up a small box, inside of which was an emergency key. He normally entered through the garage, but he didn't have his opener on him, as it was in his Jeep parked inside. He used the relic key to open the front door. He heard the car door slam and looked up to see Jennifer following him. She was reading a text on her phone when he had gotten out of the car. He hadn't expected her to come inside.

They both walked into the dark apartment. He ran back to his bedroom, flipped on a light, and grabbed a pair of running shoes out of the closet along with his blue rain jacket. He took off his sport coat and hung it up, switching it with the rain jacket. He looked around for any evidence of Becky's presence. She still had a key, so she could come back if she wanted. But there was nothing disturbed. She had come back for Racer before he left for Tennessee. She made sure she came to the condo while he was at work. She left one Post-it note, which read, "I've got the cat." That's all it said.

On the way back through the apartment, he saw Jennifer standing in the living room looking at his wedding photos hanging on the wall. She asked, "What year was this?"

"Oh, we got married in 2014." He chuckled as he looked at the photo. "I was about twenty pounds lighter in those days."

No other words were exchanged as they left the apartment. They climbed back into Jennifer's car and headed back toward the freeway.

"Oh, crap," Curtis shouted. "I forgot the prescription that Bryan sent in for me." They made a U-turn in the almost empty four-lane street, just before they made it to the freeway. They headed back in the direction they just came, looking for the 24-hour pharmacy.

Curtis walked back to the car with a small plastic Walgreens bag, carrying his prescription for the levofloxacin, a bottle of calamine lotion, a tube of hydrocortisone, and a bag of Doritos. He jumped back into the car. Jennifer pulled back out onto the street and made her way up the ramp and onto the freeway. Curtis pulled the bag of Doritos out of the plastic bag and offered her one. She rolled her eyes and said, "My dear, Curtis, you have to get off the junk food." Then she smiled and took a couple of chips from him and stuck them in her mouth. They drove in silence as he crunched away, eating his chips, mumbling with a mouthful, "This is dinner… or maybe breakfast."

As they were nearing Boeing Field, she looked directly at him, as if her mind was pregnant with thought. Breaking the silence, she asked, "Curtis, do you still love her?"

Curtis's head was spinning from all the commotion in his life over the past week. He was a little nervous about Jennifer, with what Bryan had said about her possibly having a crush on her boss. His mother was seriously sick and that was on his mind too. He had just had an affair the previous night. He had almost been the victim of a murder, at least from his perspective. He had almost disemboweled himself. He had just been told that, rather than bringing new life to the disabled poor, he would have to start helping build Frankenstein's monsters in Asia for the ultra-wealthy. He felt emotionally exhausted, too exhausted to take on a very complex question like love. Plus, now he was eaten up with poison ivy and the intense itching was at the forefront of his mind and about to drive him crazy. He even caught himself scratching his arm with a Dorito chip before tossing it into his mouth. After that, while still in the car, he began dabbing the calamine lotion onto his skin directly from the open bottle.

Normally he would feel confident that he did love Becky, but this night, driving on I-5 in the cold early-spring rain, he wasn't sure, especially with the question coming so abruptly. To buy him a little more time for thought, he asked, as if he didn't know, "Who… my mother?"

"No, Becky," Jennifer said with an emphatic tone.

"Oh," he said. "I don't know anymore."

"No one could blame you if you didn't. She stepped out of your life almost two years ago. No one would expect you to hold out hope forever."

"I know. Mack keeps making me the butt of his jokes. But you know, Nef, I've really been married to my work for a decade now. I do feel, however, that the light is finally appearing at the end of the tunnel. I know I've been saying the same thing for some time, but this time it's real. I just feel it. I do have to go to Thailand for an assignment for Joppa for a few weeks," he said, using the lab's nickname for Mack, "but when I get back, I want to focus on patients, my mom, and trying to resolve this situation with Becky."

When they had pushed through the rainstorm and rolled up in front of the small passenger terminal at Boeing Field, Curtis smiled at Jenifer and said, "Thanks," as he reached over and patted her on her left shoulder as some kind of proxy for a hug. He turned and opened his passenger door, stepped out, and closed it behind him. As he walked around the back of the car, he heard the automatic window lower on her side. He walked over to her, thinking there was something she needed to say. The heavy raindrops were hitting her face as she looked up at him, causing her eyeliner to run from the corners of her uneasy eyes.

She motioned for him to come close. The rain was noisy on the plastic pharmacy bag, which he was now holding over his head as a makeshift umbrella. He leaned over closer to listen to what she had to say. She reached up, placing her hand behind his head, and pulled him toward her face. She kissed him on the lips. She kissed him hard, putting her other hand behind his head to pull him into her, as she continued to kiss him. When she released her grip and their lips separated, she was sobbing. He stood up a bit disordered. He dropped his hand with the bag to his side, allowing the rain to soak his hair and run down his face. She looked up at him with tears and rain dripping off her chin, speaking loudly above the splattering all around them, "Dr. Eisner, I think I'm in love with you… and I don't know what to do about it." As an affront to the silence that followed, in a frantic, tear-soaked voice, she pleaded, "Curtis… you must love me back… you just have to!"

He stood still in the street obstructing the rain's long journey to the earth. He was looking at her with a smile of confusion… but no words. She grasped the soggy air for meaning, but Curtis's intent was vacant. He put the hood of his rain jacket over his head, which put his face deep within its shadow, obscuring his expressions, expressions she was so desperate to read. A car was coming from the opposite direction, and he stepped toward the terminal, out of its way.

Curtis didn't know why, but he started to cry, too… maybe out of pure exhaustion. He walked backward with a limp, toward the sidewalk with a silly side-to-side wave of his hand. He pulled his hood from his face, so she could see his sheepish grin. After the approaching car passed, he yelled through the noise of the rain hitting the pavement, "We'll have to talk about this when I get back! Take care." And he turned and darted into the terminal as fast as his sore foot would permit, as the rain had suddenly become torrential.

He entered the automatic door. He looked back at her and her Prius, which were still sitting in the street where he had left them. They weren't moving. Cars were pulling up behind her and waiting patiently, then, one by one, awkwardly navigating around her. Was she okay? He couldn't see her through the dark, the rain, and the fogged-over car windows. He waved in her direction again from behind the glass wall of the terminal, which was now coated with a distorting film of water gliding down its surface, as in a sheet.

CHAPTER FIFTEEN: THAILAND

The dark night sky combined with the soft purr of the jet's twin engines wasn't enough to lure Curtis to sleep on his return to Tennessee. There was too much on his mind. He just looked out the portal window of the small Lear onto the tops of clouds, which stretched out as far as his eyes could see. Brilliant stars were strewed across the nocturnal roof above. Beneath them, down in the rainy world below, there was a young woman whose heart was in his hands. He cared deeply for her, and he would much rather bear any potential hurt himself.

Had he really kissed her back or had he dozed off on the plane and that was all a dream… or nightmare? What did it mean? What should he do? He adored the girl. She was bright, a devoted worker, and very beautiful. Would he be a damn fool, as Mack would suggest, if he walked away from a romantic relationship with her? He just shook his head as he continued to look out the porthole. He said audibly, "Curtis Eisner, how in the hell did you turn your personal life into such a disheveled mess?"

He looked at the time on his phone, tapping the screen to stir its light. It was 1:15 in the morning. He was thinking about how just a couple of days ago, he had been in the bed of another woman—the only woman, besides Becky, with whom he had ever slept with. Then it dawned on him that it hadn't been a "couple of days ago," but rather only twenty-four hours earlier when he had been sound asleep, side by side with Sandra. This was just before all hell broke loose with Kimber's arrival. He couldn't believe it. He had sucked every drop of life out of this day, leaving it inert. It was bare, and such a convoluted day had left him feeling totally depleted, too. But now there was yet another woman in his life… or at least that's what she wanted. He, on the other hand, wanted to run away. Maybe he could have the pilots drop him off in Costa Rica? Realistically, he needed to start backing out of the sources of discombobulation in his personal life, step by step.

Divorcing Becky would be understandable to everyone… but himself. She had emotionally detached herself from his life by choice. But as a scientist, at that moment, the only question he wanted to know the answer to was "Am I in love with Jennifer?"

Sometimes people confused platonic with romantic love. The difference wasn't well-demarcated. He certainly couldn't sense the difference clearly, unlike his keen ability to sense the difference between essential tissue and supporting structures as he entered someone's spine. He didn't understand why people fell in or out of love, but he wasn't going to be in love with Jennifer, even if it took a deliberate act of will.

Yet, in a different universe, it could have happened. In a fantasy world with dark unexplored forests of giant, gnarly oaks, glistening waterfalls, and mountain castles, he and Jennifer could have ridden off together on the back of an albino unicorn and lived happily ever after. But in the real universe, the one he inhabited, to him, such a relationship was absurd. In some ways, Curtis envied Bryan because the love between those two made sense… but not between Curtis and the girl. The kiss was hypothetical to him. He had kissed her back, but maybe it was an experiment to weigh his own emotions or maybe just a primitive and simple impulse. Mostly it was reactive, automatic… without thought.

It was as if Sandra had awakened something romantic if not sexual within him, and now that it was awake, it was seeking an object of focus. It had been dormant for two years, and now released, it was like a cormorant, adrift, looking for a place to land. He felt that Jennifer deserved better than the waifish heart of a middle-aged man. She needed someone her age, with whom she could discover life together. Bryan, thirty-two, was much better suited than someone who was already over halfway to old. Outside of the past twenty-four hours, which he now only wanted to forget, Curtis had always been a rational man.

He pulled out his cellphone and wrote Jennifer a short e-mail. His plan was to save it, and when he was back on the ground, review and send it. He wanted it to simmer in the back of his mind for a few hours, to be sure he wouldn't have any regrets. He wasn't expecting cell coverage at 35,000 feet, however, when he touched his phone's screen and it lit up, he noticed the symbol for the plane's wireless network. He clicked to join it. He typed out, with his thumbs, "Dear Nef: As you know, I love and adore you very much. You are a faithful friend and co-worker, who would go to battle for me and my ideas. I am deeply grateful for that. I would go to battle for you too and never doubt that." Then he paused and looked out the window to gather his thoughts, and they were intricate thoughts that danced—ghost-like—and hid among the pillowy tops of the tall cumulus clouds, illuminated now by a weary quarter moon.

He continued typing: "I must apologize for what happened when you dropped me off. I don't know what I was thinking… to receive your kiss. To me, you're like a wonderful daughter, whom I respect too much to violate our professional relationship. I will see you in a few days, and we can talk about this if you need to." Then he deleted that last sentence letter by letter, thinking that if this wasn't settled there and then, the romantic relationship could metastasize. He pressed "SEND" at the top of the screen. He watched the little bar on his phone grow and disappear as the message fell out of the sky and back to the drizzly world below.

Curtis was stunned when he felt a lump growing in his throat. The lump raised into a fully formed grief, so much so that tears coated his eyes. After his lower lids slowly filled, a single drop tumbled down his cheek. He collected it at his chin with his right index fingertip. He examined it, like a specimen. He pondered the source of this great pain that he was now beginning to feel flowing out of his heart. It was like a lost love that never was, nor never could have been, or at least could certainly never be now.

The sun rose as Curtis's plane flew over Indiana. He felt closure on the situation with Jennifer but nonetheless was feeling her hurt… and oddly, his own wound. Yes, he envied Bryan in several ways. Besides being the perfect match for Jennifer, he could—as a PA— enjoy the love of medicine in its natural form. For Bryan, he had a career where he always exceeded society's expectations because they always underestimated what a PA did every day. However, as a physician, Curtis felt that he lived in a world where he was destined to disappoint, where he was always expected to be better, to be brighter than what he, or any mere mortal, could ever aspire to be, except for some—bigger-than-life—TV doctor from the 1960s.

When they touched down at the Tri-Cities airport, Curtis was looking out the window for his rental car. The red Civic was where he had left it. He gathered his phone, toothbrush, and shoes and headed for the car.

He wasn't sure where to go. He was hungry. He had things at his mom's house, like a clean shirt, that he wanted. However, he felt he should go directly to the hospital.

When he walked into his mother's room, she looked tired. Her hair was a mess, and she was snoring. He kissed her on the cheek and she awakened. She looked at him with startled eyes and whispered, "Wayne?"

"No, Mom. It's Curtis. I'm here with you."

When the nurse came in, she gave him the news from Dr. Kimber that her brain MRI was fine, unchanged from the previous test four months earlier. There was no evidence of a metastasis from a bone tumor or elsewhere. The nurse also reported, "I'm sorry, but you just missed him," referring to Kimber, "He asked where you were. I can call and see if he is still in the hospital."

"Oh, no thanks," Curtis said with haste.

The next morning, they prepared his mother for surgery. After the orthopedist learned that Curtis was a surgeon himself, he offered him the opportunity to come into the OR as an observer. He had no desire to watch him fillet open his dear mother, so he waited in the OR waiting room like everyone else.

The surgery took longer than expected, almost four and half hours. The surgeon came out and broke the news to Curtis. In the proverbial good news/bad news ritual, he started with the good news. "Yes, Curtis, the frozen section showed that the tumor, which caused the pathological fracture, was a chondrosarcoma. We carefully examined all the margins, and it certainly appeared to be *in situ*, in other words, had not spread beyond her femur and hip. The bad news, however, was that the tumor was so big, and we had to remove so much of her femur, that there was nothing left to attach an artificial hip to. We had no choice except to amputate the right leg." When the word *amputate* sounded in Curtis's ears, it was like an unexpected gunshot. He suddenly felt the blood drain out of his head and he sat—more like fell—back into the hard, plastic waiting room seat. Amputation wasn't anything that they had discussed as a possible outcome, although you could argue that it was implied. To the surgeon, it seemed routine. To Curtis, it was like a huge piece of his mother was gone forever, both figuratively and literally. It was personal.

The orthopedist talked about the recovery in absolute, mundane terms. It was a mechanical process of parts and pieces and prostheses. But the words were like an overheard conversation

342

coming from an adjacent room, even though the doctor was standing right in front of him. Curtis had a hard time with the language processing, as his mind was consumed with how his mother's life would be profoundly changed from this day forward. He knew that it would be months, if ever, before she could live at home, alone again. Sure, she might get over an amputation and learn to use a crutch or wheelchair, but even that process would be laborious considering the movement difficulties that were sure to follow her neurological disease. With the onset of dementia, they still weren't sure what course it would follow. If it was even moderately progressive, by the time she recovered from the amputation, she would be too demented to live alone.

Curtis never remembered seeing the doctor leave, but he was no longer there. As the cloud of shock slowly dissipated from the waiting room, Curtis felt a wave of impulsiveness. He decided not to wait on his mother to wake up in recovery, but instead to get to work, immediately.

He ran down to his car and then drove back to the memory care facility that they had visited together earlier in the week. He knocked on the door of the manager, Dorothy Carr. He explained that there had been a sudden change of plans and that his mother would also need physical assistance. She would need to enter the place sooner than later. Dorothy raised the issue that, while they had a good memory program, they were not well-equipped to handle a recent amputee and that he should look for another location for his mom. "But there are none!" said Curtis with a bit of desperation.

343

"I've looked throughout northeast Tennessee, and none are taking new patients… at least none that aren't ratholes." Eventually, Dorothy agreed but only if his mom completed a rehab program at a skilled nursing facility first.

Over the next week, Curtis had enough of the arrangements in place, that he felt comfortable to fly back to Seattle. He completed his scheduled cases for the following five weeks and handled several other pressing issues. Then he started to pack for his three-month stay in Asia. With his mother's worsening circumstances, he dreaded the trip even more.

He and Jennifer—without exchanging more than a few words about it—seemed to mutually agree to not talk about the kiss or his e-mail. It was awkward, but cordial, during the short busy weeks before his departure. She seemed to pull away. Whether it was because of hurt or embarrassment, he wasn't sure. She didn't come in his office anymore, except once to bring him a package. He grabbed her arm as she walked by and said, softly, "I'm sorry." She pretended to be puzzled and asked, "About what?" Curtis let the conversation go at that point, except to say, "We can talk when I get back from Thailand."

During his last week in Seattle, he decided to try to find Becky again. Several previous attempts had yielded naught.

All people have covert corners within their private lives, of which no one else is aware. These secrets can be as simple as the technique one employs for picking their nose. On the hideous end of that spectrum are those with dark secrets, like those who are shoplifters, peeping Toms, rapists, or even serial killers. Curtis's secret place was that he was a stalker. But he wasn't the kind of stalker driven by hate who wanted to hurt someone. He just wanted to love someone… Becky. After she had first left him, he made it a habit to drive around Seattle late at night looking for her familiar pink VW bug with the daisy stickers on the rear. He would have been greatly embarrassed if anyone knew about his clandestine self.

He figured out that Becky lived somewhere in the "U District." He was drawn back to this area night after night. He knew with her meager research assistant income, and without her asking him for any money, that her housing choices would have to be humble. If he ever saw her, he wasn't sure he would even try to talk to her, but just observe her and know that she was safe.

In the winter time, those drives late at night were typically in the rain. Curtis felt, at times, the rain coalescing the darkness into an impermeable soup of pitch. He would have only been able to see her car if it was right in front of him. In contrast with the enfolding murky void around him, the thoughts inside his head would become more clear and incandescent. During those drives, with little hope of spotting anything, Curtis worked through his thoughts about his career, his life, his loves, and even the surgery cases of the day.

But it was late spring now, and the skies were clearer and lighter well into the evening, giving him better odds for success. The night before his departure to Asia, Curtis became more determined to find her. He was prepared to drive all night until it was time to catch his 6 a.m. flight out of SeaTac. He went home after work, quickly packed his bags, and threw them into his trunk. He went directly toward the University of Washington, thinking he would walk around and find Becky, even if it meant going to every single lab and every low-rent apartment complex. As he was parking, just off campus, he saw her walking directly toward him. He would never have guessed that the inadvertent rendezvous was not a feature of chance.

She walked up beside his Jeep as he was getting out. "Hello, Curtis," she said with more warmth than she had shown him in a very long time. "What brings you to the University?"

"You do. I'm leaving for Thailand in the morning and I wanted to see you first."

"Thailand?" she asked with a muddled look.

"Yeah, Mack wants me there to supervise a new neurosurgery center he's opening. I'll be there for about three months."

"How did you know where to find me?" she asked.

"I didn't. I just guessed and got lucky."

"I'm glad you did… I mean, I'm glad you found me."

"Really? You are?" he said with a surprised look.

"Can we walk together?" She said. "I would like to show you my lab."

Side by side they walked up the sidewalk, leaving footprints in the chartreuse fir pollen. She kept her eyes straight ahead and they shared a mutual loss for words. The silence hung thickly in the air between them. Finally, Becky broke the quiet, "Curtis, I've been rough on you."

He quickly interrupted, "Well, I guess I was a selfish ass."

Her softness was interrupted with a brief frown, "Now hush for a minute. Let me talk to you. I have things I need to say, and this isn't easy."

They crossed the street and entered the main campus beneath rows of bigleaf maples that stood tall, on each side of the broad sidewalk, like a line of viridescent bumbershoots.

Becky looked at him and continued, "Curtis, I don't know if you knew this or not, but soon after I moved out of the condo, I entered an alcohol rehab program."

He felt a release of anxious acid in his stomach. He took a deep breath and exhaled slowly. "I knew you were having problems, you know, problems with drinking a lot of wine, but I didn't know… or didn't want to know… the extent of it. I'm really sorry."

Becky abruptly cut him off. "Curtis, hush! This is not about you. I have things to say and I don't want any more apologies from you right now. You've apologized enough already."

Curtis went silent. Becky continued.

"I started seeing Dr. McKenzie, a psychologist here at school as part of my rehab. He helped me recognize that I was suffering from a major depression episode—for which I had been self-medicating with wine." She paused as she took a few more steps, then added, "He also gave me insight about my relationship with you."

"Really?" he asked with an inflection of surprise.

They continued walking, quietly, side by side through the filtered twilight coming down through the broad-canopied trees. Becky gathered her thoughts as Curtis smiled. Becky was finally talking and that's all that mattered to him.

They crossed another street. As they entered the main part of campus, between concrete or red brick buildings, the big trees transitioned from maples into a forest of Japanese cherry trees, just past their bloom. The old pink blossoms, now appearing coffee-stained with age, were still stuck in the edges and contraction joints of the sidewalk.

Becky continued, "Curtis, I've felt so inadequate. I went from being an excellent graduate student in a challenging program at NYU to a nonentity. When we got here, I wasn't working; I wasn't studying, like I am now. The move had eradicated all my New York friends from my life. My only acquaintances in Seattle were the Sharks, but I rarely saw them. Besides feeling depressed, I saw myself as fat and worthless. If that wasn't enough, the move seemed to have exacerbated my migraines, which made job hunting even more complicated. Who would want to hire someone that could end up missing one day a week from a headache?"

"But, Becky, I told you to take it slow and that you didn't have to work. Your migraines aren't your fault."

"Curtis, yes, you said that, but let me finish. I didn't need to work, I wanted to. My problem wasn't simply that I was mad at you; that's why your apologies are inadequate for resolving this. It was about me hating myself. I felt like a total failure. On the other hand, there was Curtis Eisner—a brilliant neurosurgeon, a Nobel Prize winner, and a highly distinguished member of society. I felt deep down that the honorable thing to do was to leave you and to get out of your way. I wanted to pack up my depression, my migraines, and my alcoholism—into matching overnight cases—and leave on a one-way journey, dissimulating myself into obscurity."

"I'm so sorry, Becky."

She flashed him a dirty look. Then she suspended that discussion.

As they turned the corner, she pointed out, "There's my lab." It was a beautiful, modern, red brick building with glasshouses that lined the shore of Portage Bay. The water looked unusually blue under a cloudless evening sky.

She continued, "Dr. McKenzie helped me to sort out my thoughts. During one of our weekly sessions, he asked me point blank, 'Does Curtis still love you?' I told him that you say you do… but I didn't know for sure. Then he asked a strange question, 'Why would he lie to you?' I answered that I didn't know. So, Curtis, why do you love me?"

"Of course, I love you, Becky." Curtis injected. "Does love have to have a reason? I live my life in a world of science and reason and sometimes there just has to be a place of knowing… without reasons."

"Well, Dr. McKenzie made the point that you probably did love me. He also said that you were no imbecile. So, you must see something in me that makes me worth loving, even if I don't."

"Smart man," said Curtis. Then he reached out to take her hand. She let him hold it as they walked. He pulled her close to kiss her, but she turned away, saying, "I'm sorry, but I'm not ready for that."

Becky wiped away a tear. Curtis didn't understand the return to coldness. After all, wasn't she still his wife? Love stories are supposed to have a climax where they embrace and then kiss, and all is well. She did give him a smile, squeeze his hand, and say, "Okay, that's all I need to say tonight. We can talk about this more when I see you again?" He nodded.

She took him for a tour of the greenhouses and her research project, discussing her work and not talking anymore about her feelings or their relationship.

They walked back to their cars and were standing beside his Jeep. She confided in him, "Curtis, it was no accident that you found me today. I had left campus, heading home, and spotted you driving in.

I did a U turn in the middle of the boulevard and came back to find you. I followed you and parked down the street." She chuckled, "I had to run to catch up to you and then force myself to breath normally once I was here."

He gave her a smile and said, "You're silly."

She smiled back.

Then he added, "Becky… move back in with me. Please. I beg you! Let's be a couple. Let's start a family. You would make a wonderful mom."

"Shh. Stop it! You're moving too fast, Curtis. Let me think about moving back to the condo while you're in Thailand. Let's get together for dinner or something when you get home. We can talk about it then."

He answered, "Sure." Then they leaned against the Jeep and continued to talk. Curtis told her about his mother and the developments at Neurogenics. He was planning on checking on his mom in Tennessee as soon as he got back. He invited Becky to join him. She agreed to go. That's how they left it.

With things in Seattle marginally under control, it was time to fly to Asia. He arrived in Bangkok via a commercial flight. There he was picked up by a local chauffer service as he exited customs. The driver took him south ten miles, in a silver Mercedes sedan, dodging pedestrians and oxcarts with only inches to spare, ending at a small harbor in Wat Hong Thong. There, three float planes were tied up. He was instructed to board the big Grumman Albatross at the end of the dock. On the tail was painted a sea eagle in flight and the letters "PWO."

One of the pilots greeted him and welcomed him aboard. Curtis paused at the cockpit and looked at the two pilots as they were reviewing information on a clipboard. He asked, "How long of a flight is it?" To his surprise, the pilot on the right told him it would be about ninety minutes. He was expecting a much shorter trip. Then he asked the pilot, "What's the name of this airline?"

The pilot, as he was checking out the instruments, gave him a puzzled look and asked, "What do you mean?"

Curtis responded, "Well I saw a big 'PWO' on the tail, what airline does that stand for?"

"That means 'Pendleton Wellness Oasis.' We work for Mr. Pendleton just like you do. That's where we're going, you know. Now, go take a seat and fasten your seatbelt, as we will be taking off soon."

Curtis took a seat as the only passenger in the big plane, which could have held twenty. His mind started to race. So, he has a name for this place and he named it after himself? Personally, he thought "Oasis" sounded a little tacky for a medical center.

Curtis had to admit, at least from air, that the Similan Islands were gorgeous. The Andaman Sea was of such a deep turquoise that it would make the gemstone itself jealous. Coming in on a float plane also reminded him of watching reruns of *Fantasy Island*. He had a strong hunch that the TV series had been a major source of creative inspiration for Mack when he came up with this idea. Although powerful and confident in his business intelligence, Curtis saw Mack as a simple man. He seemed to have no broader thoughts inside his head than an Arkansan pencil salesman—but a very self-assured and self-serving pencil salesman.

From the air, Curtis saw a lot of construction on the island. The medical center was clearly visible as a large, two-winged stone and glass building. However, there were many other smaller buildings, all with palm thatching in the Tiki style. The plane banked sharply, as they descended through a series of corkscrew turns toward a small, blue bay with a dock. They touched the water softly, and the two big engines roared as the thrust was reversed—by the tilting of the props' blades—to slow them down.

After turning in the water, they cruised slowly over to the dock, where a worker was waiting to tie them up. Curtis was met at the float plane landing by a young, well-dressed Thai man. He was extremely respectful, addressing him as "sir." He drove him along the beach toward the hospital complex in a topless Jeep with the windshield folded down.

The warm, moist air rushed through Curtis's hair, and his clothes flapped rhythmically in the draught. The air was filled with a briny smell and a hint of spice. He noticed the color of the Jeep, and another Jeep they passed along the way, was the same deep, fern green as the plane. They turned through a security gate toward what appeared to be the living quarters.

The houses, too, were in the South Pacific—Tiki—style with palm thatched roofs. The houses sat just off the beach, around a small lagoon. When he opened the door to his unit, he found it to be, on the inside, quite modern like a five-star hotel in Scandinavia. As he walked through the living room, he found the layout to be huge, with at least 4,000 square feet of livable space on one floor.

Curtis was starting to settle in. He was unpacking his bags, putting them into the teak wood wall cabinets when a knock came at his door. He ran to the front of the house and looked through the window and saw Mack and his entourage standing on the covered porch. He moaned quietly to himself.

Curtis opened the door and smiled. Mack reached out and—oddly—gave him a big bear hug. "Hey, Curtis, son, welcome to paradise." He pulled a bottle out of his pocket with a label that said "SangSom" diagonally across it. Mack smiled as Curtis looked at the amber bottle and explained, "It's Thai rum, better than anything I've ever drank in the Caribbean, and I know you're not a Jack Daniels fan."

The two had a brief but affable meeting. Mack explained what Curtis's role would be during his stay, primary as a quality assurance agent for the company. He also wanted to have plenty of photos taken with Curtis at the facility, which Mack could later use in marketing. He would often say after Curtis had won the Nobel Prize that they should insure his face because it was worth a billion dollars.

Mack also informed Curtis that he was leaving the next day for a meeting in China but wanted to have a welcoming dinner with Curtis and all the surgeons, including doctors Takahashi, Kaur, Bidaya, and a Turkish neurosurgeon, Dr. Sarah Mustafa, that night.

The dinner—oddly—carried a Hawaiian theme, including a piglet roasted in the ground over hot coals. There were belly dancers and local Thai and Indonesian staff dressed in bright Hawaiian shirts and shorts. The whole event was set up on a beautiful beach facing to the east, with the setting sun behind them. But the brilliant red-violets of the western sky were still visible. This was the leeward side of the island, and the constant trade winds were to their backs and against the surf.

"Hawaiian?" asked Curtis, when he looked across the table at Mack. "Why not some Thai tradition?"

Mack chuckled. "Every day here is Thai day, so we wanted to make this special for our American guest. We even considered creating a Tennessee feast but passed on that due to its lack of exoticity."

In a moment, the three staff physicians arrived, followed by warm handshakes with Drs. Bidaya and Kaur. Introductions were made, by Mack, between Curtis and Drs. Takahashi and Mustafa, whom, of course, had never met before. Their conversation around dinner was social, talking about their families and life in the Islands. None of the surgeons had brought their families to Ko Pendle Island, and it was hard for Curtis to grasp why. But again, while not physically absent from Becky when he came to Seattle, she made it clear that he was emotionally absent. But the other surgeons all agreed that the work that they were about to embark on was of such significance that they could leave their own families in more hospitable places.

Dr. Mustafa was a widowed sixty-three-year-old surgeon whose two children were professionals living in Istanbul. She had come as a fellow and, saying in her excellent colloquial English, "I believe that you can teach an old dog a new trick." The jet lag was getting the best of Curtis, and he drifted in and out of a mental fog and almost into slumber every time there was a lull in the conversation.

When they got to more technical issues, Curtis had a long list of questions and tried to shake the sleep out of his head, so he could ask them. He was somewhat surprised at the level of sophistication that they had introduced to the small medical center. Most of the bases had been covered. However, Curtis's concerns weren't eased when they talked about his built-in redundancies (which they didn't think were necessary) and other quality-control measures, such as his pre-op checklist. Those issues consumed Curtis's mind before they had started their first case in Seattle. In the subsequent weeks, these same issues would come up again and again when he worked with the expatriate surgeons.

Curtis was also surprised by how far they were along in the process. They were already doing routine spinal cord injury work, including one case of anastomosis at the C7 level, just after returning from their meeting with Curtis in Seattle. Drs. Bidaya and Kaur had assured Curtis that they had done a very good job; however, they did have some complications during the New Life Assimilation process. The patient never had a full recovery, with persistent numbness and bilateral foot drop. Not being able to voluntarily lift his toes required the patient to wear foot braces behind his legs to hold his feet up. Otherwise, he would trip. The case was only three months old, however, and they held out hope for further improvement. Mack assured the whole group that Curtis would help them make it a "world class" anastomosis center, on par with Neurogenics in Seattle.

After a lively conversation, enough to keep Curtis conscious, the table was cleaned, and the waiters brought the men a choice of spirits, wine, and the best Cuban cigars. Dr. Mustafa excused herself to turn in early. Curtis was the only one remaining who didn't smoke, but he did take a small glass of port wine. They turned to face a big campfire that the staff had built on the beach, and, as a ukulele player strummed, three girls performed a hula dance. The winds carried the carbon plume out to sea and away from their eyes. They could sit, watch the performers, and observe the surf without having to shuffle to avoid the smoke. It was a splendid night, until Mack changed its temperament.

Curtis assumed that the business end of the meeting was over as small talk ensued. However, about that time, Mack turned to him and asked, "Hey, do you remember how we ended our discussion in Seattle?"

"Do you mean about me coming out to Thailand?"

"No, about my ambitions to look to the future and to offer, what you described as, body transplants?"

Curtis rolled his eyes and sat down his drink hard on the table. "Are you serious? You still want to talk about this crazy stuff?"

"Crazy? Curtis, I'm thinking ahead. We have assembled a world-class team here, and we are offering something that no one else can."

Curtis, looking angry, turned to Mack. "Really, how many candidates in the world would need a body transplant? Hum? On the other hand, we have at least two million who are desperate for what we can offer them right now, and I mean today! We need to focus."

"Curtis, like I said, I am a futurist. I see a great need for that service." He paused and looked into the air, to the left and to the right, like he was looking for something specific, but nothing was there. Then he continued talking. "And imagine, Curtis, couldn't we do a face transplant and body transplant on the same person?"

Curtis, with a puzzled looked, asked, "Who would require that much work? Who would have their hearts fail, lungs fail, kidneys fail, liver fail, and need a face transplant, too? Is there one person in the entire world? Maybe someone with severe scleroderma... perhaps."

Mack just sat in silence without even offering an answer. They watched the dancers perform and Mack puffed on his cigar. As the girls were winding down, the men watching all began to clap loudly. Mack announced to all of them, "I can have them strip for you boys if you want." When there was no answer, Mack added, "I'm serious."

Curtis immediately answered before the others had the chance, "That's fine. The Hula is great, and no stripping is required."

They were all saying good night; Mack looked at Curtis and asked him if he could escort him to his house. Curtis just wanted to lay his sleepy head down on a soft pillow. As they walked down a beach path between the coconut palms, Mack turned to Curtis and stated, "Curtis, there's one medical condition that is very widespread that takes out all the organs including the face. There are thousands, maybe tens of thousands, willing to pay a fortune, and I'm talking millions, for it. It far more common than scleroderma. That condition? It's called aging."

Curtis spun around with a severe look of confusion and asked loudly, "What the hell are you talking about?"

"Curtis, son, listen to me. Answer this question as the brilliant neurosurgeon that you are. Isn't it possible to take a nice, young, healthy body of a donor—cadaver donor of course—and give it to an older person, whose mind is still sharp but whose body is failing? Those people have an active brain living inside an old, failing body.

Is there any scientific reason why you couldn't peel down the face, switch the brains or the heads, and reattach the face to a new head?"

Curtis remained in silence with an expression of bewilderment on his own face.

Mack continued, "I've already spoken to the other doctors, and they assured me that this could be done using the Erika Procedure… and they seemed quite interested in the prospects of bringing this hope to an aging world and to stop burying all those young, beautiful donor bodies. Do you agree?"

Curtis walked out to the edge of the beach. "Mack, I think you are either drunk… mad… or perhaps both. Hell no, I don't agree!"

"Son listen to me. You've solved the great riddle of humanity, seducing nerves to regrow and to reconnect that fish you talked about back to the outside world. Now that Pandora's Box has been opened, it won't be closed again. For centuries, people have searched for the holy grail of finding a way back to youth, and you, my son, have found that path. You are the modern, more successful Ponce de León."

The two men walked side by side in silence as Curtis struggled to find the words to express his thoughts clearly. He mumbled to Mack, "You're mixing metaphors."

After another moment of silence, Curtis spoke again, "Mack, you know what my intentions were. My dream was, and still is, to restore broken people to what they once were." Before the words were completely out of Curtis's mouth, he knew he had committed a blunder of semantics. The words, which had taken so long to find, were the wrong words.

Mack, smiling big, simply said, "There you go. We really are both on the same page; that's exactly what I want, too."

"No! We're not on the same page! We're not even in the same book. We're going in two, totally different directions, Mack, and you know it."

"Now don't get all Gandhi on me, Curtis. I heard Drs. Bidaya and Kaur, who worked right beside you for a year or more, say that you saw things the same way. That you described how the person is just a fish, called the brain, living in a primal ocean, encased in our skull and spinal column. That our bodies are like the exterior of an elaborate aquarium, and the spinal cord is only the interface between the fish and the external body. Did you really say things like that to them or not?"

Curtis looked at him and said, "I've said things like that, but they're allegories, not the grounds for some monstrous creation."

"Speaking of books, Dr. Eisner. Did you ever read *A Tale of Two Cities*?"

"Of course," answered Curtis.

"Dickens is my favorite author," said Mack as he paused and took another long draw from his cigar. "The last scene, where Sydney Carton and the Seamstress are standing in queue at the guillotine, were terrifying to me. I couldn't imagine anything worse. Then one day it dawned on me, we are all in line for the guillotine. Some people say, 'Well, your death won't be that violent or predictable.' But, most likely it will be… or worse. Either I will be torn apart when my private plane plummets into the earth, or more likely, cancer will eat me from the inside out and cause so much suffering that an appointment with a guillotine would be a blessing. Curtis, all I'm asking is to delay the inevitable for a few years."

Curtis turned to look out at the beautiful surf and the rising of the full moon. He and Mack stood side by side for several minutes, their words lost to the ubiquitous marvel before them. The lunar size appeared many times larger than normal due to the magnification from the thick horizontal atmosphere. It was pushing up from the edge of the Andaman Sea like a terrestrial parturition from an amniotic ocean. Curtis remained in a meditative mode.

Mack appeared to be thinking—more like hoping—that Curtis was pondering what he had been saying and seriously considering becoming a central part of this new venture. Curtis was giving serious thought to whether it would be wise at this juncture to explain to Mack that he was leaving Neurogenics altogether as soon as she had the cash to buy out his contract. He was a third of the way there. He was also thinking about how badly he wanted this crazy conversation to end so he could go to bed.

"Beautiful moon, ain't it, son?" They stood silently waiting until the moon was fully birthed. The Andaman Sea was flirting with them, its soft rhythmic waves moving up the sand, one after the other without pause. Mack eventually broke the silence when he turned and said to Curtis, "Wasn't it you who also quoted some great Greek philosopher, like Archimedes, that the human soul wasn't connected to the body but floated independently? That's all I'm saying, son. We have the right to restore the youth that age has taken. Age is a disease like any other disease and deserves a cure, too. It's the brain or the soul we must fight to preserve."

"No, it was Pythagoras who came up with that idea; it is called metempsychosis." The two men stood watching as the entire moon drifted away from the horizontal edge up into the night sky. Now there was a shard of darkness expanding between the yellowish disk and the sea. Curtis turned and faced Mack. The moonlight enhanced Mack's aging features, his ruddy skin, and, despite his pony tail, the bald top of his head. Curtis said softly without emotion, "I'm leaving Neurogenics."

Mack sighed and shook his head, then reacted with a bit of sarcasm in his voice, "Well, you don't say. After all we've done to help build your enterprise, to give you the damn Nobel Prize, where you get all the damn credit and we foot all the bills. You must have won the lottery, son. Really, how did you come up with $11 million? You owe Thomas at least that much if not more by now."

"I will find a way out of this mess. I don't need to raise the entire amount. Other, more philanthropic organizations, like the Mayo Clinic, are interested in my work. I'll stay here in Thailand for my full three months because I do want the patients to do well. But I'm not going down this path with you and your crazy doctor friends. This wasn't my dream."

"You're naïve, Curtis."

"That's what I keep hearing, but I would rather be naïve than a part of this foolish game to make a buck."

"Everyone is out to make a buck; that's where you're most naïve. There are no philanthropic organizations on this planet. That's a boyish fantasy. Curtis, you are making a huge mistake… a mistake that just might come back to bite you in the ass." Then Mack gave one of his infamous belly laughs and started to walk away.

"Be careful walking back in the dark," shouted Curtis. His caution for the man was sincere, after his four or five glasses of Jack Daniels.

Mack looked over his shoulder and bellowed back, "I'm not afraid of the dark… the damn dark's afraid of me!" He chuckled as he turned and continued walking back through the trees. Mack disappeared into the moon shadow of the palms, and Curtis continued watching him until all he could see was the red glow of the cigar that appeared with each draw of the old man's breath.

CHAPTER SIXTEEN: COREPLANT

Curtis had a way of converging all his mental energy into his work. It was habitual. He made creating the best possible outcomes for patients his sole purpose for the duration of his time in Thailand. He worked side by side with Drs. Bidaya, Kaur, and Mustafa. They seemed highly skilled, and there was no reason that they couldn't be successful in the Erika Procedure, except that they all had the tendency to cut corners during their preparation.

What bothered Curtis the most was that Dr. Kaur was often willing to lie to cover his tracks. If Curtis came in to the case late, as he often had to do because he was just finishing a case with Dr. Bidaya or Mustafa, he would ask the team, "Did you go over the pre-op checklist?" Dr. Kaur would always say, "Of course." Then later Curtis would find out that they hadn't.

The checklist was an important step to the surgery in Curtis's mind. It included things like testing the primary and backup 3-D printers, loading all the relevant MRI scans in the virtual viewer, and inventorying the supplies. The CCWs were also to be turned on and tested before the incision was made. More than once, a failure of equipment during the procedure or a missing instrument demonstrated to Curtis that the pre-surgery checklist had not been done.

Curtis talked to both doctors several times about this, and they promised to do better. Drs. Bidaya and Mustafa seemed to make some effort but not Dr. Kaur, who carried a lackadaisical attitude.

Curtis wanted to understand the situation and try to figure out if it was the Indian culture or something within Vihaan's own personality. He finally had a moment of insight when one of the OR techs, Chaem, pointed out to Curtis that she thought the problem was the "girls."

"What girls?" asked Curtis with a puzzled look.

Chaem went on to explain that Mack hadn't only provided the surgeons with nice houses, personal chefs, money, and alcohol, but the male surgeons also got girls. These were girls that Mack brought in from Bangkok. Chaem called them "street girls."

"Do you mean prostitutes?" asked Curtis with a bit of apprehension in his voice.

Chaem started to blush, and she added, "Yes, prostitutes, but we call them 'street girls.' Dr. V"—her nickname for Dr. Kaur—"likes the young ones, and when they are with him, he comes to work late. So, we don't have time to do the checklist before the surgery."

This disturbed Curtis immensely but didn't surprise him. "How young?" he asked.

She smiled and seemed to blush again. "Very young."

"Like teenagers?" asked Curtis, with raised eyebrows.

"Oh, maybe younger."

"Twelve?" asked Curtis with growing uneasiness.

"Maybe… or younger," answered Ms. Choi.

Curtis was then deeply disturbed over this new information. He promptly left the OR and marched in a heavy pace as he searched for some private space to make a call. He tried to call Mack first, but Mack never seemed to answer his phone when he was out of town. He went home and had dinner, but he didn't eat much due to a nervous stomach. Then he waited, watching the digital clock until it was 10 p.m., which would translate to 7 a.m. in Seattle. Immediately he called Thomas.

"Thomas!"

"Yes… what's up?"

"We have a huge problem here."

"Like what? I just saw Mack when he came through Seattle on Friday, and he said you're being a big help and things were hunky-dory. What's changed?"

"Mack is supplying the surgeons with prostitutes as part of their compensation."

Thomas waited a few seconds in a contemplative silence. "Well, those surgeons are adults, and Thailand isn't America, so they may do things differently there."

"Really, is that all you can say? Seriously? Thomas, it appears that Dr. Kaur likes them young, like children. This can't go on!"

Thomas was quiet.

"Thomas are you listening to me?"

"Yes, Curtis! Just focus on your work and don't entangle yourself with Mack and the way he does his business and let me look into this."

Then there was silence again, so Curtis said, "That's it? That's all you got?"

Thomas continued, "No, we can't allow child prostitutes on the island if we're going to associate with Mack. We'll eventually separate our companies as soon as we can return his investment. But please don't bring this up to Mack yourself."

"What really should concern you and Mack—as if the fate of the girls isn't enough—is that Dr. Kaur is letting his nasty habit influence the quality of his work. He comes to the OR late and is disorganized because of the girls. Someday a patient is going be hurt, and this whole thing is going to blow up. Mack is going down, and I think he's going to take us with him. He's already spread the word through Asia that 'Dr. Curtis Eisner, Nobel laureate' is part of their team. Even if you have no moral regard for girls, surely you will care about the reputation of Neurogenics or the quality of the work. I'm damn concerned about my name being associated with this mess but even more concerned about the kids."

"Okay, Curtis, I'll talk to Mack! He's passing through here again in a couple of days. Then I think he's going back to China and back to Thailand before you leave. But you just stay out of this issue, and I will deal with it."

Curtis thought for a moment and then responded, "Thomas, you knew about this, didn't you?"

"Curtis, like I said, let it go. I will take care of the situation, and no, I didn't know about the young girls." He paused and continued, "Curtis, I'm telling you again, as your employer, stay out of this! It doesn't matter how, but I will take care of this. Do your job there and come back to Seattle."

"Thomas, I'm getting the hell out of here on the first plane, but I'll meet with the team first. If I can find the girls, I'm taking them with me, too."

Thomas just sighed, and Curtis hung up the phone.

Curtis kept an eye out for young girls on their island. He had seen a couple of girls, ages nine or ten, before and had assumed they were the daughters of staff or patients. Never in his wildest imagination did he think they could be street girls.

Curtis met with Vihaan Kaur that evening. Dr. Kaur denied the story... at least at first. Then he became angry, something Curtis had never seen from the quiet man before. The conversation eventually led to Vihaan shouting, "This is none of your damn business," as he slammed his fist down on his kitchen table.

Curtis worked on booking a flight to Seattle. The first flight with open seats was a week away. In those seven days, he packed up his stuff, watched over a couple more surgeries with Dr. Mustafa, and was diligent in watching for any sight of a child on the island. There were none that couldn't be accounted for as family members of adults on the island. Apparently, they had sent the street girls back to Bangkok or kept them in hiding, waiting for Curtis's departure.

One evening, Curtis was sitting in his house looking out over the sea. The chef had just left, and he was finishing a great dinner. He allowed the girls—once again—to come to the forefront of his mind. Then, out of impulse, he walked down to Vihaan's house and knocked on the door. There wasn't an answer, but he could hear music, oddly Steely Dan, playing in a back room. He knocked several times, and then reached down and found the door locked. Then he banged on the door as hard as he could. Eventually, Vihaan came to the window in a bathrobe. He opened the door and looked at Curtis. "What the hell do *you* want?"

Curtis pushed past the man and ran to his bedroom. It was empty. He opened the closets and ran to the guest room. There was nothing out of sorts. Finally, Vihaan shouted, while pointing toward the door, "Get out of my house!" As Curtis walked past him, he said in a normal voice, "You've become a madman. All of you are madmen."

Curtis returned to his own house, poured himself a drink of Thai rum, and went out to sit on his deck. He looked out over the beach. In a moment of self-doubt, he asked himself, "Am I really the lunatic?" He rubbed his face and started to backtrack on his thoughts. He reflected on Vihaan's tardiness and the conversation with Chaem Choi. She seemed honest and informed. He really did remember seeing a couple of young Thai girls on the island in previous weeks and seemed to remember Vihaan walking with one of them on the beach. He assumed it was his daughter visiting from India, but to think about it now, her skin was much lighter. Surely Curtis wasn't just imagining all of this, was he?

Curtis eventually felt a—displaced—wave of peace come over him. The peace grew out of the satisfaction that he had done all that he could to redeem the situation. He considered going to the police in Bangkok, but he had already heard about how the police there often turned a blind eye to prostitution, even child prostitution. He read that they were often paid to look the other way, sometimes being paid by the kids' own relatives who didn't want a disruption in income. Sometimes the police were even paid in flesh or drugs. His peace was also coming from the thought that he had only about sixty more hours before he left the island. He felt tired and went to bed.

The next morning, his phone started to ring. It was five in the morning. He normally got up at 5:30 a.m. and made a dash to the OR, eating some fruit on the way. His only thought regarding this early hour phone call was that they must have had to take a patient back to the OR and needed his help. He picked up the phone. It was Mack on the other end. Curtis sat up in bed. To his surprise, Mack announced that he was back on Ko Pendle. He said to him, "Uh, Dr. Eisner, we had a deal, didn't we, son, that you would come out and spend three months with my staff? Unless I forgot how to count, I think you have only been here seven weeks, and now I'm hearing rumors from Thomas that you are leaving. So, when are you coming back to finish up your promised time?"

Curtis wrestled with the thought of bringing up the claim of child prostitution on the island, but Thomas had made him promise that he wouldn't. So, Curtis wanted to put the best spin on the purpose of his leaving. "I think I'm done here. The surgeons know what they are doing... they just need more discipline, something that must come from within. Dr. Mustafa is coming along fine. She has a lot of good experience."

"Curtis, son, I need to talk to you. Stop by the beach bar on your way up to the medical center, and I'll be waiting for you."

After showering, Curtis grabbed his backpack and flashlight and started up the beach path. The sun must have been slowly approaching the horizon from the other side of the world, as it was getting brighter and brighter to the point he could put the flashlight away before reaching his destination.

There was Mack sitting outside with an amber drink on the rocks in a clear glass. The bartender, who normally served only coffee, tea, or fruit drinks this time of day, asked Curtis what he wanted. "A fruit smoothie and a cappuccino would be fine."

Mack studied Curtis up and down like he was sizing him up. "So, I got this call from Thomas that you were upset over hearing that there were young girls out here shacking up with our good doctors. Well, I knew I had to fly back to straighten this out. Curtis, son, good God, I wouldn't let something like that happen here. I mean, if Drs. Bidaya and Kaur wanted to visit the girls, or boys…" he added with a chuckle, "… in Bangkok, that's none of my business and should be none of yours. What they do in their private lives is, well, private. You told me to stay out of your personal business when I asked you how you and Rebecca were getting along. Same applies here."

The bartender handed Curtis the tall glass filled with a reddish thick paste with a straw. He began to drink from it. It had this strange but delightful taste of strawberries, kiwifruit, and a nutty barley. As he sipped, in his mind, he felt that Mack was lying to him. He just didn't care anymore… about the lies. He just wanted out of there.

"So, Curtis, my man. Can I persuade you to stay another month to finish up your work?"

Curtis, shaking his head, said, "Nope. My mind is made up. I've got a flight to Tokyo in two days and then Seattle. I need to check on my mom in Tennessee, after stopping to check on my team. You really don't need anything else from me here."

Mack was sucking on the ice cube from his empty glass. He spat it back in and looked out over the sea and back at Curtis. "Okay, son, I will let you go. But I do want you to do one thing for me. I want you to spend tomorrow with Dr. Takahashi and his team. Then I would like to meet with you for dinner at my house tomorrow night."

Curtis agreed to the deal. The next day, he went to the north end of the medical center, the transplant unit. Dr. Takahashi was waiting for him. He was an intelligent and straightforward man. He spoke English like an American and, from what Curtis was told, could speak German and Spanish with equal fluency. That morning, Curtis scrubbed in on a case where the doctor was transplanting two cadaver ears and a large piece of hair-bearing scalp tissue onto a young man who had been severely burned in a motorcycle accident in Kathmandu. He was part of the royal family, a nephew or something like that, and they sent him to the Medical Oasis for the family had considered as the best treatment in the world.

Curtis, as a surgeon, was fascinated by this surgeon's skill and precision. His hand was extremely steady, especially for a sixty-eight-year-old. After the surgery, Dr. Takahashi told Curtis that Mack wanted him to see something. Curtis followed him to the rehab unit. There they met a man from Kuwait, named Ahmed Khouri. He was lying in a recliner, and the physical therapist was working with his facial movements. Curtis could tell that the man had had a face transplant because the motor movements were slow and weak. However, oddly, the man also had an external metal fixation ladder around his neck, the type that Curtis used to stabilize the spine after the Erika Procedure. While his head was mostly shaven for the procedure, the stubble hair grown revealed a blondish color, and his complexion was quite light for a man of Arab heritage. As they walked away, Curtis asked, "So what procedures did this man have done?" Dr. Takahashi seemed to ignore the question, so Curtis asked in a different way, "Obviously, he's had a face transplant, but what's with the external fixation of his cervical spine?"

Dr. Takahashi looked at him without speaking as he pushed the swinging doors which exited the NLAU. They took a couple more steps, and he looked at Curtis and replied, "He's our third collaborative case."

Curtis, looking puzzled, simply said, "Explain?"

"Come up to my office."

The two men climbed the flight of stairs up one floor and walked into Dr. Takahashi's very large office suite, looking directly out on the sea. It was decorated in a mixture of Japanese ink-on-silk paintings and French Impressionistic oils on canvas. The furniture was distinctly Japanese with a chabudai and pillows on the floor in front of a typical European wooden desk and upright chairs. Dr. Takahashi took off his lab coat and hung it on a wooden hanger in a methodical way that reminded Curtis of Mr. Rogers. Then he put on a yukata over his scrubs.

Curtis took a seat at the desk, and Dr. Takahashi walked over and then motioned for Curtis to join him at the chabudai. With both sitting on cushions, legs folded, Takahashi began to talk. "This man, Mr. Khouri, is a seventy-nine-year-old man who had multiple organ failure."

With those few words spoken, Curtis's mind started to run wild with nervous anticipation. Certainly, the man that they just visited couldn't have been more than thirty.

Dr. Takahashi continued, "His kidneys were failing, his heart was failing, his liver was failing. It was a great case of a good healthy psyche, or man, inside a failing body. His son came to us and asked for help. He had been followed by the Cleveland Clinic at their site in Abu Dhabi and in Cleveland. They could offer only palliative care, as he wasn't a good candidate for multiple organ transplantation. However, Drs. Bidaya and Kaur reviewed his case. We thought the gentleman would be a great candidate for corporis-transplantation, or what we are calling our 'Coreplant' Procedure."

Curtis placed his face into his hands and began to shake his head back and forth in a gesture of disbelief. Dr. Takahashi paused for just a moment to observe him and then continued, "The primary hurdle, of course, was finding a good donor specimen. The patient's extended family found the body of a young Swiss man who had been declared dead at the Kuwait City Hospital. I think he drowned while jet skiing in the Persian Gulf. He was resuscitated on the beach, but not before suffering an irreparable brain injury. His family were prepared to take him off the ventilator as the EEG showed no viable brain activity. That's when we intervened."

Curtis still had his hands over his face. He mumbled, "Did the family know?"

Dr. Takahashi asked, "Did they know about the donation? Oh, of course. The hospital had them sign a release of his body for organ donation and cremation. They cremate his brain, which is the soul."

Curtis sat quietly with his eyes closed.

"Are you listening to me?" asked Dr. Takahashi.

Curtis said with a sigh, "Yes... yes, I'm listening to *everything*."

"So, we did the usual tissue matching, blood type, and others, and he was a close match. With modern anti-rejection drugs, of course, we don't need to have exact matches any more. In the future, we may even find with the Coreplant Procedure, and the help of the blood-brain barrier, that we may need little in the way of anti-rejection drugs."

Curtis dropped his hands from his face, tilted his head back to look straight up, and whispered, "God no... this can't be happening."

Dr. Takahashi paused momentarily to stare at him and then continued, "Oh, yes, this is happening... so, we brought the donor corporis here to our center. We left the specimen on ice and a mobile ventilator. Dr. Eisner, it was a beautiful thing. Any student of physiology would be amazed at the work that we did."

Curtis had covered his face with his hands again, and a couple of tears were running down his cheeks. Dr. Takahashi ignored this behavior as a trivial distraction and spoke to him like Curtis was sitting upright listening soberly... even though he wasn't.

"Drs. Bidaya and Kaur joined me, and we had a team of about twelve in the Coreplant suite. First, I opened the scalp of the donor corporis cutting transversely from ear-to-ear. I carefully dissected and brought forward the facial structures, just beneath the subcutaneous fat layers, like I do in a face transplant. In this case, I could avoid taking muscle tissue as we would use the recipient's own cranial muscles. This simplifies preserving facial expressions. Some cases may require donor muscle tissue, too, and eyes. But then I carefully cut the pair of facial nerves, each pair of three branches of the trigeminal nerve, the accessory nerve, and the vagal nerve. We found that it is best to cut them ten millimeters from where they exit the boney skull and, in this case at least, above the muscle layer."

Curtis was still looking up at the ceiling, eyes open and speechless.

"Curtis!" Dr. Takahashi said as he reached out and touched Curtis's arm. "It was beautiful; you would've loved to have been there." Then he chuckled. "So, as I was saying, we moved the facial flap forward and then did the same on the posterior side. There I only had the greater and the cranial branch of the lesser occipital nerves to dissect. We then tied off the internal and external carotid arteries, just superior to their bifurcation. With the posterior, occipital flap then peeled back and secured, we removed the skull and its contents. We separated the head from the neck at the C2 level, clamping the vertebral arteries. I then moved to Mr. Khouri and repeated the same procedure. However, when we cut the carotid arteries below the bifurcation and we then connected Mr. Khouri's cranium and contents to our portable heart/lung machine. When have our own four-way, out and in flow tubing to supply the carotids and vertebral arteries. In a well-orchestrated move, a move that you would have been proud of, Drs. Bidaya and Kaur and I moved the cranium containing the brain of Mr. Khouri, which remained attached to the heart/lung machine, to the donated corporis and worked to merge the two. I cut Mr. Khouri's internal and external carotids, one by one, and attached them to the donor body's arteries. Connecting the vertebral arteries was the most tedious part of the whole procedure, requiring the splitting and removal of C2, and then rejoining it around the joined arteries. It was very complicated, and your team did a marvelous job in connecting each of the major nerves as I joined all the major vessels. You can't even see a wound site because I hid them in the hair and behind the ears."

Curtis spoke for the first time in a while. "It's not my team. I am *not* part of this madness. God help us all!"

Dr. Takahashi smiled. "You have an amazing team that you should be proud of. So, Drs. Bidaya and Kaur moved in and started the process of creating the nerve couple device by mapping each of the major nerves and using the 3-D printer for the connector. They placed the connectors on each nerve and the spinal cord on the corporis side of the connection. We then placed the skull, with the Atlas vertebra, on top of the C2 vertebra of the donor corporis. I think you know the procedure going forward, as it is just like all your other nervous anastomosis procedures. Dr. Mustafa came in toward the end to relieve Dr. Bidaya, who was fatigued during the long case. We then created the external fixation for the cervical spine. I then took back over and connected the trachea and esophagus and rolled the donor face and scalp back over Mr. Khouri's cranium and his attached musculature to the donor's subcutaneous structures to preserve facial expressions." Dr. Takahashi finished talking and looked at Curtis, who was now lying back, completely on the floor, looking up at the ceiling, speechless.

Dr. Takahashi got up and left the office, returning with a tea pot and two cups. He proceeded to ignore Curtis's behavior and poured some tea like it was a normal conversation.

Curtis eventually sat back up. He looked at Dr. Takahashi and said, "Please tell me that this is some type of cruel joke that someone is playing on me."

Dr. Takahashi smiled. "No, Dr. Eisner. You're a funny man. Mr. Pendleton said that this was his eventual plan when he built this facility. I thought you would be excited about our accomplishments."

"So, you're telling me that Mr. Khouri is walking around, or soon will be walking around, inside the body of some poor Swiss bastard?"

"Oh, the Swiss man had been dead for a long time before we got his body. But, yes, Mr. Khouri is alive and doing well with a new body, and he is extremely excited. His organs are functioning well. To him, it is like a gift of life and a gift of youth. It is a beautiful thing."

"Did you say that there're more?"

"Oh, yes, Dr. Eisner. This is our fourth case. Our first case died in post-op, but this is our third living case. The others have done quite well."

"But this would be an extremely complex surgery, and you have actually done it? You really pulled this off?"

"Oh, yes, Dr. Eisner. It is very complicated. It took our team of four great surgeons and many technicians over twelve hours to complete."

"Why are you doing this? Have you all gone completely mad?"

"Of course not." Dr. Takahashi began to chuckle again as he sipped his tea from his yunomi, holding it with both hands. He looked up at Curtis after he sat his tea bowl down, with his face still supporting a broad smile. "This is just the next step in mankind's long progress to eliminate suffering and disease. We here at Ko Pendle share the same dream you have. Can you imagine the immense potential of this? The hopes of living in a young, healthy body when you are your seventies or older? This is an incredible breakthrough that rivals the discovery of penicillin. Dr. Eisner, you brought this to the world, and you should feel very gratified." He chuckled again and added, "It is also true that Mr. Khouri's family paid ten million dollars for the procedure. Each surgeon took home $1 million for a very hard day's work, and the center got the other $6 million."

Curtis felt ill and his own soul seemed to be aloof. The world around him was no longer making sense, and he just wanted to escape. If he couldn't leave the whole world, he at least wanted to run from the world that Mack had created in Ko Pendle.

CHAPTER SEVENTEEN: ALTERCATION

Curtis's bags were packed, and he was counting down to the moment when his float plane would carry him from this place and off on the east winds, back to Bangkok, Tokyo, and then Seattle. He had just a few more hours on the island. Ahead, too, was the dreaded dinner with Mack.

He arrived at Mack's large, modern home via golf cart, which was driven by a young, silent Thai man. The property sat on a western, rocky part of the island, which he had never seen before. Just north and south of the house were tall, limestone cliffs that the islands were famous for. Jetting out from his place, connecting directly to the house, was a very long dock reaching all the way out to the deep waters where Mack's 280-foot yacht, *The Lolita*, was berthed.

He knocked on the door of the house and a Thai woman, dressed in the stereotypical black and white "French maid" outfit, greeted him. That seemed unbefitting for a Thai tropical island. She took him into a room surrounded by glass overlooking the sea. The room, while visually astounding, smelled of old cigar and that familiar sent of Mack. He had noticed Mack's unique smell early on, but it took several visits with the man to finally figure it out the source. It was a bad blend of body odor and Old Spice Aftershave. It this room, it seemed to linger in the still air or on the furniture.

On a small table, beside his "assigned" chair, sat a goblet of SangSom on ice. Curtis knew it was SangSom because the bottle was opened on the bar. He realized then that he had tasted Mack's gift and really didn't like it. He was not a fan of spirits in general. But Mack, being Mack, had assumed that he liked it, and that was all that mattered to the man. People like Mack, so thought Curtis, lived within a closed universe of their own conventions. "Is there anything else I can get for you, Dr. Eisner?" she asked in rather good English.

"No, thank you." He smiled at her.

Curtis sat in the living room, alone, for almost an hour. He could hear Mack in the back of the house talking on the phone. It was an odious tone. No one came out to speak to him. In his native Tennessean culture, this behavior would have been considered rude. He stood, walked over to the windows, and looked out over the waters where the sun lazily rested, propped up by the Indian Ocean gales. It was indeed one of the most beautiful places he had ever visited. If Mack and his madness were removed from the equation, he could see Becky and him living here and running an Erika treatment and training center. He would want as many neurosurgeons as he could find to become proficient in the procedure and to spread the cure around the world.

He watched a boat full of fishermen slowly moving before the dusky sky, navigating across the surface of the low-setting sun, like silhouettes or a scene from a shadow theater. As they worked their nets, the feeling of disappointment—once again—began to envelop his spirit. Were there some magnanimous mistakes he kept making that allowed his dreams to keep steering off course? He felt that any other neurosurgeon with this same dream would not be in this predicament. Somehow, if someone else had been in his shoes, they would have found a way to get a residency match with a huge university or someplace like Mayo Clinic or Johns Hopkins instead of Apple Health. Their dream would have been realized without a complexity of patents and owing so much money to different entities.

When Becky was still conversing with him, back in their New York days, she would always say, "Curtis, this is life. Life is hard and uphill for *most* people. You're not alone in your struggle. But you grapple more than others because you try to do very hard things."

In the foreground, Curtis watched workmen scrubbing the sides of *The Lolita*; they, too, looked like stick-figure silhouettes against the bright—burnt umber—backdrop. Eventually, the woman in the maid's outfit came back into the room, intruding upon his contemplations, and said, "Dinner is served, Dr. Eisner."

Curtis entered the grand dining room and was seated in front of a gourmet-looking salad with small pieces of smoked baby octopus arms, and a glass of white wine was poured by a young, muscular man. Curtis sat in the empty room waiting for another twenty minutes. Eventually, Mack walked through the door. "Hello, Curt, how are you?" he asked in a dry, formal voice.

"Fine. Yes, I am fine, and yourself?"

Mack took a seat, although not across the table from Curtis, which would have been conducive to a good conversation. But he sat at the end of the table, forcing Curtis to turn hard to his right to speak to the man five feet away. Mack spoke, "Oh, I'm dandy."

Mack rang a bell on the table, and the maid returned promptly. Mack asked in a stern voice, "Where's the damn bread?"

The lady blushed. "I'm sorry, but the first rolls were slightly overcooked while we waited for you. I know that you don't like them that way. I am just finishing another set, and they will be out in just a moment." She bowed and returned to the kitchen.

Mack chuckled and drank an amber drink from a small clear glass, which he was carrying—until then, unnoticed—in his hand. Then he spoke, "Damn help. You just can't get good help these days in Asia." Pointing his index toward Curtis, he added, "There was a time, not long ago, that they made the perfect household servants. I may look for a Nepalese woman; I heard they work their asses off for nothing and never complain." Taking another sip and swallowing, he said, "I need to look at some photos of them first because my maids need to be good to look at, too. Never met a Nepalese woman, and I honestly don't know what they look like." He took another sip from his drink and sat it down. "Do they have rings in their noses?" He chuckled. "Or around their necks?"

"I don't know. Well, not neck rings, maybe nose rings. But I heard that they are quite beautiful as all Nepalese people are. You have a Nepalese family staying here, on the island… with their son, who has been receiving treatment." Curtis noticed, for the first time, that Mack's eyes were quite bloodshot. He took a deep breath thinking that a confrontation would eventually come this evening. He certainly didn't want to start the dispute over a tangential issue of the role of maids or the repulsive way that Mack treated them. But he did say, in her defense, "Well, anyone can burn rolls if they aren't careful. I know I have before."

Mack gave him a harsh stare and didn't respond. They sat in silence for a moment as they both started to eat their salads. Mack interrupted the silence with a comment that seemed to be in response to the Nepalese family comment by Curtis. "I don't fraternize with patients or their families."

The maid brought in a basket of steaming rolls. Curtis looked at her and smiled. "Thank you, they look wonderful." Mack didn't acknowledge her presence.

When Curtis's throat was clear, he looked back at Mack. "So, this is an interesting side of the island. I didn't realize that the west was so rocky, in contrast to the beautiful beaches on the east side."

Mack, taking a bite of a roll and then speaking—muffled—with a mouthful of food, "Yeah. When I was deciding where to build my own house, I first wanted to be on the beach. However, the only place to moor my boat close to shore was in the deeper water here on the west side. This is the windward side, with constant trade winds; it is also the most worn side of the island, with rocks, cliffs, and deep water hugging the shoreline. I treat *The Lolita* like an extension of my home, and it is nice to have her fifty yards away. I also don't want that damn sunrise coming in through my windows so early in the morning."

Mack paused to finish his second roll and to take another drink. Then he yelled, "Toey!"

The maid came into the room. "Yes, Mr. Pendleton?"

Then he said, in a somewhat softer voice, "Hon, we're ready for dinner." The young woman left for the kitchen.

"As I was saying," Mack continued, "I don't want that morning sunrise in my window because I'm up at ungodly hours. Do you know what it's like to run a business empire that's in virtually every time zone on the planet?"

At first Curtis sat in silence, not realizing it wasn't just a rhetorical question. Mack kept staring at him with anticipation until he answered, "No, I wouldn't know what that's like."

"It's terrible. They're calling me every damn hour of the night. You just can't get good managers like you used to. I pay these sons of bitches half a million a year or more to run something. Still, they have to bug the hell out of me."

The maid brought in a beautifully prepared dish that looked like a ground meat with spices over rice and garnished with what appeared to be mint leaves. Curtis smiled at her and asked, "What's the name of this?"

The woman smiled back. "Oh, this is pad krapow moo saap, a famous Thai dish. I will bring southern-styled fired chicken for Mr. Pendleton. You can have that if you do not like Thai food."

"Oh, I love Thai food."

She returned with a large bowl of what looked and smelled like Kentucky Fried Chicken. Mack was watching Curtis looking at him, as he dished up three pieces of chicken and a scoop of macaroni and cheese onto his plate. "I had her learn to make chicken just like the colonel." Then Mack smiled and added, "I know insiders in Louisville who gave me their so-called secret recipe. It's amazing what people are willing to do when you wave a few bucks in front of their noses."

As they were finishing their meal, with little talking, Curtis was contemplating when to bring up his concerns. However, Mack surprised him when he looked up and said preemptively, as if he was reading Curtis's mind, "If you have something to say to me, wait until I have finished my meal. We can go into the cigar room and talk later. Hateful conversation during dinner gives me indigestion." So, Curtis remained quiet throughout dessert and coffee.

When dinner was finished, they walked back into the same room that Curtis was in earlier. The space was now overlooking a brilliant sky, a palette smeared with fuchsia and vermilion, absent of the sun, which had been drawn completely beyond the horizon by Africa's evening. They sat in over-stuffed, gray leather chairs facing the

389

window with a round, tall table between them. Mack padded the side of his chair and winked at Curtis, "Elephant hide... real elephant hide."

Curtis looked astonished. The two men then turned and looked to the west. The ship workers were now gone. A few of the lights were on inside the massive yacht. Mack looked at him and said, "Gorgeous place, isn't it?"

Curtis smiled and voiced his agreement.

After lighting a cigar and offering Curtis one, which he declined, Mack turned to him and said sharply, "So, my man, Dr. Eisner, you're still leaving us?"

"Yes, tomorrow I have a plane out of Bangkok."

Mack rolled his eyes a bit and said with a bit of sarcasm, "No, son, you said the other night that you're not only leaving the Pendleton Restorative Oasis, but you are leaving Neurogenics as well?"

Curtis first asked, "'Pendleton Restorative Oasis'... is that your name now? What happened to the 'Wellness' in the name?"

"It soon will be the official name. The Wellness Oasis will apply to my other island resort that I am developing."

Curtis continued, "My work at Neurogenics is done. They're up and running. They have trained staff, and I don't think they need me anymore. As you know, my heart has always been with helping all people, not just those with means."

"Well, as Jesus said, 'You'll always have the poor among you.'"

Curtis interrupted, "You're often quoting Jesus, but do you really know anything about the man?"

He pulled the glass from his lips. "Son, I'm from Arkansas, and we quote Jesus… do you have a problem with that?" He raised his eyebrows, in anticipation for an answer.

Curtis shook his head in the negative.

Mack leaned over, placing his face close to Curtis. "So, tell me, son, how did you come up with the $11 million that you owe Thomas? What's your secret?"

Curtis smiled and leaned back away from Mack and his cigar breath. "I don't need $11 million. I have over $2 million now, including the Nobel Prize money. However, once I won the prize, I had many suitors for my talents. Mayo Clinic came back with an offer. While previously their board wouldn't approve a $9 million buy-out for my work, now they approved it. I assume having a Nobel laureate on staff and a one-of-a-kind spinal cord anastomosis program was worth it for their reputation." As soon as the words were out of his mouth, Curtis felt he had said too much. He didn't know how, but he figured that Mack would eventually use his words against him.

This news seemed to make Mack very upset, and he sat back hard in his bloated chair, spilling the remainder of his drink. He looked directly at Curtis but yelled, "Toey! Toey! Damnit, where are you, girl?"

The maid came running into the room in a rush. "Get me another drink... hon."

To Curtis's surprise, the Jack Daniel's whiskey bottle and ice were just four feet away at the bar, but she quickly got him a new drink and cleaned up the mess on the floor.

Mack lifted the drink to his lips and sipped with a shaking hand. He sat his drink on the round table. He said in aloud, annoyed voice, "Curt, you're a damn fool! With what you discovered and the reputation that you have in the world, you could've been a billionaire, too, if you just knew how to brand yourself. You could've had a line of women stretching out to that damn," pointing out the window, "piss-pink horizon. Women love the smell of money, but you just don't get it. There're many men like me that would love to be in your shoes."

"Mack, I don't think *you* get it! And please stop calling me 'Curt.' My name is Curtis. I don't want the damn money! I live on $60,000 a year right now, and I'm content with that. Why would I need more? Here's what you don't get." Curtis paused, the two men stared at each other, and he then continued, "There's a boundary over which we shouldn't cross, and you've crossed it. This so-called restorative center is your narcissistic mirage, not an oasis. You created a for-profit, bizarre head-transplant program that dehumanizes people into machines and machine parts. This isn't a Fantasy Island utopia... this is nothing more than Doctor Moreau's island of monsters! I want nothing to do with this mess, and if you try to associate my name with this place I will sue you for millions!" Curtis was feeling his own anger building, and each of his words was like a step on a staircase, taking him higher and higher in intensity. He didn't like to have emotions take over his faculties, but they were an overpowering force at this point. He was shaken and scared—not of Mack but of losing total control and saying more things he would regret.

Mack sat back in his chair and thought for a moment. He said in a rather soft, maybe intoxicated, voice. "Curt… oh, I mean, Curtis your highness"… pausing to chuckle… "you're the one who's a chump. I've three, maybe four—if you count Sarah—great surgeons who see things exactly the way that I do. They get it, fool! I don't know who the hell Dr. Morrow is or what he's saying, but this is the future. There's now a real hope for old men like myself, of rediscovering that youthful and healthy body and maintaining ourselves. Do you realize what my mind and my money could do in the body of a twenty-one-year-old good-looking body? I would have *everything*. I would have a house full of gorgeous eighteen-year-old women, who really loved me and not just the toys I buy them."

The big man turned to look out the window, which was now framing a significantly darker sky. Without making eye contact with Curtis, Mack said something that he would only say in a drunken state. It was a clear change in tone, as if he was opening a door into an inward chamber of his identity. "I just want to be loved for *me*… who loves a seventy-five-year-old man anymore? I look like a walking corpse." He turned and looked at Curtis. "When you're my age, you have nothing, even if you own everything. I don't even

393

have a mama anymore to love me unconditionally. All men share this want and this dream, and they'll pay millions or maybe hundreds of millions for it. This is the ultimate cure for what really makes us ill. Maybe I don't have a mother, but this is my motherlode."

Quietness filtered back into the room. Toey stepped back in to turn on the lights as darkness had overtaken them without their perception. She refilled Mack's glass and offered Curtis more wine. He covered his glass with his hand, smiling at her. She left.

Curtis said, "It's Moreau, Dr. Moreau, an H. G. Wells creation."

Mack looked totally confused. "What the hell was his creation… my motherlode?"

"Never mind, you're too drunk to comprehend." Curtis finished his own drink. "I think I'm done here, and I will be seeing you Mack." Then he started to stand up.

As Curtis was walking toward the outside door, Mack added, "Oh, there's one more thing, son." Mack said, with a slur. "I've recruited Jennifer Baker from your lab to come and manage our lab here."

Curtis spun around with a deep frown on his face. He squared up with Mack, looking him in the eye and leaning in his direction with an angry scowl radiating from his face. Mack, still sitting in his chair, looked like a walrus -king on his Neptunian throne. Curtis walked toward him, asking, "What … the … hell … are you talking about? Jennifer would never come here!"

"Oh, I beg to differ, Curt. I have a signed contract with the girl."

"What did you do to her?" asked Curtis as he continued walking toward the man in his throne.

"Well, for starters, I offered her 200 grand a year, a beach house, and a lot of respect as a lab manager. Yeah,"—a creepy smile swept across his face—"she's a nice piece of ass… with a brain, too. I like that in a girl. She'll give me something to look at. Something to fantasize about and who knows, maybe to touch."

Curtis tightened up both of his fists and stepped toward Mack. He was feeling a sudden resurgence of rage and shouted, "She would never accept that, she thinks you're a creep!"

Sitting back in the overstuffed chair, Mack started to laugh and to laugh hard, the kind of silly belly laugh that only a drunk can muster. "You moralistic phony! I know about your affair with her, and the scratches you got on your face when her boyfriend beat the hell out of you. That was no damn poison ivy." He laughed harder as Curtis's face drew more taught and red.

Curtis allowed the word, "What?" to slip out from his pursed lips, displaying total confusion.

Mack laughed even harder, pausing to say, "The clincher, my boy Curt, was when I had your man Thomas tell her that you were leaving Neurogenics because she—now—made you feel very uncomfortable. Ha, ha, ha." Mack almost fell out of his seat because he was shaking so hard as he laughed with his eyes tightly closed.

395

"What are you talking about?" whispered Curtis with a contorted look of confusion on his face. Then, out of impulse, he dove right toward Mack, tackling him. The heavy, sodden man didn't have the balance to stay in his chair and the whole thing turned over with Curtis on top of him. Curtis's hands could not fit around Mack's fat neck, so he grabbed handfuls of his flesh on each side of his throat. He squeezed with intensity and a look of rage on his face, a look that Mack had never seen before in the man. It was a rage that Curtis had pent-up inside him for over two years. Curtis was sure that he had no intention to strangle the man to death, but he was just letting a primal impulse run its course.

Mack was trying to shout, but the force of Curtis's hands on his larynx prevented him from making any audible sound. Then he began to slap Curtis's ears and slap them hard with the palms of his open hands. Curtis felt a painful pop in his left ear and had an intense ringing in it. Finally, out of desperation, Mack kicked the table, with its two "rocks glasses"—with ice still in them—sitting on top. The table crashed into the floor with a loud sound, with broken glass and ice spilling across the tile. Soon, Toey came running back into the room and shouted, "Oh, my God!" as she observed the two men on the floor struggling.

The petite maid didn't have the strength to pull Curtis off her boss or even dislodge his fingers from around his neck. Mack was starting to turn a bluish hue, and the expression on his face was turning from one of anger to one of fear.

The maid left and came back with three Thai men. One was the man who poured the wine, and the others came in from outside. Possibly they were the ones working earlier on *The Lolita*. They grabbed Curtis. Two pulled on him as one tried to pry his fingers off Mach's portly neck. The fingers were peeled off, and, with the force of the men behind him, Curtis launched backward, landing on the floor with the two men under him. The men quickly rolled on top of him and held him down, waiting for further instructions from Mack. The third man ran back into an adjacent room and then returned with something in his hand, which he quickly put under his waistband.

Mack sat up on the floor, rubbing his neck, the look of fear slowly draining from his face and being replaced once again by the look of anger… and the color of rage. He was rubbing his neck and looked over at Curtis. The look of fear had now transferred to Curtis's face as the three men kept him immobilized. Mack stood up and walked toward him.

"You goddamn son of a bitch! So, you were going to kill me? You pathetic, little man. No damn fool lays a hand on me and lives without regret!" Mack kicked Curtis hard in the ribs, feeling like he had broken a couple of them as Curtis let out a loud moan.

Mack just looked at him, grinding his teeth in wrath, and added, "You sorry son of a bitch! Do you know who you are dealing with here? I could make you disappear off the freakin' planet like Earhart, and no one would ever know what the hell happened to you."

Curtis was looking up at him, still in a state of moot fear. He did consider that Mack probably had caused the "disappearances" of other men like him before. In a way, Curtis no longer cared. But he did want to warn Jennifer to stay away, and that was his goal of survival.

Mack continued, "However, I'm going to let you live because I cannot stomach the thought of murdering a man of your talent."

Mack looked at the young Thai men and back at Curtis like he was trying to decide what to do with the restrained doctor. "Take him outside, boys, and show the man some discipline." Then he looked back at Curtis, "And you, you son of a bitch, I could have made you the most loved man in the world… and one of the richest, but now I will ruin you… you bastard! Get your damn pathetic ass off my island, and I never want to see your narrowed little mind again!"

The three men dragged Curtis across the tiled floor toward the door. On the way, they passed the maid. She looked worried. She said something in Thai to the men, and one of them yelled something back at her in a sullen voice.

One of the men opened the front door and the three dragged him out onto the deck. Curtis had no clue what was about to happen. The men talked briefly between themselves, and then one wrapped his arms around Curtis's chest from behind him, squeezing his thorax, causing Curtis to squeal from the pain from his freshly damaged ribs. Then one man grabbed each leg, like they were going to carry him. The man, with his arms around his chest shouted something in Thai to them. The men on each leg started to pull his legs apart until it hurt. Then the man holding his arms around his chest dropped one arm, reached behind himself. He pulled a telescoping metal bar out of his waistband, snapped it to its full length, and struck Curtis in the testicles with the full might of his strength. Curtis felt an incredible pain, like he had never felt in his entire life. The men then threw him off the porch into the bushes, causing him to land directly on his back. He screamed in pain. He could hear Mack belly laughing just inside the door.

The big man walked out and stepped off the deck, still rubbing his neck. He hovered over Curtis, who was curled up in a ball with a red face grimacing in agony. Mack bent over and spit on Curtis's face. Curtis tasted the bitter flavor of cigar in his mouth, which had been widely agape due to his screaming.

Mack snarled. "Don't even think about going to the authorities, asshole. I write the laws here, and I am the only authority." Mack turned and escorted the three Thai men back inside his house and closed the door.

Curtis lay in the dirt for a few minutes, as he was too weak to stand. He felt like he was about to lose consciousness from hurt. However, at the same time, he had a terror that they would come back for him and beat him even more. He pulled himself up on a small banana tree and got to his feet, but he wasn't sure he could walk. Each time he swung out his right leg to take a step, the pain in his groin was absurd… beyond the level that Curtis had thought a human could bear. He struggled to find his way through the brush and back to the road, walking and stumbling the two miles back to his side of the island and his house. The arduous journey took several hours. He lay behind the undergrowth whenever he would see the lights of a car or golf cart. Several times he had to drop to his knees and rest, as the pain of his groin and his ribs had drained all the potency from his legs. He vomited once, and it went all over his shoes. The waning moon, just a sliver, was rising over the east side of the island, giving him just enough light to re-orientate himself toward home.

When Curtis made it back to his house, he slowly stepped onto the porch and fiddled with his keys to open the door. He was still worried that someone would be inside waiting to kill him and throw his body, tied to a stone anchor, into the deep Andaman Sea. The cruelty of Mack convinced him that he wouldn't give murder a second thought if it offered some advantage to the billionaire.

He collapsed on his bed without pausing to pull down the covers or take off his dirty clothes. Throughout the night, Curtis lay awake between short respite naps. The constant throbbing of pain in his groin made a restful sleep impossible. The intensity of it moved beyond his groin, into his whole pelvis and up the right side of his back like burning fire. The pain at the center, in his testicle, was grinding and tearing, as if a giant drill was turning and digging slowly into his flesh. It was constant, not letting up, even for a breath. When he did inhale, it caused excruciating pain in his chest, but he forced himself to breathe and to breathe deeply. He hated the thought of standing, but he forced himself to get up once to get a tray of ice from the freezer and place it on his swollen scrotum, tray and all. There was nothing, not even an acetaminophen or paracetamol, in the house to take for pain.

He looked at the clock, watching the green, digital numbers slowly parade through the night—minute by minute—at a funeral's pace. In the predawn glow of the sky, the only analgesia that he could find was in the release of suffering through his loud moans. He was scheduled to take a float plane at 9 a.m. to Bangkok and then catch his international flight to Tokyo at three in the afternoon. He couldn't imagine how he could do it in such pain and being unable to walk.

He did force himself to get up again. Knowing that he wouldn't be able to carry a suitcase or even pack up his bag, he collected his essentials: cellphone, billfold, toothbrush, and his passport. He would have called someone on his cellphone, but there was no reception on the island. He lay in bed clutching his essentials, enclosed in a zip-locked bag in his right hand. He waited for someone to come and take him to the seaplane port, thinking that maybe they could help him walk. But no one came.

He listened carefully at nine, and there was no plane landing. The roar of the engine as it reverse-thrusted was normally easily to hear from Curtis's house. He heard the familiar sound several times a week… but not on this morning.

Curtis spent the remainder of his day alone, lying on his bed. He drank the water from the ice tray as it melted. He was trying to figure out the relevance of this new development. Had Mack cancelled his pickup? How was he supposed to get home? He spent the next four days on his back, sipping water and occasionally snacking on cheese, pickles, and a few other items he found in his refrigerator. His scrotum had swollen to the size of a baseball, and it turned black with old blood coagulating inside. As the hours passed, still, no one came to check on him.

On the third day, he tried again to walk. He stuffed the plastic bag of possessions inside the back of his pants with the top of the bag sticking out the top, which he wrapped under his belt to secure it. He looked in his closet, hoping to find a broom handle for support. He did, however, find an old cricket bat—obviously left by a previous tenant—which worked even better. As he walked slowly across the compound, using his makeshift crutch for support, he looked for anyone who could help him. Eventually, he saw one of the gardeners trimming and pruning a palm tree. Curtis walked under the man and looked up, "Do you speak English?"

The man, when he finished cutting a palm branch, climbed down the tree and wiped his hands off on his pants. He looked at Curtis and said, "A little."

Curtis asked him how he could get to Bangkok. The man seemed confused that a Western man would be asking *him* such a question. Curtis told him that he came in on a seaplane, but none were available to take him back. The gardener explained that there was a national ferry system that connected all the islands. It only stopped on Ko Pendle upon demand because it wasn't part of their normal route. That's how the employees got on and off the island.

The gardener escorted Curtis down to the harbor and into the harbormaster's office. The two Thai men spoke in their native language for a moment and seemed to be having an argument. Finally, the harbormaster spoke English for the first time and said to Curtis, "The ferry only passes this way every other day. I can call them, and they will stop here tomorrow morning. They will need 1,038.15 THB in cash."

"Will they take US dollars?" Curtis asked.

The harbormaster answered, after thinking for a moment, "If you can give me fifty dollars, US, I can buy your ticket." Curtis agreed to the inflated price.

The next morning, Curtis caught the ferry after making sure his phone was fully charged. The passenger ferry did stop, and it took him north to Port Blair. On the ride over, he sat outside on the ferry to feel the cool air off the sea. It hurt to breathe, but somehow the fresh air made it a little less laborious. From Port Blair, Curtis secured a spot on a diving tourist boat that would take him back to the mainland the next morning. He had twelve hours to wait in Port Blair. He walked down, in a shuffle, to the Golden Buddha Beach Resort. He lay on the beach that night collecting a few moments of sleep. There were no rooms in the resort available and, for a "tip" of $20 US, the groundskeeper promised that Curtis could sleep in peace on a lounge chair on the beach. Curtis was skeptical, but it was his only choice.

Once lying on the beach chair, Curtis suddenly remembered to turn on his phone, and thankfully he had service. He immediately called Jennifer.

Not thinking about the inconvenience, but only the urgency, he called at three in the morning Seattle time. Jennifer, recognizing the number, with hesitation, answered with concern in her voice, "Hello."

"Hey, Nef… are you okay?"

"Of course, why do you ask?"

"Nef… were you really thinking about coming to Thailand to work? You know that Mack is a jerk."

There was a long pause. "Why would you say that? Did they tell you I was coming?"

"Yes. Mack did."

"Uh, well," she stumbled in her heavy-eyed thoughts. "I only agreed for a year or two. The money was so good that I could return and finish art school without working… I can handle myself around people like Mack."

"Nef, I'm sure you can. But, I know that Thomas and Mack have lied to you. I've never felt uncomfortable working around you. That's bullshit. Mack is a piranha…don't trust him!"

"Why would they lie to me?"

"Nef, Mack and his cronies just beat me almost to death, and I'm trying to find my way back to Seattle on my own. They're up to no good here."

Another long pause followed, then she asked in a bewildered tone. "What are you talking about? Are you okay?"

"No, I'm hurt pretty bad. I think he seriously considered killing me out here." He answered through the static of a tattered connection.

"Is this some type of joke? They really *beat* you?"

"No, Nef, it is no joke. Yes, they beat me. I'm telling you, don't trust the man." Then the phone connection was lost.

It took Curtis another three days to find his way to Bangkok by a bumpy national bus and then secure a flight back to the US. This time, he had a direct flight landing in Los Angles. The only seat available was for first class at $8,000. He would welcome the extra comfort, but he still cringed when they put the payment on his credit card. He had to wait another twelve hours to get a flight back to Seattle. He had no clue what was about to happen next.

CHAPTER EIGHTEEN: RECOVERY

Curtis was sitting in LAX, contemplating his next move. A menagerie of thoughts and feelings had consumed him since he lay awake in pain that first night after the altercation. Anger, fear, relief, disbelief, optimism, urgency... and hate. He methodically considered each step going forward. Everything had changed. His immediate concerns were to separate himself from Neurogenics, find a way to protect Jennifer, reconcile with Becky, and check on his mother. The hopes of moving his program to Mayo Clinic in Rochester, Minnesota seemed quite hopeful but hinged on several legal factors about patents. In their previous talks, just prior to his departure to Asia, it seemed that his original dreams could be fulfilled there. But many questions remained. How would Thomas take his leaving? How would Thomas respond to the assault by Mack's cronies? Would he fight over his patents? Was Thomas involved with Mack's so-called "Coreplant" program? Should Curtis make any more attempts to sabotage the program before he left? Should he go forward to the media, if not Interpol or other organizations, about what was happening in the Similan Islands? There were so many things to think about and so many things to do. He was bone-weary, and to start a big and nasty legal attack seemed daunting.

However, at that moment he was sitting in Terminal Six at LAX and had nothing to do. There was no action he could take in that moment to help resolve any of his problems. He had left his clothes, his laptop, and all his reading material in Thailand. He purchased a new charger for his phone from a vending machine in the Tom Bradley Terminal.

He was also worried about his groin. The swelling was slowly going down, but not fast enough. The pain was still severe while walking or twisting. He could even sit on a toilet without having to bite into his arm to keep from screaming. He was sure that he also had fractured ribs. He realized that his left eardrum was ruptured because his hearing was diminished in that ear, and he had only experienced air-pressure equalization in his right during his flights' ascents and descents.

He hit the power button to his phone and allowed it to boot up, now that the battery was eighty percent charged. He could at least start to check emails. His inbox was, oddly, silent from Neurogenics. On a normal day, he would have twenty emails from the company server.

He called Jennifer again. She reassured him that she was backing out of the contract with Mack. But she wanted to know more. Curtis kept saying to her, "We'll talk about it when I'm back."

Curtis decided to call Bryan.

"Hey, boss. How's it going?"

"Bryan, listen. I'm at LAX heading home and will be in Seattle tonight."

"Oh… I thought you were in Thailand for another month or so."

"Well, that was the original plan. But Mack and I have had a falling out, you might say. He's creating some crazy programs for head and face transplants that I don't agree with. Then I found out he's bringing prostitutes, possibly child prostitutes, to the island and all this led to a nasty confrontation and… I guess, to be blunt, he had some men beat the hell out of me."

"What! Mack had someone intentionally beat you? Head transplants? Prostitutes? Wait a minute! What are you talking about?"

"I'll explain more when I see you. Yeah, I got the hell beat out of me. I mean, in a way I started it by choking him, but then he escalated it a level. Anyway, I'm hurt. I know the last time I came in wounded you helped me out. Right now, I'm sure I have a ruptured eardrum, but I doubt if we can do anything about that. I also have some broken ribs, but again, there's not much to do about that. But I am a bit worried that I have a smashed testicle and may need to see a urologist. As my best friend, and someone whose medical judgement I trust, I would be most grateful if you could check me out or help me make an appointment with someone who could. Your general medicine training was more recent than mine."

There was a long pause on the other end, then Bryan spoke, "I would be happy to do anything for you. However, my expertise is in the neurosurgery operating room. I will find someone really good who can look at you." There was another pause, and then Bryan spoke again with anger in his voice and began to ask questions like a rapid-fire machine gun, "So that cocksucker did this to you? I hate that man. He's a big pile of narcissistic bullshit. Head transplants? Are you freakin serious! Was Thomas a part of this? Are you going to the police?"

"Settle down for a minute. Right now, I just need to get home. Don't worry about the particulars. We can talk more about this in Seattle."

"Surely, you're going to the police," Bryan said.

Curtis responded, "Mack is living in his own micro-kingdom, so I don't think there's much we can do about him from the states. I don't know how much Thomas knows about all of this. Has he said anything to you?"

"Nothing," answered Bryan.

"It's odd that, since our big fight, my e-mails from Neurogenics have gone silent, like someone pulled the plug on my account. But know this, Bryan. If I set up a deal to move to Mayo, I will make sure I bring you with me. Would you be okay living in Rochester, Minnesota?"

There was a silence on the other end of the phone. "Bryan?"

"I'm just thinking about how I would like to march up to Thomas's office and punch that dickhead in the face."

"Mayo?" Curtis asked again.

"Oh." His mind tried to refocus on Curtis's question. "I would consider it an honor to keep working with you and see your original dreams fulfilled. Minnesota, so I hear, is cold."

Curtis was sensing more to his hesitation and added, "I'll bring Jennifer, too, if she will come."

"What's that got to do with me?" Bryan asked with a sense of detachment.

"Bryan, I honestly think you have a shot with the girl. I know she had this idol thing with me, but she'll get over that."

"You really think so?"

"Absolutely!" Curtis implied that he knew something, or Jennifer had said something that supported his great confidence. But he based his intuition on the notion that he would, hopefully, be restoring his relationship with Becky, and that would put an end to Jennifer's infatuation with himself. He continued, "One more thing, Bryan."

"Yeah?"

"Stop calling me 'boss.' Just call me Curtis… okay?"

"Sure thing, uh, Curtis."

Curtis called Becky next. She didn't answer, so he sent her a text: "I'm coming home early and will be arriving at SeaTac at seven in the evening on a Delta flight, DL 2596, from LA. Text me when you want to get together."

Curtis was prepared to take a taxi home to Ballard. When he turned his phone back on, after arriving at the gate in Seattle, he got Becky's text: "I don't know if you have baggage, but I will meet you at baggage claim number four, the one for your plane." He felt such a relief, almost like the old times between them were beginning to turn back into reality.

Curtis came down the escalator into baggage claim, leaning on his improvised cane. Below, next to the limo drivers holding up electronic signs with names like "Mr. Kulongoski" lit up on them, stood Becky, Bryan, Jennifer, and the entire New York Sharks with balloons and a big welcome sign. His eyes became teary, and he came around hugging each one, limping as he walked.

Someone pointed at his cane and asked, "What's that?"

"A cricket bat… I think," answered Curtis. "Who knows, maybe it is a paddle, like the one a nun would use to beat a disruptive kid."

It flashed through his mind that maybe Bryan or Jennifer had spread the word about him getting beat up and his tongue and cheek comment about the bat was being taken too seriously. What concerned him the most was, if he left Neurogenics, what would happen to these wonderful people? Would they keep working for Thomas? What if Thomas continued to have a business relationship with Mack? If they knew that Mack had been such a jerk, and Thomas and Mack were still partners, Curtis was afraid that they would all resign. What would then happen to the program and all the patients who had hope for the first time? But those thoughts quickly left his mind as he focused on the people in front of him.

Over the subsequent months, Curtis was a busy man. He planned a trip to Rochester to meet with the neurosurgery team and then one to visit his mother. But then he had to reschedule those trips when his testicular pain persisted and worsened. An ultrasound revealed that his right testicle was dying. In surgery, they found that the major artery to the organ had been severed and the tissue was necrosing. It wasn't savable and had to be removed. The surgeon said he had rarely seen such a severe blunt trauma before, and the consequences could mean that Curtis was now sterile. A sperm count in six months would be helpful. It was upsetting news to him, as it had always been his dream to be a father… the great father that he never had. He foresaw a time, as soon as things settled down in Rochester, when they could start a family. He longed to have a little boy and to hold that boy on his lap and to reassure him daily that he loved him to pieces. But a little girl would steal his heart even more. Part of him felt a rage toward Mack. But having a total disdain for the man, it was hard to add any more repugnance than he already carried.

His meeting with Mayo went very well. They were excited for the potential of working with him. Curtis was concerned about potential jealously between the other surgeons because they were spending millions of dollars on him. But, to his pleasant surprise, they all welcomed him to the team with open arms.

All didn't go as smoothly as he had hoped, however. Curtis had one
setback when he met with the legal team at the end of the week. As
he feared, the Mayo lawyers were concerned about the patents,
which Curtis had turned over, first to Apple Health and then to
Neurogenics. Neurogenics had entangled the patents with Mack's
corporation. If Neurogenics wouldn't be willing to share those
patents with Mayo, the result would—in an ironic twist—be that
Curtis wouldn't be allowed to perform the Erika Procedure ever
again. It wasn't as if he couldn't do the same precise surgical
technique of cutting and arranging nerves, skin, and bones. It
became illegal to patent a purely surgical procedure in the United
States in 1996. However, the supplies, tools, and certainly the
pharmaceuticals (such as their neuro-growth factor solution), were
patentable. He would therefore be forbidden from using the axillary
supplies or the bridge matrix. Those carried the bulk of the patents,
and without those the surgery could not succeed. One of the
lawyers remarked that Curtis should have known better a decade
ago not to relinquish his patents. Yet, Curtis pointed out that Mayo
would require the same surrender of all rights to the procedure.
They concluded that if Neurogenics put up a fight to avoid sharing
the rights with Curtis, it would be a real problem. Curtis would have
to create a different approach and a new kind of growth factor
solution. That wouldn't be so difficult, as Curtis had already seen
ways to improve the procedure, including the neuro-growth factor
solution. However, to have FDA approval for the new procedure,
including improvements in the solutions, he would have to endure
years of IRBs, clinical trials, and published papers. Mayo's only hope

of ever getting insurance reimbursement, thus opening the door for those without unlimited personal resources, was having FDA approval. It was a labyrinth of logic. While the FDA's involvement was the national safeguard against dangerous or ineffective treatments, it stood in the way of offering effective treatments to those most in need.

At the end of the legal meeting, the chief lawyer looked at Curtis and asked, "How's your personal relationship with Thomas? If he's a good friend, I think he'd be willing to come to an agreement. If you share the same vision of seeing as many people as possible find a cure, I think he would be cooperative and share the patents with you. Don't you?" To which Curtis shrugged his shoulders.

Curtis dithered in his verbal response. Then he answered, "Well, historically, Thomas and I have been close. However, since I announced I was leaving Neurogenics, our relationship has been awkward at best. I honestly don't think I've spoken to the man, even by phone, in weeks."

The lawyer smiled. "Well, you need to play the role of a diplomat and start to thaw your relationship with him. If he wants to put up a legal fight, then Mayo would have to reconsider their offer. If he demands a royalty payment every time we do the procedure, or if we must buy all your supplies from him, at an inflated price, that, too, would make this acquisition much more difficult." The lawyer thought for a moment, observing the sour, contemplative look on Curtis's face, and added, "But surely the man will be thinking of all

414

the people we can help and that the number who need help are so many that we wouldn't hurt the business of Neurogenics."

That night, in the hotel, Curtis awoke at 2:35 A.M. in a cold sweat. He felt the delicate task of getting the patents resting heavily upon his shoulders. He also had haunting thoughts of Ko Pendle. Were the Bangkok girls still coming? Who would protect them? Was the Coreplant program continuing? If anything, Curtis's opposition to the program was congealing. While Mack and his team were clearly motivated by money, they were justifying their plan on rational terms. Some would argue that there was a rational merit, a real hope for the failing human body. But the step from healing SCIs to Coreplant was a leap across a giant chasm, from which there was no return. Pandora's Box had not been fully opened... yet. A handful of cases does not constitute a trend. It is when it, like face transplants, becomes normal that the box becomes unshuttable.

There, in his humble room in the Khaler Grand, Curtis made a commitment to himself that he would not leave Neurogenics without his patents and without making sure the Coreplant program had been terminated and the girls were safe.

From Minnesota, Curtis flew to Tennessee to visit his mother. Becky few directly from Seattle, and they met at the Nashville International Airport, rented an Impala, and drove across state. In the car, the conversation started cordially. Curtis was genuinely interested in what was happening in Becky's life since they had been

415

apart. Eventually, he came to the point of asking her to move back in with him and join him in the effort of restoring their marriage. Still Becky was hesitant, but it was more of a habitual hesitancy.

She looked out her window, studying the rock cuts of the freeway through the clearly defined layers of taupe sedimentary shales. It reminded her of sitting in her Grandma's kitchen on Long Island, as a little girl, watching her making apple butter stack cake. Then she was thinking about the layers of years of her life, one put down on top of the other over a circle of seasons. She focused on the layers since she met Curtis. She felt bad about how she had been treating him. Through the rains of winter and the sun of summers, she had walked alone, first by Curtis's neglect, and later by her own will. She honestly wanted to break that cycle. Her musing was scattered when Curtis looked at her and asked, "What are you thinking about?"

She unveiled her entire daydream and then added, "I was reflecting on something Dr. McKenzie said. He kept saying to me that I have to start visualizing myself as worthy of your love."

"I think I like this Dr. McKenzie. Of course, you're worthy," responded Curtis. Becky continued staring at the layered bedrock beside the highway, putting her forehead against the glass of the passenger's door. Curtis's words seeming to fall on an impenetrable heart. But she did want to believe them.

Curtis pulled the car over on a Cumberland Mountain overlook. They got out and walked up to the stacked-stone safety wall that separated the parking lot from the top of a cliff. Curtis sat down on the wall then spun around to dangle his legs over the void. He looked down at the ground, several hundred feet below, while Becky was enjoying the view of the landscape in the distance. She said softly, "Be careful, Curtis. I don't like heights."

"Becky," he said looking down at the tops of the trees below, "do you remember your first day in the lab… back in New York?"

"Of course, I do," came her immediate response.

He turned and looked far over his right shoulder and directly at her, "Well, the first time I saw you… I immediately fell in love with you and have been hopelessly in love with you ever since. It may not be rational, to fall so quickly and hard, but it just happened." He waited for a response, but only silence filled the temperate air between them.

Curtis turned back around to face the void below and continued to speak, but now with his back to her, "I don't know what to do to fix this, Becky. Will you please help me make this good again? Please?"

She sat down on the wall beside Curtis but facing the opposite direction away from the abyss and toward the car. Still engulfed in quietude, there was only the wind of that high place.

Curtis asked, while still looking down, over the valley, "How many times do I need to say I'm sorry, Becky? One hundred? A thousand? A million? I *will* say it a million times if that's what it takes… seriously. I could start now. I'm sorry, number one. I'm sorry, number two. I'm sorry, number three. I'm sorry…"

"Stop it!" she finally said shaking her head back and forth rapidly. "The problem isn't your lack of sorrow. It is something within me," pointing at her chest, "that *I* must overcome."

"Why does this have to be so complicated?" he asked with some harshness in his voice. She didn't answer him.

Becky stood and walked away from Curtis, down the stone wall toward where the sun was now in control of the western sky. She turned and looked again out over the inspiring vista. He stood up from the wall and walked on the top of it, with his arms stuck out like a tight rope walker, toward her and then put his arms around her, resting his chin on the top of her head. She reached up and grasped his left hand in front of her and held on to it, in a rare show of affection. She turned around and looked up at him. Tears were streaming down her face. "Yes, Curtis, I do love you, but I don't know what to do about it. You deserve better than me." They just stared at each other, with her looking up at him at a steep angle. She added, "And would you get off that stupid wall, so I can talk to you face to face?"

He jumped down, and they stood eye to eye, his arms over her shoulders, his fingers interlaced behind her head. Becky, now looking down at the ground, broke free of his arms and walked a couple of steps away. She looked over the vista again. She continued, without eye contact, "When we first moved to Seattle, I stopped feeling anything. I had anesthesia of the soul. I drank a lot of wine. I drank alone. It was through my alcoholism that I eventually found help." She turned and looked directly at him. "But it hasn't been easy. Curtis, I'm messed up. It's not fair to you to have me this way. That's why I never came back. I wanted to come back when I was well and when I was a better person… and I'm still not. I can't bear to let you go and divorce you, but that would be the decent thing to do. So, you see, I'm stuck. I'm living in purgatory."

He walked up beside her and leaned into her. She looked into his eyes, which were now teary.

She spoke again, but in a softer voice, "When I was in Catholic school, we learned that Saint Augustine had a lover. They even had a son together. But since he was from a far higher social status than the woman, they could never marry. As great as the saint was, he could not send her away because he loved her so much. Finally, she left him, even though she was deeply in love with him, too. In that act, Augustine said that she was much greater then he was because she had the courage to do the noble thing, something he could never have done."

"Becky, you're stuck with me." Curtis sniffed. "I want you just the way you are. I'm not above you." He shook his head, "God knows I'm not better. Please come home to me, just who you honestly are. We can fight to make this better, together. Come to Rochester with me; we can find excellent help for you there. I don't care if you were a cutter, anorexic, psychotic, or whatever… I'm dreadfully in love with you, and I can't help it. I can fix broken spines, but I would never be able to fix my broken heart if you left me. My love for you is immutable."

She laid her head on his shoulder. She looked up at him, and they shared a long and deep kiss. Both were shaking with the rhythm of the sobs coming from deep within each of their cores.

Curtis took Becky's chin with his fingers and turned her head to look at him. Then he spoke again, "The noble thing for you to do is to be by my side and soak up my love for you because it has no place else to go." She gave him a crooked smile of half-belief. Then he added, "I'm an expert in what is noble... remember, I won the Nobel Prize."

Becky chuckled and stepped back, wiping the tears off her face with her sleeve. She said softly, "Curtis Eisner, you are so corny. And cutter? Do you really think I would hurt myself like that?"

"No." Then, with a second thought, he said, "I don't know. My point is, whatever has happened, I can accept that." They both sat down on the wall, and Curtis pulled her around, throwing their legs over the lichened stones so they were both looking down on the treetops. She kept her eyes shut and let him hold her tight to help repose her acrophobia.

There they sat in silence, holding hands—feet dangling over the edge. Within that solitude, the soft autumn wind was rustling the dehydrated, yellow and orange maple leaves around them. A distant roar visited them up through the cracks of silence between the rustle. They both looked directly below them and saw—for the first time—a river flowing over the layered rocks 200 feet below. In its course, it made a sudden plunge over a small fall, where a thick layer of the sedimentary stone abruptly ended.

Curtis seemed to have something on his mind, Becky could sense it. She asked, "Okay, Curtis... what is it?"

He had a melancholic look. His eyes teared up again. "Becky, I've had my problems, too. I feel that I must tell you what I've done."

Becky seemed anxious and started to shake her head with a nervous anticipation of what was to come.

"Becky, look at me." She looked up, taking her eyes off the ribbon of silvery waters below.

"I'm very sorry, but I did something terrible while we were apart."

"Curtis, I'm not sure I want to hear about this."

"I must tell you, Becky. I'm very sorry, but while we were apart, I was unfaithful to you."

As soon as the word *unfaithful* came out of his mouth, Becky put the palms of her hands over her ears and shook her head hard, saying, "Shah, I don't want to hear this!"

Curtis pulled her hands down and held them in his. He was looking closely into her eyes from a distance of a few inches "Becky, I have to tell you and you have to listen! I'm seeking your forgiveness."

Becky responded with strain, "I'm going to pretend you never brought this up."

"But, Becky, I need your forgiveness… do you understand? You have to listen to my confession."

With tears running down her rosy cheeks again, Becky responded, "No, I don't. I don't have to hear any of it."

Curtis was speechless, and puzzlement filled his face.

She added, "Denial… maybe that's the coward's way of forgiveness."

Curtis decided to let it go, but his need for clemency was left unsatisfied.

It was over an hour later, while on I-40 just west of Knoxville, that Becky's suspended curiosity resurfaced. In the middle of a Jon Pardi song, playing softly on the pre-set radio of the Chevrolet, she asked in a lenient voice, "Was it Jennifer?"

It crossed Curtis's mind that there were a variety of ways to honestly answer the question. But if denial was the path she was choosing, he decided to keep the answer succinct, "No… no it wasn't." The subject was never brought up again. He wanted to tell her how he had scurried about in the dirt like a piglet, scared out of his mind when Kimber was after him. That he, too, was a coward. But the story, like so many stories, had to remain untold.

The trip to Tennessee was productive in many ways. Curtis checked on his mother to make sure she was well-taken care of, and she was. Her memory wasn't that much worse, and she was getting around with a walker and, when she was tired, a wheelchair. She asked

Curtis to take her home. He reassured his mother that when he settled in Rochester, he would buy a big house and bring her home to live with him.

When Curtis and Becky returned to Seattle, she started the emotional process of moving back home again. On the work front, he knew that his only way out of the contractual imprisonment at Neurogenics was to make nice with Thomas. Yet, he also knew that Thomas—at least—had knowledge of what had happened in Thailand, even if he was not an active participant. But, through a conscious effort, he buried his ill-feelings as best as he could.

Curtis started a process of meeting weekly with Thomas and the Neurogenics lawyers. They kept coming to the impasse where Thomas was refusing to relinquish or even share the patents. The lawyers did bring up the idea of allowing Curtis to do the procedure, however, Mayo Clinic would have to purchase the patented growth factor soup from Neurogenics at hefty price of $20,000 per case. Additionally, they would have to purchase all the equipment, such as the nanotube matrix printer and its accessories from Neurogenics. The Neurogenics lawyers kept trying to say that this was the reasonable compromise. Curtis remembered that the Mayo Clinic lawyers indicated a royalty arrangement or a restrictive purchase contract, such as the Neurogenics lawyers were asking for, would be a deal-breaker, so he rejected that. His perfect compromise was where both Neurogenics and Curtis, himself, would share the patents equally. Then Curtis would relinquish his share of the patent to Mayo Clinic. Then they could produce their own—endless supply—of the neuro growth soup as well as create their own printers and mapping devices, with the help of MIT. The discussions seemed to stall out before reaching that point.

One evening, Curtis and Thomas had a long talk over glasses of Persian-black-market, Shiraz wine, which he had just brought back from a trip in the Middle East, long with small cloth bags of salted, dried cherries and nuts. As they snacked, Curtis demanded to know the status of the young girls at Ko Pendle and the Coreplant program.

Thomas spoke with great confidence, "Curtis, I promised that I would take care of everything. I got in touch with a humanitarian group in Thailand that rescues street girls. They work with a group of 'untouchable' policemen, who can't be bribed. They did an inspection of Ko Pendle and threatened to evoke their visas if they were ever caught bringing prostitutes of any kind out there. Mack had no idea I was behind that raid. I can't promise that some of the physicians, or any of the staff, don't visit them in Bangkok during their personal time. But we don't need to worry about Mack being behind such deeds."

"What about Coreplant? Is that still operational?" asked Curtis.

"It's over. All of it. I do have leverage over Mack. Our contract says that all I must do is offer him a repayment of his investment, plus interest, and he has to revert control of Neurogenics back to me. I have almost enough money to do that. I told him that if he didn't want me to buy him out, he had to shut down the program. So, he

424

did. He even bought out Dr. Takahashi's contract and he has returned to Osaka. So, there's no more Coreplant or any type of transplant program. Everything is focused on bringing Erika to the world." Curtis tried hard to believe him.

In the meantime, Curtis kept doing the procedure for the cash-paying patients coming to Neurogenics. He also kept pressing ahead to refine the procedure and to increase the quality control. He was preparing Clayton Emerson to step in as the permanent chief of neurosurgery services at the company. He had, intentionally, left Clayton out of the loop as far as the mischief going on in the Thai operation. Dr. Emerson knew that Curtis had been beat up in Thailand, but he had no idea that it was by the hands of the Neurogenics' main investor. He assumed it was by a gang of backstreet thugs and robbers in Bangkok.

Curtis's intention was that Clayton could just focus on helping patients on their Seattle campus. He was planning on debriefing Clayton, to some degree, just prior to his departure to Mayo Clinic. It was for Clayton's own safety. However, Curtis wanted to be careful as to avoid Clayton becoming so disillusioned that he would leave the company too. If Clayton left, simultaneously with Curtis's leaving, there was a chance that the whole Seattle treatment center would collapse.

Back on the personal front, Becky finally moved back into the condo in Ballard, but she wanted to have her space, so she slept in the guest room. Curtis didn't understand her motives but was willing to move at her pace.

Curtis made it clear to Jennifer that he and Becky were getting back together. He also made it clear to her that he deeply valued her and wanted her to be part of his team in Rochester. She wasn't sure she would make the move. She was considering going back to art school to escape the crazy world of the business of modern medicine. Bryan had agreed to join him in the move, and everything hinged on the patent agreement. Despite the hurdles, at last Curtis had some real optimism that everything was going to work out great in the end. However, Dr. Eisner's optimism was proven to transient.

CHAPTER NINETEEN: RECONCILIATION

It only took a few months before the discouragement began to seep into the edges of Dr. Eisner's soul once again. On one hand, the Mayo Clinic's offer still stood and was supported with great enthusiasm in their neurosurgery department. However, the stalemate between him and Thomas over patent rights seemed to be going nowhere. They eventually stopped talking altogether. Curtis refocused on the daily cases and building his relationship with Becky, allowing Mayo Clinic and Minnesota to slowly drift away from this cognizant mind.

Then, one morning, Curtis had a call from Thomas. Spontaneous calls, unlike the early days at Neurogenics, had become a rarity from the man. "Hey, Curtis, come up to my office this afternoon. I think there's a way we can break this logjam."

Curtis's mind was too focused on the two cases he had on his schedule that day to give the request much thought. At the end of the day, he and Bryan were rounding on their post-op patients. Bryan asked him if he wanted to go out for a beer, and only at that point did he remember Thomas's request.

"I would love to, but Thomas wanted to see me." Curtis looked at the time: 6:30 in the evening. "I doubt if he's still here, but if he is, I should see what he wants before I commit to a beer."

Curtis called Thomas's phone, and to his surprise, he was still in his office. He directed Curtis, "Come on up."

Curtis knocked on his door, and Thomas motioned for him to come in. It was a bit reminiscent of the early days when they would sit in his office after hours and dream together. In some ways, their dreams came true… in some ways, not at all.

"Can I get you a drink?" asked Thomas.

"I'm craving a tea… a cup of old-fashioned English black tea."

Thomas walked over to his bar, put a tea kettle on the burner, and turned it on. While the water was heating, he poured himself a rum and Coke. He looked over at Curtis and asked, "When's the last time you had contact with Mack?"

Then he turned his back toward Curtis, as he poured the hot water over a teabag in a cup at the bar and waited for the answer. The steam rose from the cup like Old Faithful's overture.

Curtis felt a cold chill rise up his spine. He rubbed his face and asked, "Why do you ask?"

Thomas turned and walked toward him with a drink in each hand, "So, when was it?"

"Well, it was just before I left Thailand about fourteen months ago, you know, when he tried to have me killed. Why do you ask?"

Thomas took a seat across the coffee table from Curtis. He sat their drinks down and leaned back in a relaxed state, crossing his legs. "Curtis, as I've said before, I'm deeply sorry about what happened in Ko Pendle." He paused to sip his rum and Coke, and continued, "I will first ask, is there any chance that you'll change your mind and stay with Neurogenics? I mean, you have all your wishes. The Coreplant Program is history. What would it take to keep you? More money?"

Curtis asked him, "How long is your contract with Mack good for? You said you were about ready to buy him out."

"Well, Mack gave us a lot of money to get on our feet. Our contract is good for five years. He's paying me a good royalty on the Erika patents in Thailand, which is a sustaining amount for us. His team there is bringing Erika to Asia and the Middle East." Thomas sipped his drink again. "I know the man can be a little rough around the edges, but he means well, and his surgeons are doing good work."

Curtis let out a sigh, while shaking his head, "No, he's a greedy, narcissistic pig! There's nothing he does that is *well* intended. He considered having me killed, and that's more than a little *rough around the edges*. He only wants what's good for him, and he's a very dangerous man."

"It does no good to sensationalize things, Curtis. Remember, you assaulted him first. He does have the right to defend himself."

429

The two men sat in silence for a moment, and then Thomas spoke again, "I think you'd find Mack to be a changed man now." He looked Curtis directly in the eyes and leaned in his direction. "I don't know if you know it, but Mack's dying."

Curtis looked stunned as a hush settled over his demeanor. He finally spoke, "Dying? What are you talking about?"

Thomas leaned back again on his couch. "He has cirrhosis. He stopped by here a few weeks ago, on his way home from the National Institute of Health. They probably have the best liver program in the world, but they couldn't help him."

"I'm surprised he isn't looking for a handsome twenty-year-old man to transplant his brain into. That was his dream."

"Well, like I said, he shut the Coreplant program down. He did so willingly, because it wasn't going as smoothly as they had hoped. I'm no physician so I can't understand what it was, but there were complications during the recovery process. So, it wasn't a viable program from the start. Now, Mack is facing the same mortality as a penniless bum."

"So, what has this got to do with me?" asked Curtis.

"Curtis, Mack feels horrible about what happened to you. He has somewhat, literally, come to Jesus as he's faced death. He wants to make amends for all the wrongs he's done."

"So, you're saying that he's apologizing and wants me to forgive him?" asked Curtis.

"Something like that. He has asked me many times how you're doing and if you still hold a grudge. But I think he wants to tell you himself. I have grown to like the man. I have nothing but pity for him now. I think he's harmless as a Teddy bear. It would mean a lot to me if you'd speak to him."

Curtis rubbed his face and sat back in the chair, "I don't know, Thomas. That's asking a lot of me. I mean, the man considered killing me. He may have ruined my chance to become a father. Only time will tell." Curtis shook his head and then looked up at Thomas, "Is he coming by Seattle any time soon?"

"As far as I know, he isn't travelling anymore. But he could be here by teleconference in a minute." Thomas looked at his watch "It's now nine in the morning out there, and I think he's available."

The thought that ran through Curtis's head was that he wanted to keep warming up to Thomas until he got his patent agreement. He hated the idea of talking to Mack as part of that warming up process… but if he had to, he would rather do it now and get it over with. "Okay, get him on the screen, and I'll talk to him."

It took only a few minutes for Thomas to call Mack and to get him set up on his desktop computer. Curtis stayed to the side as Thomas spoke to the man. Then he announced, "Hey, Mack, I'm going to switch you to the wall screen so that you can speak to someone here in my office."

Thomas clicked on a couple of buttons and then the large wall screen flickered. There was Mack's face, looking swollen, jaundiced, and older than Curtis remembered. He appeared to be sitting on a deck chair. On the small, round table beside him, sat a glass with amber liquid. Mack spoke first, "Well, I can't believe it; it is our golden goose boy."

"Hello, Mack," said Curtis in a business-like monotone.

"How are you, son? I hope my boys weren't too rough on you."

Curtis didn't know what to say so he just sat in silence trying to mollify the anger within. Mack spoke again, "Remember, son, it was you who tried to kill me first." Then he gave his trademark belly laugh, followed by a series of wet coughs.

Curtis said in a self-restrained tone, "No, I wasn't trying to kill you. I was just angry. If I had wanted to kill you, Mack, I would have." Curtis's tough words even surprised himself.

"Really?" Mack chuckled. "It doesn't matter anyway, son. It looks like Jack is killing me now." He lifted his glass, "Here's a toast to Mr. Daniels." He sipped and then smiled. "As Thomas, here, may have told you, I'm not sure how much time I have left on this earth, so I'm going back and making peace with all the people I've hurt. So, I'll ask frankly, will you forgive me?"

Curtis questioned Mack's probity, but had to respond to the request. Could he forgive the man? Wasn't he the madman who

432

wanted to create monsters? But once again, his mind stumbled across the fact that the only way out of Neurogenics was through the patent offer. The way to the patent offer might be through a token offer of forgiveness. Now, if anything, Big Mack looked more pitiful than big.

"Okay, Mack, I'll forgive you."

"Thank you, son. I do appreciate that." There was an awkward pause. Mack filled the conversational vacuum by adding, "You may not know it, but you have been my hero since I first read about you in *People Magazine* about ten years ago. I respect you more than about any other person on this earth. Therefore, your forgiveness means a lot to me." The two men stared at each other through their monitors, each wearing bewildering looks on their faces like odd-fitting spectacles. Finally, Mack spoke again, "I want to show my appreciation by sending you a nice gift in the next few days."

The two men said their farewells and the connection was shut down. Thomas looked at Curtis and said, "Thanks. That'll mean a lot to Mack, and I'm also grateful."

Curtis had almost forgotten about Mack's offer of a gift until the following week when Thomas summoned him back to his office again. After taking a seat, Thomas reminded Curtis that Mack had been working on a six-star private spa on another Similan Island, now called the Wellness Oasis. He had started it before he ever broke ground on Ko Pendle's medical complex. Now the resort was near completion. Mack's gift was for Curtis to have twelve weeks of pampering at the spa, all expenses paid. Mack had remembered that Curtis said he was dreaming of a day that he could take a few months off to rest. This would be the sabbatical that Curtis had longed for. Thomas said that he and the lawyers were drawing up an agreement to share the patents. He added that going on this long rest would give Curtis a chance to renew himself and to leave Neurogenics on good terms.

"Really? You are really going to give me my patents back?"

Thomas said, as the ends of his mouth turned up in more of a smirk than a smile, "That's what I said isn't it?"

"And, you're really asking me to go back to Thailand after what happened the last time I was there? Are you insane?"

Thomas responded with a look of surprise on his face, "Curtis, this spa has nothing to do with the medical facility. It's on a different island. You won't have to see Mack on this trip if you don't want to." He gave Curtis a disappointed look and then added, "He really has had a change of perspective. It's like Paul on the road to Damascus. He has become a very compassionate man. We both know how you've worked your ass off for ten years. The only vacation I've ever seen you take is when you went to care for your mom... and we know that wasn't easy. Give Mack a chance to make up for the way he's treated you by accepting this gift."

Curtis got up and walked to the window with a feeling of bewilderment. He looked down on Seattle and studied the people

434

and the streets. Without looking back at Thomas, he said almost in a whisper, "Have you ever noticed that Seattle is not on a true grid? The blocks are rhomboids, not squares or rectangles."

Thomas seemed a little frustrated by this tangential distraction. "Yes, Curtis. You told me that before. What does that have to do with anything? It won't affect our property value if that's what concerns you."

"The rhomboids correspond to a much bigger reference point--the whole universe."

"So?"

"Maybe, we, too, must have some outside reference point to make sense of who we are." Thomas was so confused by those words that he decided to ignore them.

Curtis looked back at Thomas, "I just can't imagine ever being back in Thailand... for any reason. What if I pass on this gift?"

Thomas had a deep scowl on his face. "Curtis, it would tell me that you're still bitter, and I'm wouldn't want to part ways with hard feelings between us. I would view your willingness to accept this gift as your way of forgiving Mack... and me."

"You? Is there something I need to forgive you for?" Until that point, Thomas had not admitted personal guilt about anything. Thomas didn't answer, so Curtis continued, "So, if I don't go, the patent deal's off? Is that what you're saying?"

"Curtis, you were just talking about big principles of life or something like that. Well, I have principles, too. I won't dissolve this business relationship on bad terms. This trip will be our peace treaty. Then you'll come back all rested, and we'll have the patent papers in order. And then you can sign them, and we can go our separate ways."

"So, a spa you say?" Curtis asked as he turned away from the window. His instincts were giving him warning signs. Could he trust Mack again? Not fully.

Thomas added with some enthusiasm in his voice, "Curtis, the place is beautiful. I went out there about six months ago. Raymond has been there several times. I was pampered like a monarch. It was fantastic! You'll stay in a beautiful beachfront villa. You'll have a gourmet chef who will make very good tasting and nutritious meals three times a day. You'll have a personal trainer to get you back in shape. You'll have a personal psychologist and spiritual adviser. You can get daily massages, acupuncture, anything that you want. It will all be centered on you. This is the best sabbatical anyone could imagine, and it is time to take it. A month stay there for a paying customer would be over $50,000. It's a good and decent gift."

"Could I bring Becky?"

Thomas seemed to stagger in his focus for a minute and then responded, "Maybe. It's set up for single participants, so their

436

recovery won't have distractions. But I could ask Mack for an exception."

Curtis's reason for accepting this gift wouldn't be the allure of rest and pampering. If Thomas was being honest with him, and he wasn't sure he was, it could speed up the process of leaving Neurogenics. However, more importantly, it would give him one last opportunity to find out if Mack's evil diversions had been shut down or not. He wasn't sure how he could, safely, find out, but being on a nearby island he might have easier access to information. He had unfinished business in Thailand. At the same time, he had vowed to himself that he would never return. Curtis rubbed his face. The choices, to go or not to go, grappled deeply within his mind. He looked back up at Thomas, asking, "So, I won't be expected to visit Mack or have any contact with him?"

Thomas said with confidence, "None. Not unless you took the initiative. This I promise."

With hesitation in his voice, Curtis finally replied, "Okay. I'll accept his gift. When do I leave?"

Thomas had a big smile cover his face. He answered, "That's fantastic! You're doing the right thing." He cleared his throat and gathered his thoughts. "I want to give you three weeks to finish up all your loose ends here before you take off. I'll have our lawyers put together the details of the patent sharing agreement while you're gone. We will communicate directly with the Mayo Clinic lawyers, so we get everything right. We can sign it when you get back. Then you'll be a free man to go to Mayo or wherever you want."

When Curtis went home that night, Becky was there. It felt good to come home to her again. He told her of his plans to accept the gift. She was stunned when he told her his plans.

"Curtis," she said, with a tone of disappointment, "this was a big choice to move back in with you so that we could have time together, and now your work is taking you away again… and this time for three months? I'm feeling a bit of déjà vu." She paused for a minute. "I also can't believe you would go anywhere near Mack." She walked away into the kitchen and started working on dinner, shaking her head.

Curtis followed her and helped her make a salad. "Becky, I'm not going to start saying I'm sorry again… so I won't. I did ask Thomas if I could bring you and he's looking into it. But, we have three weeks together before I leave. I will cut my schedule back during this time. I see this trip as an important step toward closure. It'll speed up the whole process of getting out of Seattle and starting our new lives."

Becky didn't say much, but instead worked on separating frozen chicken pieces. She looked up at him, "There is no way I could take even two weeks off right now, and still finish my PhD before we leave Seattle." She paused to wash the chicken pieces off under warm water and looked back at him again. "I'm also worried about you. What if Mack tries to hurt you again?"

438

As they continued making dinner, Curtis shared the entire conversation that he had had with Thomas, including his reassurances. Then he confided in Becky, "I have another reason I'm going. I must make sure that Thomas is telling me the truth, that no one is being hurt at Ko Pendle, neither the girls as sex workers nor the patients as part of some grotesque procedure. I must see for myself that this is really over. Otherwise, this will haunt me for the rest of my life."

They enjoyed a good dinner out on their short deck, just off the kitchen, like the old days. Sitting across from one another— both heads turned toward the water—they ate silently. They looked out over the canal and watched the beautiful parade of boats coming and going. Becky allowed the topic to drop.

The next morning, Becky was up first. She was emptying the dishwasher when Curtis came out of the bedroom, dressed for work. She put her arms around him and laid her head on his shoulder. Then she looked at him. "Curtis, I've had time to think about this trip. I'm okay with it. I don't like it… but maybe it's best. I want you to do it for you. Get as much rest as you can and come back refreshed and ready to start our new lives." She kissed him and added, "But please be very careful. I don't trust Mack or Thomas." Curtis promised he would take caution. That ended the discussion.

Bryan was totally against the idea when Curtis told him the next morning as they were scrubbing in. "Are you crazy? Don't do it, Curtis!" He said in a stern whisper as people were coming and going through the pre-op area. "I don't trust that asshole," referring to Mack, "as far as I could throw the behemoth."

Curtis invited him to the Flatstick Pub after work, so they could discuss it more. He called Becky first and invited her to join them, however, she couldn't make it. She had to work on a research paper.

Sitting over two mugs of dark, artisan beers, Curtis looked at Bryan and said, "Hey, there's some things that I want to tell you… and I want you to keep this to yourself. These things pertain to why I want to go back to Thailand. I don't want Becky knowing about this or she will worry herself sick."

Bryan looked concerned and nodded, implying that Curtis had his trust.

Curtis continued, "Thomas has assured me that Mack is deeply sorry for having his men assault me." He rolled his eyes a bit, with a grin. "I'm not so sure I agree with him on that one. But he also assures me that Mack's experimentation with exchanging body parts and allowing sex workers onto the island have stopped. He says that they are only doing the Erika Procedure on SCI sufferers, wealthy SCI sufferers I must add. I can live with that. I can focus on those with less financial resources when I set up my program at Mayo." Curtis sipped his beer and cleared his throat. "Bryan, you know that I want to get to Mayo as soon as I can. My going back to Thailand to take this sabbatical, somehow, Thomas has tied to getting my patents. That is one reason I think I must go. But, the

440

most important reason is that I must, personally, investigate the medical facility and see what's happening there now."

Bryan frowned, tasted his beer, and said, "Curtis, they were bad to you, in more ways than just beating the hell out of you. You told me that Mack suggested that he could have had you killed. I see a lot of danger lurking in those islands. I'm not sure how you can investigate it and still stay safe."

"Bryan, I've put a lot of thought into this. I'll play along with the sabbatical thing. Who knows, I may even enjoy it a bit. But I'll be nosey and try to find out as much as I can. If my curiosity is not satisfied from the spa, I'll take an unannounced trip down to the medical center. To do this, I'll go up to Port Blair and rent my own taxi boat, so I'll have a way out. I'll also hire some bodyguards to go with me. I've been investigating this online and—do not breathe a word about this to anyone—I found that off-duty police officers and soldiers are often hired by celebrities and—who knows—maybe drug kingpins, to protect them while in Thailand. I would bring a couple armed bodyguards with me and pretend that I wanted to say my goodbyes to Mack. I'll visit the medical center and talk to the supporting staff. They were always truthful with me. They'll let me know if there are any girls or Coreplant patients on the island. I will make sure that things are well there, and then I can come home and live in peace."

Curtis finished his beer in one big gulp. He continued, "Would he really want to hurt me more, simply because I'm leaving Neurogenics? He has what he wanted. He has my Erika Procedure, my golden egg as he calls it. He has my reputation for his brand, which he wanted. My leaving won't threaten any of those things. I'm sure that the best patent agreement I can get with Thomas is a patent sharing arrangement. No, I don't trust the man, but what motive would he have for hurting me now?"

Oddly, Bryan stirred the foam of his beer with his finger as he thought. Looking up at Curtis, he added, "But I'm concerned that once you get to the spa, it could be a trap or something. Then you'd be stuck. You told me how Mack had cancelled your pick up after they assaulted you and you had to find your own way back. Mack is not a human… he's a pig."

"Yeah, I've thought about that too. I want to take a satellite phone with me, if I can find one small enough to hide. Then I can call you if I think I'm trapped. You must remember, too, that, due to my own lack of discipline, I did provoke the assault last time. I've always had a good reign over my emotions, but I've noticed that my fuse has gotten shorter over the past few years. This time, I won't let that happen."

Bryan was shaking his head, "No, I'm not buying it. That's no excuse for what they did to you."

"I agree, Bryan, that it doesn't excuse their response, but what I'm trying to say is that I will be more disciplined this time. If I spot trouble, I'm not going to fly off the handle and start choking someone. I will remain calm and get a hold of help. I promise."

442

Bryan responded by telling Curtis that his clear position was that going back to Thailand was a bad idea and he didn't support his decision. However, if he was going despite his protest, then he wanted Curtis to let him work on the technical part of his safety. If he couldn't persuade him not to go, he at least wanted to do his best to keep him safe.

Just before his departure to Thailand, and after he had wrapped up all his work at Neurogenics, Bryan stopped by the basement research office. He brought Curtis a bottle of his favorite microbrew. The basement office was still Curtis's preferred place to be, unless it was in the OR. He was hoping that being home with Becky would soon be his place of peace, once the awkwardness had passed.

Bryan sat on Curtis's old couch, and they reminisced for a while about the New York days as they sipped their beers. Then, again, he warned Curtis to be careful in Thailand. When they were done talking and saying their goodbyes, Bryan pulled out a wrapped gift from his backpack. He handed it to Curtis and remarked, "Here's a little travelling gift."

Curtis just looked at it.

"Open it. I have to show you how it works before I leave."

Curtis tore the paper off the small box and opened it. Inside was a small, burnt-orange, device that looked like a small cellphone with a short, stubby antenna. Bryan explained that it was a satellite-based, backcountry GPS and texting device. Bryan would be monitoring it on his laptop and would know exactly where Curtis was at all times. They could also send limited text messages through the satellite system. There was also a panic button on the device. If Curtis pressed it, a text would be sent directly to Bryan's phone and would include the GPS positioning of the person holding the device. Bryan then explained, "I would immediately be on my way with my posse." He instructed Curtis to send him a text on October sixth, five days after his arrival. Bryan said, "Just let me know it's okay there, and I can stop worrying about you. Then send me a short text once a week just to say you're okay."

"So...you have a posse, Bryan?" asked Curtis with a big grin on his face.

"Hey, man, don't forget that my older brother Dan played football at Yale. He was a linebacker. My younger brother, Allen, the runt, of the family, was a Navy Seal. And my little sister Chloe, well... she's the toughest one in the family. She has a black belt in in Kyokushinkai. From what I've told her, there's nothing else she would rather do than kick Mack Pendleton's misogynist— womanizing ass. Yeah, you can say I have a posse."

Curtis chuckled and thought Bryan was being a little melodramatic, but he took the device and put it in his duffle. "I think I can find a way to hide it." They hugged and said their goodbyes. Curtis felt good knowing that Bryan would be watching over all the clinical issues at Neurogenics in his absence, and over his own safety from a world away.

Curtis contacted the lawyers at Mayo and gave them an update that they had finally reached a patent-sharing agreement. The lawyers, of course, wanted to see it before Curtis signed anything. He assured them that they would. He explained that he was taking a vacation and wouldn't consider signing it until he was back in three months.

Curtis felt peace as he walked out of the Neurogenics building on the first day of October. It was unusually warm and sunny for Seattle this time of year. The snows in the mountains had barely started their gentle reversion back down toward the lowlands.

He felt satisfied that the previous four years weren't wasted years, as he had brought his techniques to perfection there. He tried to do the math but figured that he and the team had brought the ability to walk and move back to over a thousand individuals. That was still only scratching the surface of the more than two million people in the world who could benefit from their treatments. It was still Curtis's dream to have an anastomosis center in every major city in the world. He was hoping that Mayo Clinic would be a launching place for this dream. Curtis wanted nothing more than a full-throttle proliferation of the cure.

It was an uncommon practice for Curtis, but he made it his intention to focus on himself while on this trip, with his investigation into Mack's Medical Oasis on the back burner. After a decade of eighty-hour weeks, not to mention the daily grind of inexorable stress, he was ready to be pampered, even though it would be peculiar at first. It would take a gigantic effort to keep his mind off things back home, but he was ready to try. He did look forward to exercising, eating right, and getting back into shape.

Curtis felt a flash of déjà vu when he arrived at Suvarnabhumi Airport in Bangkok. But the familiarity also carried with it a slight ill feeling. He walked past the place where, fifteen months previously, he had lay on the floor in pain, waiting for his flight to get him out of the country. He felt his palms go sweaty, and his heart began to race. He had hoped he would never see this place again… but here he was… back where he promised himself he would never be. A feeling of regret and uncertainty rushed through his mind.

Rather than taking Mack's seaplane, which was an option, he took a local Thai airline to Port Blair. It was a small, wheeled prop that wrestled, powerfully, with the headwinds the whole way, leaving him a bit nauseated. Once on the ground, he ventured into a tea shop, where most of the seating was outside. After a cup of black pekoe, he asked the proprietor about security guards for hire. In his rustic English, the man reported that he had heard of them, but didn't know any. As Curtis was paying his bill, the man ran his hand through his cropped head of coal-black hair and said, with a hesitant voice, "Check at the tourist police department, they may know where to find one… you know, a bodyguard."

Curtis thought that was an odd place to find out about private security, who, he assumed, worked in the shadow world, a

446

world he wouldn't think the official police would condone. He knew that policemen worked as private bodyguards, per his research, but he assumed that you had to meet them in a bar or back alley. Maybe he had watched too many Humphrey Bogart movies. But to his surprise, the officer at the front desk, a Captain Atitarn (according to his name badge), said that he, himself, worked as a private bodyguard when he was off-duty. Curtis wrote down his name and phone number on the back of one of his own business cards. He later loaded the number into the directory of the satellite device. Captain assured him that he could come up with at least one more body guard, if Curtis was to need them.

From Port Blair, he took a private speed boat taxi service to the Pendleton Wellness Oasis Resort. At the dock, he met a young Thai man who checked him in. He was well-groomed, wearing tan pants, a white shirt, a forest-green blazer, and a polite smile. They rode together across the beautiful island on a narrow, paved road in a golf cart to Curtis's private beachfront house. The houses there had a more modern, rustic-industrial theme of concrete, corrugated steel, and glass. But it was beautiful and well-designed. Inside, the house was simple but comfortable. There was a basket on the table with flowers, a bottle of Curtis's favorite wine, and an assortment of Spanish tapas, which Mack knew was his favorite snack. At least there was no bottle of SangSom on the table. This indicated to Curtis that it was possible that Mack really was trying to be nice to him. A card was attached to the basket with a handwritten note,

"Let me know if there is anything you need. Your friend, Big Mack."

Curtis poured himself a glass of wine and went out on the deck overlooking the white sandy beach. The evening air was warm and damp. It smelled of the sea and a touch of spice, which, he now realized, was from the blooming Phalaenopsis flowers he saw in front of his house. He suspected it was their second blooming of the year as the autumn had been quite warm in Asia. He put back the teak, cushioned deck chair into a reclining position. He listened to the roar of the waves, evenly spaced about fifteen seconds apart. He allowed the jet lag to slowly draw close his eyes. Before drifting into a sweet somber, his mind fell prostrate into lenient thoughts of peace. He sensed that brighter days were heading his and Becky's way. This was nearing the end of an arduous chapter in their lives. He was sure she was back with him for good. His work in Seattle was done. There were no demands on him now, other than to find rest. He drifted into the transcendental kind of sleep that only good peace and a bit of jet lag can bring. But just before dozing, the haunting of concern came back to the forefront of his mind. He hoped all was well in the Andaman Sea, but he wasn't sure.

CHAPTER TWENTY: RENEWAL

Curtis awakened into a dopy world where the lines between thoughts and dreams had lost demarcation. A place where the senses from the external world and the impressions from the imagination merged. He could hear rhythmic sounds, but what were they? Jet engines outside his portal window? He opened his eyes, but at first it made no difference. With the sun now far over the horizon behind him, and the clouds blocking any celestial bodies, the darkness of the night was comprehensive.

He sat up. He felt dizzy, as he normally did after a long flight. He looked around and his eyes caught a few small lights far out on the sea. Another light was coming from a digital clock inside his house as a petite green glow. He couldn't tell the time from this distance. He pulled out his cellphone, which on this cell-tower-less island would only serve as a clock itself. He hit the power button, and the battery image with a red line at the bottom showed up. Then the whole phone, like a reflection of the night, went dark.

He stumbled to the glass slider, which he remembered having left open. He bumped into it, as now it was closed. He fiddled around with the edge until he felt a handle. He opened it and went inside and found a switch on the wall. The bright living room lights were blinding at first. The clock on the wall reported *3:16* a.m. in digital letters. He now felt awake, so awake that he knew that his long nap would last him for the day or at least until the afternoon.

On the stone kitchen island, beside the welcoming basket, he found a formal-looking notebook with the embossed lettering on the cover, "Dr. Curtis Eisner Renewal Program." He was surprised, not realizing that there was a pre-planned program to his relaxation. It seemed too efficient.

He opened the notebook and began to read. Fortunately, there was nothing on the schedule for the first two days, allowing him to adjust to the new time and sleep pattern. His first meeting was on the third day, and it was titled "Medical Examination and Goals Setting." Immediately after the physical exam and for each morning after that, he was scheduled to meet with a Dr. Ben Pearle for "Psychological and Spiritual Renewal." After each two-hour morning session with Dr. Pearle was a three-hour meeting at the gym with his personal trainer. Then he was scheduled to have a vegetarian lunch at the beach kitchen. In the afternoon, massages were scheduled and finally *Beach Therapy*. Curtis had no idea what Beach Therapy was, but it would eventually become his favorite part. Additionally, a chef was assigned to Curtis who prepared all his house meals, breakfast, and dinner.

The introduction letter described how each person's schedule was carefully tailored to meet his or her personal needs for renewal. The letter also explained that there would be other participants at the resort; however, to support an atmosphere of peace and quiet, the staff strongly discouraged guests from socializing or even speaking to one another. According to the information booklet, a vow of silence was a key part to the recovery. The island was also established as an electronic-free zone. There would be no phones, radios, TV, or any sound that did not directly come from nature. They were instructed to "listen to nature and its voice of peace."

Upon reading the schedule, Curtis had a feeling of optimism. Maybe this whole experience was, indeed, an altruistic gesture by Mack. This could be what his tired soul really needed. It would be a good closure to his years at Neurogenics. But was that just wishful thinking? He made a personal vow not to allow his suspicion to dwindle, even if things were going well.

On the morning of the third day, Curtis showed up at the assigned office for his physical exam. A kind Thai physician went over the details of his medical history. He did a careful physical exam, and then he drew blood to check on all his vital organs. He performed a treadmill test to look at his heart. Besides a modestly elevated cholesterol level and a missing right testicle, no other problems were discovered. From that station, he went to meet Dr. Pearle.

The psychologist was a short man, maybe five foot five, apparently of Chinese–American descent, who wore a perpetual soft smile and spoke kindly. His office was in a plush and comfortable suite overlooking the beach. He served Curtis a cup of tea and, after a brief period of small talk, dove into Curtis's personal history. He started to draw from the well of Curtis's memories, starting with his preschool years, working his way up through his life until the point his father left them. Curtis felt comfortable with the psychologist from the beginning, as if he had cast a spell of trust over him. It seemed to be a gift of the man's disposition. Within days, Curtis started to talk about things that he had never even shared with Becky or his mom. Things about feelings, dreams, and fears.

They ended the third session with Curtis explaining that he had hated his father for decades… until he found out that he had left his mom for another man. Then he felt more compassion for the man, and he wasn't sure why. Maybe it was because he realized that the marriage to his mom was a sham from the beginning. He married his mother because of the imposed social mores of the 1960s and 1970s. His father had finally tried to find his true self. This made Curtis less angry than imagining a father who dumped his mother because she was getting older, less attractive, and he wanted a new, younger chick. He always felt some guilt that, if he hadn't come along, his father would have stayed with his mom. Now he understood that he had nothing to do with his leaving.

He shared with Dr. Pearle that this preconceived notion of his father chasing skirts in his office was one of the reasons he despised Mack. From the beginning, he saw Mack as an arrogant womanizer. He had thought his dad was the same… but not now.

From the "mental gym," as Curtis thought of it, he went to the "physical gym." There he had a Thai trainer who went by the name Bono (like the singer). His real name was long and something like Bojing Honghuig Chen, but he gave the Western people the permission to just use "Bono." He was tough on Curtis, wanting to get his BMI down from twenty-seven to nineteen, and he wanted to do it quickly.

Bono worked Curtis hard with weights, aerobics, followed by more weights. The three-hour sessions ended with an exhausting three-mile run on the treadmill. Their goal was to increase that to seven miles by the end of his stay. But Curtis liked the exercise. He had been a casual runner in college, but then the long sixteen-hour work days had stolen that time from exercise. He just didn't like running on a treadmill and asked if he could do his run on the inviting beach, but oddly Bono said no. The reason he gave was that, throughout the day, other guests were having their beach time, and running along the beach could distract them.

Beach therapy for Curtis was a time that he was simply lying on a beach chaise and drifting in and out of sleep, between moments of meditation, while listening to the natural sounds, which only a beach could offer. The rhythmic waves, squawking of the gulls, and the whispering of the wind, were all there was to hear. Day by day, the thoughts of work, troubles, and past mistakes (such as the night at Sandra's cabin and his chronic neglect of his relationship with Becky) started to fade from his mind, and more of a nothingness started taking their place. He did feel the stress draining from him day after day, like the nasty water out of a vagrant's bathtub, circling and disappearing down the drain.

The beach therapy time always began with a deep massage from a muted Thai man or woman. They never said a word to him but used hand motions to tell him what to do. He was never sure if they just couldn't speak English or if it was part of the quiet tranquility that the place tried to maintain.

The chef served tasty but extremely low-calorie meals three times a day with no in-between snacks. Curtis did become hungry and stayed in that state for his entire stay on the resort. But he did lose weight rapidly, and that he liked.

Curtis was making progress on many fronts. He felt more at peace than any other time he could remember… at least in recent years. With no TV, Internet, or phone service, he felt completely cut off from the outside world… which seemed like a good thing. He did have Bryan's device, which he had hidden in between the mattress and box springs the night he arrived. He had only taken it out on October sixth to send his text to Bryan: "All is well. Looks and feels like a resort. No sign of Joppa."

His most recognizable progress was what came out of the gym. He lost five pounds of fat in the first week at the resort. By a few weeks later, he would start to see biceps on his arms like he had never seen before. He was feeling better about his physical self.

The isolation wasn't bothering him the way he thought it would when he first read the introduction notebook. Part of the isolation was broken up by the long morning sessions with the psychologist, where he shared the intimate details of his life as a cathartic exercise. He talked more than he would have with a therapist back in Seattle, because his words were so pent up, with the code of silence for the other 23 hours of the day. Even Bono was a man of few words. After the first couple of mornings, the trainer gave Curtis a printed list of exercises to do and which order to do them in. He then sat at a table, watched, and took notes, or worked out himself.

There were other people at the resort, whom Curtis had seen only from a distance, never close enough to converse with. He did notice four men and one woman who seemed to be guests as well. They were escorted to the beach each day, about the same time that Curtis was. He could look down the beach and see the others, also stretched out on their chaises about fifty yards apart.

One afternoon as Curtis was entering his time of bliss, the beginning of the second week mark, he went out and took his position on his reclining chair. His qualms about Mack were almost extinguished through the spell of tranquility, and he had almost forgotten his vow to himself to be cognizant of treachery.

He saw, out of the corner of his eye, a young lady—obviously, his masseuse—approaching, carrying her supplies. Because it was the routine to do the massage treatment in silence, he didn't even make eye contact with her, except for a brief smile. The young woman worked hard on his back and thighs. After a hard workout, he felt so good and would drift in and out of sleep.

The masseuse pulled on him to roll over, and she started to work on his face, neck, and chest. He briefly looked at her through the slits in his eyelids. Then he closed them again. The November sun was especially bright that morning, making it difficult to keep his eyes open for very long. It was unseasonably warm, too, like a solar oven over his pale—previously rain-soaked—skin. Feeling the warmth soaking into his bones, he thought of the face of his masseuse. Something about her face felt familiar to him. He thought that maybe she was the one who worked on him the first day. But that wasn't right.

He went into his semi-doze state again with the image of her fixed smile in his mind. As he was just ready to fully snooze again, he suddenly realized that he had seen the woman at Mack's house. The one in the French maid's outfit. What was her name? He thought hard. He went through the alphabet, "Andrea, Betty, Candy, Debra," and so on. Unfortunately, his little alphabet exercise only brought up American names, and he didn't know many Thai ones. It wasn't until he got to the letter "T" that something clicked.

The masseuse laid smooth, flat stones onto his eyes to hold his lids shut. Each masseuse had a similar technique, sometimes using stones, sometimes sea weed or cucumbers. Then her name suddenly came to him. *Toey.*

Opening his eyes abruptly caused the stones to tumble off. He looked directly at her and caught her carrying an odd grimace. Was she working that hard on him that she had to frown? Curtis didn't think so. His eyes met hers directly. She tried to look away, toward the surf, but she couldn't. Her eyes were drawn back to his, and they became moist with emotion. They both remained in a muted state. Curtis was now more curious than anything. He thought to himself, what's with the scowl?

The silence broke when a tear was set free from her eye and dripped onto Curtis's cheek and ran down to his lip. He, as a reflex, quickly wiped it off with his bare hand.

The woman blushed and, breaking her silence, said in a panicked whisper, "I'm so sorry."

She started to grab her supplies to run away, and Curtis reached out and clutched her left wrist with his hand and held it firmly. "Toey?"

The young woman pulled against his grip. "Toey… what is it?" He asked.

She finally jerked away and ran from him, toward her golf cart parked on the road. She laid her massage supplies in the back and quickly climbed into the driver's seat. She drove the cart away.

Curtis looked up and down the beach. There was nothing but silence, broken only by the thunderous sound of the waves breaking on the white sand. He closed his eyes again and could hear a high-pitched squeal. He peeked between his lids and saw a white-bellied sea eagle circling overhead. He had learned about the birds during his previous stay and had watched them feeding daily from his office window. The creatures, like the wind, were unmindful of his presence. He turned his head and looked to the right and to the left. He could see his usual "neighbors" lying in silence on their cots, yards away.

He lay back down. But that brief experience with Toey was a wrinkle in his serenity, a crinkle that he hadn't witnessed until now. His suspicion was suddenly reawakened. He had to—once again—remind himself that his secondary mission, after being pampered, was to check on the state of things in Mack's kingdom.

It was another week before the young Thai lady rotated again as Curtis's masseuse. At first, he said nothing. He waited patiently until he turned onto his back and faced her. Just before she laid the stones on his eyes, he whispered, "Toey, it's you, isn't it?"

She seemed alarmed but stayed silent.

He asked again, "Toey?"

She then tried to whisper without moving her mouth. She continued working on massaging his face and temples. "Yes… it is me. . . but I must not talk."

Curtis assumed that the silence was just part of treatment scenario at the resort, and he, as a guest, had the ultimate control of his experience. Or did he? Why did Toey take it so seriously? Would she be punished, beaten, or fired if she talked? These thoughts passed through Curtis's head in a matter of seconds. "It's okay, Toey. You can talk to me. Are you okay? You seem upset and sad."

"I can't talk. They're watching" she whispered without disturbing her rigid smile. She tried hard not to move her lips.

Curtis raised up his head and looked around. "Who's watching?"

She gently pushed his head back down. She whispered again, "I mustn't talk, they're watching."

Curtis gave up trying to communicate and, instead, lay on the couch with a puzzled look on his face, beneath the stones now covering his eyes.

When Toey was done, she removed the round stones. Her eyes were filled with tears. She whispered the words, "This place isn't for you. It's for them." She looked at the road when she said *them* and then continued, "This isn't a resort... it's a farm."

Then she collected her things and walked away, back to her golf cart.

Curtis never saw Toey again, but he ruminated on those last words of hers, over and over for the next week. Sometimes his mind would get the words mixed up, and he would fight to restore them to their proper order. But he kept asking himself, what does that mean? Why did this bring such distress to Toey?

Curtis had started his trip with some doubts about Mack and the gift that he had so generously provided. But so far, the experience was very positive and providing the restoration that he needed. He was even starting to feel a genuine gratitude toward the billionaire. But now, there were doubts growing in his mind. This new uneasiness haunted him constantly. He had always been a puzzle solver, and here was a puzzle without resolution.

What is the *farm*, in this context? Were Toey and the other employees working rice or sugar cane fields? Were they slaves? Mack seemed to turn a blind eye to sex slaves, so it wouldn't be surprising if he was using slave labor on a farm. But growing what? But, she said this place wasn't for *you*. Who's the *you*? Was it Curtis himself or the other guests in general? Were they going to have us work the fields, too? Then the obvious thought came to him, a thought that he was trying to suppress. Were the other guests here to have their parts harvested, like cattle on a meat farm? "Good God, no! This can't be," he said aloud. No definitive answers came to him. Not from the warm breeze, not from the rhythmic surf, not from the white-bellied sea eagles, and not from within his own intellect.

A few days later, he was lying on the same cot on the same beach but with a different masseuse. He started to think about Mack's, supposedly now defunct, Coreplant program. How far had it advanced before it ended? Thomas had assured Curtis that it had been shut down. But, had it? Was the program's demise caused by Mack's new repentance? Had it been laden with technical complications as Thomas had said? If it had continued, it must have evolved into a clandestine project. There was nothing in the papers or scientific literature about it. "Surely not," whispered Curtis audibly to himself.

He had done some preliminary investigating before leaving Seattle. The Pendleton Restorative Oasis had an informative website. It said nothing about any procedures, except for the Erika Procedure. He searched for Dr. Takahashi's presence and he was not mentioned on that website, but he did find his name with the University of Osaka. He was back, so it appeared, to doing routine restorative plastic surgery and a rare face transplant. All that research was consistent with what Thomas had told him. But now Toey had brought a new disturbance to the quietude and flood of doubts.

The masseuse finished, and he was left on the beach, alone. In his solitude, he began to meditate in his usual manner. Within minutes, the proverbial light went on. As Curtis thought of the word "farm," the horrible and terrifying thought came to him. Was there any other explanation except that the other guests were being groomed as organ transplant donors? The only question was, did they know it? Were they suffering from some terminal illness, and they were there to relax before they donated? But they all looked so healthy. Were the other guests just livestock destined for the butcher like at the Jonesborough Farmer's Cooperative? Where healthy people walked in one end and organs came out of the other in coolers. It certainly wouldn't be the world's first black market organ procurement program. Other groups had even taken kidneys from people whom they had kidnapped off the streets in India or Kenya. China had a robust organ procurement program, too. In China, people with money could put in an order for a kidney, liver, or heart. They had a huge data base of potential "donors." When a match was made, and the donor was a political prisoner, they executed them and took their organs. If they weren't already incarcerated, they were quickly arrested and given a speedy trial. They were hastily executed... and the organs procured.

Curtis asked himself again, were these just paranoid thoughts? Why would Mack take the chance of letting Curtis enjoy the benefits of the spa while other guests were there to be harvested? He literally shook his head to make these jumbled and scary thoughts go away, like shaking a rock out of an empty shoe. He wanted to pretend all

461

was well and return to the peaceful bliss, which he had been enjoying so well up to this point. He invited the mother sun to warm him with her comfort, and a fragile smile returned to his face.

However, the clearing of his mind did not take. He couldn't put the dreadful thoughts completely away. Anytime his mind was not preoccupied, the bad thoughts slowly dribbled back into his head. Lying alone on a quiet beach didn't offer him the luxury of distractions of a busy office. He started to ruminate again. He looked down the beach and saw his neighbor lying on his cot, either sleeping or in a deep meditative state. Curtis sat up on the foot of his chaise and looked out to the sea. For the first time, he wondered if he, too, was being watched. He looked over his shoulder to the left and right and saw no one, except a gardener working along the road. If this experience was only for the guest's benefit, then no one would care if he approached his neighbor. However, if anyone tried to interfere, then he knew that something was seriously wrong.

Curtis stood up and stretched. Then he walked toward his neighbor's cot. He looked up and down the beach to see if any employees were watching, and he didn't see any, even the gardener was no longer there. He arrived next to the cot, and the man was lying on his belly, fast asleep, softly snoring.

"Hello," said Curtis in a loud voice. "Hello," he said again.

The man was startled and raised up his head with an arched back. He looked up at Curtis, squinting out the bright afternoon sun. "Oh, hello," he said with an Australian accent.

The man rubbed his face and rotated over onto his side, facing Curtis. For the first time, he noticed the man's appearance. He was young, probably still in his twenties. He was remarkably handsome with deep blue eyes and long blond hair teased into dreadlocks. You could also tell the work with the trainer was paying off for him, even more than it was for Curtis's middle-aged physique.

"Hi, I am sorry to bother you, but my name is Curtis Eisner, and I'm one of the guests."

The man looked around and asked, "Should we be talking?"

"Why not? Whose business is it if we talk to each other?"

The man shrugged his shoulders. "Well, I was told that I should talk to other guests for the sake of tranquility."

"I've just have a couple of questions for you" said Curtis. "How did you get here? Are you a paying guest?"

Curtis sat down on the loose, dry sand in front of the man with his legs crossed to listen to the response. The man sat up and dropped his legs over the side of his cot and started to tell his story. He was a surfing pro on one of the outlying islands. One day he noticed a man watching him; the man came up and asked him if he wanted a very easy job for good money. He went on to explain, "Then the dude told me that he was working for a new resort. I was sure he was going to try and hire me to teach surfing lessons. I get those requests all the time. They end up paying per class and not per hour. So many classes are canceled, especially during the off season, that you can't make a living that way. But that's not want he wanted me to do. The man explained that the resort hadn't opened to the public yet. So, they needed some young, energetic, and good-looking—his words not mine—people to just come and take advantage of the perks and treatment. All I must do is blog about it, and eventually they may use me in some of the PR material. In exchange, I get an attractive salary and get to live like a king."

"But there's no access to the Internet here," said Curtis.

"Oh, I know. I put it on a thumb drive and they upload it for me. I think Dr. Pearle has a private Internet connection by satellite, or at least someone does."

Curtis asked, "Really? So how long have you been here?"

"Three weeks."

That was a week longer than Curtis. Yet, Curtis was the first person he had spoken to. He added that a couple of the people that were there when he arrived were now gone.

Curtis looked up and saw one of the staff pulling up on the road in a golf cart. He then—hastily—stated, "Hmm, it looks like they are coming for us. So, one last question, what's the name of your blog?"

"Oh, it's simply called *Sand-dude at the Pendleton Resort*. I've gone by the name 'Sand-dude' since I was a kid growing up across from the beach in Byron Bay. You know, in New South Wales. That's Australia. You can find the web page at Sand-dudeblogger.com."

Curtis turned to walk away as the staff man was closing in. Then he looked back at Sand-dude and faced him while walking backwards, "The blog's online now, isn't it? I mean, if I went online tonight I could find it?"

"Sure." Then the distance between them and the sound of the surf forced Sand-dude to yell, "But you don't have Internet service here… do you?"

Curtis didn't answer but turned and walked toward his own cot. The staff member came up beside him, "Is everything okay?"

"Yeah. Fine."

"Oh, sir, we ask you to respect the privacy of the other guests. This is a place for private contemplation, and privacy is to be respected."

"Oh, okay. I'm sorry. It won't happen again."

That evening, after Curtis had his dinner and his chef had left, he reached in between his mattress and box springs for the satellite texting device. He was one day early for his scheduled weekly check-in with Bryan, but the days weren't written in stone. He turned it on and let it boot up. He turned on the texting application and typed out the message, "Everything here is still okay, but something has come up. Please go online and look up a blog called 'Sand-dudeblogger.com.' Read it and tell me your impressions." He hit "send" and the device waited until the satellite was overhead and uploaded to it. Then he turned it off, stuffing it back between the mattress and box springs.

Curtis went about his typical schedule the following days, only being slightly more observant about his surroundings. He did get a text back from Bryan the following night, which simply said, "No such site." Curtis felt a chill go down his spine. He still wasn't sure if his growing ill-feeling was justified or not. It could be the site was down or, somehow, Bryan got the address wrong. However, Bryan was pretty tech savvy and should have figured it out. Thomas had accused Curtis's lack of trust in Mack as an unjustifiable bias. Maybe it was now some type of paranoia that came on during a period of rest after a long period of stress… and the memory of Mack having him seriously beaten almost to death. He even briefly thought about discussing these things with Dr. Pearle, but then he thought about the fact that the psychologist was a Pendleton employee… so he quickly dismissed that thought.

By the end of the week, he was once again on his beach cot for the time of meditation and rest after a very hard work out. He saw Sand-dude come and take his place on his cot. The masseuse was quickly at the man's side. Curtis watched and waited until the beach was clear. He walked down to him.

"Hey, Sand-dude."

The man sat up. "Oh, hi. Did you get in trouble the other day for talking to me?"

"Oh, not really. The employee only asked me to not bother you. But I had some more questions for you." Curtis sat on the sand in front

466

of the man like he had the last time. "First, did you know that your blog wasn't up on the Internet?"

The man looked perplexed. "How would you know that?"

"I had a friend check it out back home, and he said there was no such thing on the Internet as your site."

"Well, that's strange. I mean, I write it on my laptop every day and Dr. Pearle says he uploads it to the blog server. He even gives me a list of comments by fans. I try to respond to each one. I don't know why your friend can't find it." He was quiet for a moment as he shook the sand out of his hair. Then he looked back at Curtis with a puzzled look. "How did you communicate with your friend? Do you have cellphone coverage here?"

Curtis looked up and saw a golf cart coming down the road. He ignored the question because he had little time and didn't have the luxury of creating a convoluted lie to cover his method. "Crap! Hey, I have one more question before I go. When are you done here?"

"I'm not sure. Like I said, they are paying me well, about a grand, US, a day. I'll collect the money when I leave. So, I'm in no hurry. But they told me that I could be here for a couple of months. I'm making the most of it and am in the best shape of my life and have never eaten as healthy as I have here. The only problem is," then a big smile came across his face, "I didn't bring my board."

Curtis looked up and saw a man walking toward them. "Okay, Sand-dude, I'll talk to you later." Then he stood up, turned, and walked fast toward his own cot. That was the last time that Curtis ever saw Sand-dude. The next day, he had disappeared from the beach for good.

A few days later, Curtis made a slip while he was talking to Dr. Pearle. He brought up Sand-dude, saying, "There was a man I met on the beach and he's gone. I miss him, and I only talked to him twice."

Dr. Pearle asked, "So what did you talk about, you and this Sand-dude guy?"

"Oh, he told me about his blog that he was assigned to work on, but oddly that site is not online." Curtis immediately knew that he had made a big blunder because it was Dr. Pearle who was supposed to be uploading it to the Internet.

Dr. Pearle cleared this throat, took off his black-rimmed glasses, putting the tip of the earpiece against his lips, and asked with methodical wording, "So, how did *you* know that his site wasn't up?"

Curtis deeply regretted bringing up the whole issue. "Oh, I had a friend back home check." He felt himself digging the hole deeper.

Dr. Pearle looked closely at Curtis, leaning forward, "So, we use isolation from the electronic world as part of our rejuvenation process. How did you communicate with your friend back in the states?"

Curtis paused and thought. There was no lie that would make sense in this context, at least a lie that he could come up with on the spur of the moment. So, he said, "I'd rather not say." He felt that was about the dumbest thing he could have said.

Dr. Pearle stared at him for a moment—in a contemplative state. Finally, he sat back up and put his glasses back on. He flashed Curtis a big smile and ended the conversation.

After his gym workout and lunch at the beach kitchen, Curtis went out to take his place on his beach chaises. He looked to the north, toward Sand-dude's cot. It was still empty. He had never witnessed a fellow client just disappear before. After beach therapy, Curtis returned to his house. When he came into the door, he sensed someone had been there. He just quite couldn't put his finger on why he felt that way… but he did. He went into this bedroom and opened his drawers. He was obsessive about rolling his socks up into balls and laying them in rows. The rows were not in line as they were that morning, or at least he didn't think so… but again, he wasn't sure. Sometimes he left them out of order.

He then rushed over to the bed and reached under his mattress and grabbed the satellite communicator. It appeared as he had left it. He turned it on. He waited to see if there was a message from Bryan, hoping that Sand-dude man's site was up, which would remove some of Curtis's angst. The device came on with no problem but couldn't find the satellite's signal.

Sometimes there had been a wait for several minutes until one of the Iridium satellites was overhead. But the device, on that evening, couldn't find one after searching for twenty minutes. The little search symbol kept spinning without connecting. What did that mean? Curtis felt that he would have to be a little paranoid for him to think that someone had come in and tampered with it. Or would he?

CHAPTER TWENTY-ONE: PINNACLE

Curtis was confronted with his conflicting thoughts each morning as soon as he opened his eyes from sleep. This told him that even during the night, his subconscious mind was in pursuit of the right interpretation. There was no one, objective sign that was indicative that something was awry at the resort. It was a general feeling. There was Toey's odd response and disappearance. But that could be accounted for by her just being a disgruntled employee. After all, she wasn't very happy with Mack and his cronies the night they beat him up. Maybe by "farm" she meant that she was working hard like a poor rice field worker in Thailand, but was it only a metaphor? It could have also meant something far more sinister.

Then there was Sand-dude's disappearance… but that could be explained as his time being up. But Sand-dude gave no hints that he was preparing to leave.

It was possible that the texting device couldn't find a satellite because it had changed its orbit, or solar flares, or bad weather… somewhere. Maybe the device's batteries were low. Curtis found himself living in two minds. He thought it was time to challenge the situation in a way that would force an illuminating response.

He considered his options off and on for several days. Then he concocted a plan. One afternoon, while lying on his beach cot, he took a stroll. He walked down the beach in the direction of Sand-dude's empty cot. He passed it and kept on walking. He had a glimpse of someone else on a cot another fifty yards away. As he closed in on that person, he saw the infamous golf cart coming down the road. He tried to ignore it. The cart came to a stop and a young man exited and came walking briskly toward Curtis, yet a hundred yards away. Dr. Eisner picked up his pace into a jog, as did the man, now seventy yards behind him. Curtis eventually made it to the person on the cot, who was a woman. She looked up at him and then sat up, wrapping her towel around her, being a bit startled. About the time he was about to speak to her, the young man arrived. He was breathless, yet had stamina enough to jump between them, "Excuse me, sir, but please do not disturb the other guests!"

Curtis pushed past the small man to get closer to the woman. She stood up with a look of perplexity rapidly filling her face. Curtis only then noticed that she was a remarkably beautiful young woman. She had short, brunette hair, dark-olive skin, and striking cobalt-blue eyes. "Excuse me," said Curtis as the young Thai man was pulling at his arm.

The woman answered "Yes?"

The Thai man was trying to reinsert himself between Curtis and the woman. Curtis gave him a hard push to the side again and said to her, "I just wanted to meet you and tell you my name is Curtis." Curtis reached out his right hand to shake hers. When she took his hand, she felt a piece of paper stuck in his palm. Then she reached up with her left hand to sandwich his hand between hers and to keep the paper from falling when he pulled his hand away.

472

"My name is Mona," she said.

The young Thai man inserted himself once again, between the two of them, saying, "Sir, we must respect the privacy of the other guests. I insist that you go back to your spot."

Curtis looked back at the woman and smiled as he walked away, being escorted back to his cot by the man.

Curtis noticed Mona opening the note and reading it. Curtis had prepared it that morning in the anticipation of contacting another guest on the beach. The note simply said, "Please meet me here tonight at 21:00 as I have something important to talk to you about." He decided to use military time because it was more universal. Thailand ran on a six-hour clock, which he found very confusing.

Curtis went through his normal afternoon routine and returned to his house for dinner. After dinner, he sat in his usual fashion in the living room reading *Treasure Island*, which came from the house's library of classic novels. The chef, who went by the name Chaow, was finished cleaning the kitchen, and he asked Curtis, as he usually did, if he needed anything else. Curtis said a polite, "No, thank you."

He continued reading but also watched the clock. During his six weeks on the island, he had only ventured out at night to sit on the beach in front of his house. He had never tried to explore the island, which was kept very dark. There were no streetlights, and the main facilities, such as the gym, were not lit up. He wasn't sure where the other houses were, as there was enough vegetation around each one to shroud their presence. The houses came without any source of portable lights, such as a flashlight. His phone was now dead, as the power source (a strange 260 volts) and the electric receptacle were an eccentric type that Curtis had never seen before anywhere in the world. He had no adapter for any electronics, and it seemed planned that way.

He knew the beach, where the "beach therapy" sessions occurred, was north, and his house faced the east. When he got to the beach, he turned left and started walking. From riding the golf cart back and forth each day, he estimated the distance to be about one and a half miles one way.

It was a moonless night and the stars, under a sky of high thin clouds, were negligent in their assistance. He could see the lights of ships, in a queue, along the horizon, but otherwise there were no landmarks. He had an audible reference point of crashing waves on his right, and on this night, the sea seemed more angry than normal. A stiff and cool breeze was blowing in off the surf, which was atypical, as the normal winds came from the west. The breeze carried with it the smell of fish. He assumed that at least one of the boats with lights on the horizon was a fish-processing boat.

He walked as a blind man, listening to the waves for guidance and dragging his toes in the sand as not to trip over something, like driftwood or a coconut. He was just hoping that there would be some indicator when he got to the beach therapy area, such as one of the cots. What he didn't anticipate was walking right into a chain link fence at full force. Not only did it make a lot of racket, but it about knocked the breath out of him. He followed it toward the sea, and, oddly, it disappeared into the water. He turned around and then walked away from the sea and the fence continued up, toward the road through thick underbrush. In frustration, he decided to climb it without any benefit of sight. He hoped it wasn't tall... but it was. It made no sense to him to have such a tall fence dividing the island, but it was a good fifteen feet up. Then he felt barbed wire at the top. He was glad it wasn't razor wire, or he would have been severely cut. He rethought his plan. Could he make the climb over? Would Mona still come if she was faced with the same obstacle on her side?

It was about that time that he heard a noise below him. Who was out here this time of night? It quickly dawned on him that it could be the woman. It could also be a security guard coming for him.

"Mona?" he shouted.

He heard a giggle, "Yes... who put this damn fence on the beach?" she replied, speaking English but with a rather strong accent that Curtis didn't notice earlier.

"Which side are you on?" asked Curtis fumbling around at the south-side of the top of the fence.

"I don't know. Hmm... if you're facing the water... I guess I'm on the right side of the fence."

"Hang on." Curtis climbed back down, landing on the same side he had climbed up on. He wasn't sure how they had missed each other, despite the lack of light. He just realized that she may be housed to the south of his house, and he assumed it was to the north because her cot was over a hundred yards to the north. He realized now that chain of logic made no sense. He worked his way back down the fence toward the water, feeling his way along the cold metal links. Then he felt her warm hand clutching the wires. He stopped and reached out with his right hand and felt her arm. "I hope this is you."

She giggled again. "Yes. I've never seen it so dark anywhere."

"Thanks so much for coming to meet me. I have some important questions for you. Can we sit down and talk a minute?"

"Where?"

"Right here," said Curtis as he dropped into a sitting position on the sand. He felt her plop down in front of him and her foot sliding to rest on his. Rather than pulling his away, he left it in place, so he could be aware of her presence, even though he couldn't visualize her. He leaned back against the fence, using it as a backrest.

"I'm sorry, but I forgot your name," she said.

"Oh, it's Curtis, uh, Curtis Eisner."

She asked, "And you have some questions for me? I think I have some for you, too; otherwise, I wouldn't have come."

"Yes, I do." Without stopping to think about offering to let her go first, he spoke, "How did you get here? Are you a paying guest?"

"No, I am staying here for free. I'm working here. I'm from Bangkok."

Mona paused for a moment. Now that Curtis's eyes had fully adjusted to the dark, he was starting to see her silhouette against the white of the breaking surf. Her head was turned looking back at the sea, and then she looked toward him. "Do you have a cigarette?" she asked.

"Uh… no." Curtis chuckled. "If I had a cigarette and a lighter, I wouldn't be fumbling around here in the dark like a blind man. So, you're obviously a smoker."

"No, not really. Okay, sometimes. Like when I'm stressed, and I'm stressed now. I would love to have a damn cigarette."

"So, how did you get to this place from Bangkok? I mean, if you're working here, who hired you and what are you doing? I mean, besides lying on the beach and getting massages?"

"It's a long story. I'm a model in the fashion industry. My agent called and asked if I wanted a gig at a new beach resort operated by Aman at Patong Beach. It sounded like a fantastic job where I would come and enjoy the resort, and it paid 35,000 TBH per day. It sounded too good to be true. They said that when I was done they would do a lot of interviews with me and photo shoots. All of this was for their public relations."

"Aman?" asked Curtis. "What's that?"

"It is one of the top resort companies in this part of the world. But I'm not sure if this resort is owned by Aman. I haven't seen any signs." Then she added, with a rising inflection in her voice, "Is it?"

"No," said Curtis. "At least I don't think so. I think it's owned by Mack Pendleton, an American billionaire. I'm not sure where Patong Beach is, but I am pretty sure that we are in the Similan Islands."

He couldn't see Mona's facial expressions in the dark, but the silence told him that she was confused.

"Oh, my God!" said Mona in a whisper as if to herself. "I started to get a little confused when I first got here. Things weren't making sense. Then I began to worry that I had been taken in by a sex trafficking group. But now I know they're lying to me... and I don't know why."

"Has someone assaulted you or done something else to give you the impression that it was a sex trafficking operation? I mean, I wouldn't put it past Mr. Pendleton."

"No," Mona answered. "But models, in Bangkok at least, have to always be leery that a so-called 'job' is really a sex trafficker."

"But you took this job anyway?"

"Being a model is highly overrated, unless you're some type of supermodel. I mean, I've done shoots in New York, Paris, Milano,

478

and Dubai; however, I still support myself by working in my mom's flower shop." She snickered and continued, "At the flower shop… I make potting soil out of ox poop." She giggled again, which morphed into an outright laugh. "The money these people offered was very good, and it was hard to turn down."

"Really?" Curtis said with a doubtful tone.

Mona added, "Plus I know how to handle myself."

They sat in silence for a couple of minutes, and Curtis added, "When I saw you on the beach this afternoon, you didn't appear to me as Thai."

"Actually, I'm Pakistani. My father came to Thailand to work with the UN when I was a little girl. My mother got me involved in beauty pageants in high school—against my wishes I may add—and that's where a modeling agent spotted me. My real interest was in sports. There wasn't a women's cricket league when I was in high school, so I got involved in triathlons and—to please my mom—modeling."

"So, what's with the brilliant blue eyes… surely your parents aren't both Pakistani?"

"Actually, they are. We are from the Kalash Tribe, and many of us have blue eyes. Some say it's from Alexander the Great's soldiers' DNA." Then she chuckled, "But who knows. There're even theories that we are descendants from the Aryans. You know, the super race that Hitler was so found of. I mean, the real Aryans did

479

conquer Pakistan." She paused for a moment and continued, "It's funny that our blue eyes caused us to be the underclass in Pakistan, but when we came to Thailand, we found that blue eyes were highly appraised for their beauty. My mother, especially, loved that about our move, and she never wanted to go back."

"So, Mona, how long have you been here… here at the resort… and how long are you staying?"

"I've lost track of time, but I think I've been here at least six weeks. They told me that they wanted me to stay for six to twelve weeks, and I'm anxious to go home now. I miss my family."

"Have you asked them to let you go?" he asked.

"I have. But they said it is in my contract to stay until they are finished fine-tuning the resort, and if I break that contract I will not receive any of my salary, which they are holding until the end, and I must even pay them back for my stay here. I don't have that kind of money, and if I tried to borrow money like that from my dad, he would be furious." She paused for a moment and then added, "It's also tempting to stay here as part of me wants to believe them. Where else on the planet can you get paid so much to exercise, eat right, and lay on the beach?"

They both sat in silence for a while. Curtis turned to lean his back further into the fence for comfort. Mona did likewise. Side by side they were looking to the south, toward the direction they had both come. Mona finally spoke again, "No, one thing's for sure, we now know they're lying to us. That's a big problem." After another long pause, she asked again, "Are you sure you don't have a cigarette... somewhere, maybe back at your house?"

Curtis chuckled. "No... I don't have a cigarette! I've never smoked." He chucked again. "Actually, I tried to smoke a pipe a year and a half ago and coughed my head off. It wasn't pretty." They sat in silence, both assuming the other was in deep thought. "Yeah, you're right," Curtis added. "We're at a junction now that we must do something to push them to show their hand."

Curtis was considering how much he should tell Mona. Finally, he spoke, "If they aren't involved in the sex trade, the other horrifying business they might be in is harvesting body parts for transplantation."

Mona, not taking him seriously, began to laugh. "What are you talking about?"

"Listen to me. I'm a surgeon. I was working on techniques for regrowing nerves that ended up helping Mr. Pendleton. He took my ideas and created a hospital on another island, where they were doing transplants. I wouldn't put it past him to be doing something as horrible as stealing body parts for transplantation. It wouldn't be the first time in history that this has happened. There's a huge black market for body parts, especially in Asia, and it has gone even to the extreme of harvesting organs from living people. China has been doing it for decades. They have timely executions of inmates who are good donors for paying customers."

"But why me?" Mona asked.

"Because you're gorgeous and athletic."

Curtis could sense her shock, even though he couldn't see her. He sensed it in her deep breaths and her restlessness to find a comfortable position to sit in. Finally, she spoke, "But… I don't understand. They could get my kidneys or my heart, but they couldn't take those things that they would see as beautiful. The kidneys of an ugly person are just as good as those from a model, maybe better. Constantly starving yourself, like we have been known to do, can't be good for the kidneys or any organ."

"Mona, it's complicated to explain, but I think Mr. Pendleton may have found a way to do just that, to steal someone's beauty."

"So… are you saying that when they're done with me that I'll be either disfigured or have someone else's face on me?"

"No, Mona. You'd be sacrificed in the end."

"You're scaring me! I would think that you're crazy saying those things, but something isn't right here, and I am really getting frightened." There was a pause and she added, "Damn, what I'd give for a cigarette!"

The two of them sat for another hour, until the very front edge of dawn was crawling upon the eastern horizon. The sunrise was hazy on this day, and you couldn't make out the sun, only its light. They agreed that it was time to act. Curtis discussed escape plans, and the most available one was for one, or both, of them to swim to the shipping lanes, which were at least two miles off the beach. That's where he could still make out the boat lights. There they could look for a ferry or fishing boat. But he couldn't imagine the unknowns of the Andaman Sea. Were there sharks? Poisonous sea snakes? In Puget Sound the tides could be quite brisk, enough to carry a power boat away against its will.

Curtis wasn't a good swimmer, and he knew that he couldn't make that swim without some flotation device. Mona was confident that she could make it, and she offered to swim with him. She swam in the ocean many times for triathlons and longer distance races. But both realized that it would be dangerous to escape by swimming together. They had lingering doubts. The whole ordeal just seemed too bizarre to be true. Curtis insisted that they be one hundred percent sure before they risked their lives, and swimming would put him most at risk.

They also agreed that Mona should go first as he saw her as being in the most jeopardy. He didn't see his worn-out, soon to be forty-six-year-old body as a subject for harvesting and assumed that he was here simply to rest… and not ask questions. But if he learned too much about the operation, he wouldn't put it past Mack to make him disappear like Earhart, as he once threatened.

Mona disagreed about him not being a transplant donor candidate. She raised the question that if they weren't looking to harvest organs from Curtis, too, why were they getting him in such good shape? Maybe they wanted him for more than just his body. Curtis had never entertained the thought prior to that point. He could imagine being murdered, especially if he knew too much, but never considered himself as a donor, too. Of course, he had heard of stealing someone's identity for financial gain. But this could be an operation to steal his total identity for some other gain. Such an assumption made his blood run cold. His lips searched for words, but there was nothing in the English language that would suffice.

The plan was completed, and they reviewed it, making sure they were coordinated in their thinking. The next day, Mona would ask Dr. Pearle to have her taken home. She'd insist that she would leave even if it meant giving up all her money and breaking the contract. She would be aggressive in her demand. Maybe that's all it would take, and she'd be sent home in a few days with no questions asked. Problem solved. Curtis promised to pay off her debt at the resort if that happened.

Mona agreed that she would meet Curtis at the fence at 1 a.m. the following morning. She would inform him about the outcome of her meeting with Dr. Pearle. However, if they refused to send her home, Curtis would see her off for her predawn swim to get help.

When he got home that night, he reached under the mattress and pulled out his satellite texting device. He tried to use it one more time. But again, it stayed in search mode, without finding a satellite signal. If he had a way to contact the outside world, this juncture would have been the right time to contact Captain Atitarn in Port Blair. The fact that the satellite device was no longer working was a bit disconcerting and threw an unanticipated wrench into his contingency plans for a safety net. He recognized that the scary thought of someone having come in and tampered with it could just be a brush with paranoid thinking. He felt that if he waited one more day, he would know the truth.

CHAPTER TWENTY-TWO: THE RECKONING

The next day, Curtis saw Mona being escorted to the beach a hundred yards away in the usual fashion. Between them—to his surprise—was a new man on Sand-dude's cot. Curtis didn't want to stir up more concern from the staff by walking down to either one of the sunbathers. Mona's session with Dr. Pearle was scheduled for right after the beach therapy, so the situation was still in suspense. She glanced down in his direction. He smiled but was likely too far away for her to read his facial features. He left first, looking down the beach to see Mona resting on her chaises as if she didn't have a care in the world.

That night, Curtis slipped out the slider door, which faced the beach. He was anxiously waiting for the verdict. Was Mona to swim or not? He felt nervous for her. The previous night, he had counted 1154 steps between his slider door and the fence. He had counted then, knowing that he would have to retrace them back to his house in the dark. On this night, while not as dark as the previous, the step count was helpful. He focused on the numbers as he walked.

After about thirty minutes, with the step count being accurate, he found the fence. He estimated that it was very close to 1 a.m. He whispered for Mona, but only the waves answered him. The winds were gentler this night, once again from the west, but cooler. He couldn't detect fish in the air, only that familiar surf smell, almost the same as it had smelled on Long Island, when he and Becky would take day-long picnics at Jones Beach. He sat against the fence and felt the calm of the moment, not knowing if it was the calm before the storm, or the end of fear itself.

He thought of Puget Sound, with its strong, unique smell, which was—he was told—related to the sea grass, especially a variety called "Sea Lettuce" that was exposed during the low tides. So, the cool breeze and the smell of surf on this night clearly evoked the New York days. The stars were out and brilliantly sewed across the dark navy-blue sky like a patriotic banner. However, he would exchange the long sunlit days on Long Island for this starry night. Even the grey and rainy days of Seattle felt glorious compared with this uneasy moment.

He rattled the fence, which was their signal that the other one was there. Still he heard nothing in response, save the crashing of the waves. The thought of having to swim through and past those waves terrified him. He waited fifteen minutes and repeated his signal… still nothing. Over and over he repeated until it must have been at least 2:30 a.m. Fear was seeping in from the sea and he felt it at his core like a cold fog. His first thought, of course, was that something must have happened to Mona. Most likely, that wasn't a good something. But the second thought was that she was one of them, and now… he had been baited for a trap. He had to leave. He decided to follow the chain link fence away from the beach and try to reach the road. He frequently stumbled over vegetation, which grew along the fence. He continued to bushwhack his way through the undergrowth. He came to a clearing and then found the hard asphalt. He slipped down the road, to his right, in the dark. He worked his way, step by step, back toward the main campus.

Curtis walked for what seemed like a mile. The campus was utterly black… and as silent as interstellar space. The light of the brilliant sky of stars helped him barely make out the outline of the narrow blacktop. Standing in the silence, near to what he thought was the main building, he noticed a quiet, buzzing sound in the distance. The sound was coming closer, so he jumped behind a cluster of elephant ear plants and stooped. In a moment, a three-wheeled Tuk Tuk van came down the road and passed him. Then it turned to the left and took a side street, one that Curtis hadn't observed before, between the gym and the beach kitchen. It disappeared behind the buildings.

Curtis followed the vehicle from a distance while walking on the narrow street. He saw the little truck back up to a small cinderblock building, and he heard two doors open on each side of it and then close. He tried to head for the bushes to hide himself but struck something hard and sharp with his shin. Feeling intense pain, he stumbled across the pavement as he swallowed his scream. After the pain had diminished, he looked carefully, and it appeared he had walked into a wheelbarrow beside the road, now on its side. The noise of his crash didn't catch the ears of the people at the truck, much to his good fortune.

Curtis lay on the ground holding his leg, as the pain slowly dissipated. He felt sticky blood on his fingers. The fumbling around in the dark was too reminiscent of the night he had jumped out of

Sandra's cabin window or the night he had crawled the two miles back to his house with a smashed testicle. But now he even saw those horrible nights with envy.

He stood up and tried to walk. He noticed that the people were now inside the building and the lights were on. He walked quietly across the sand and peeked inside one of the two small windows. The window in front revealed an empty room, but he could hear noise coming from inside, so he knew they were still there.

He walked to the back of the building and peeked in that window. From that vantage point, he could see through an inside door two people working in an adjacent room. They were busy and active, but he couldn't tell what they were doing. In a moment's time, they came into the large room directly attached to the window in which Curtis was peering. He ducked down and peaked just above the sill. The lights in that room came on.

Now he noticed in that room was a big, galvanized, metal box. It was rectangular, like a large planter, or perhaps... a coffin? The two men rolled a stretcher in and on it was—confirming his vilest nightmare—the naked body of Mona. Was she dead? He felt an awful numbness come over him and then terror as he spontaneous whispered, "Oh, my God." Up until that point, it all seemed to be a silly dream or game, but now it was real and a horrible nightmare. The instinct was to reach out for help, but there was none to be reached. He was cut off from the outside world, and he realized how ill-conceived his plan was of using the satellite device as his only safety net. He knew, too, that the act and intent that had brought Mona harm would quickly do the same to him if he didn't escape. He now felt his whole plan of coming back to Thailand was stupid. He had grossly overrated his ability to find a way out and should have listened to Bryan.

His palms became sweaty. He was trying to decide what to do, and he felt an overwhelming urgency. Then he noticed a bag of IV fluids laid across Mona's abdomen with a tube running to a catheter, entering a main vein behind her right clavicle. This reassured him that she was at least alive. You wouldn't put an IV in a dead person... except to infuse embalming fluids. But embalming would make no sense if they only wanted her as a donor.

Curtis watched carefully, and he could see her breast delicately rising and falling, indicating breathing and confirming his hope of life. Yes, at that moment she was still alive, but what could he do to save her? He had no chance of fighting the men like some hero in a movie. One of them had a gun in a holster on his belt. Curtis had no weapons, just his meek surgeon's fists. He was in better shape now, but no match for two men, one of whom was armed. His only chance to save her was to wait them out. He longed for Bryan's posse, but was denied a way to summon them.

He watched carefully, hoping that they would leave her, and then he could break in and rescue the woman. He would have to carry her, which would put him at a great disadvantage. But she wasn't left alone. The two men lifted her and laid her in the metal box. They spoke, and one left the room, then the building. Curtis heard the familiar door of the little truck squeak open and close. Then it suddenly drove away. The man in the room with Mona—obviously not realizing he was being watch—gazed upon her naked body with what appeared to Curtis to be a licentious intent. Then Curtis watched helplessly as the man pulled out his phone and took photos of her naked body. "Damn creep," Curtis mumbled out loud to himself. The last horrible thing he did was to touch her. Curtis couldn't make out where he was touching her because she was inside the box, but he could tell that it was likely sexual. He wanted to scream for the man to leave her alone. But such a scream would seal both their fates. The man in the room was the man with the revolver.

The other man returned in the truck and came back in with a cart carrying two large, black plastic bags of crushed ice. They laid a semi-transparent sheet over her—sparing only her face—and then emptied both bags directly over the sheet. They spread out the ice like they were covering freshly caught fish, and Curtis figured they had been doing exactly that in their previous careers. That's all he needed to see. It confirmed to him that Mona was going to be harvested for her parts or even Mack's gruesome Coreplant program. But nonetheless, it was going to be a murder—his worst fears being graphically realized. How could he have been such a fool? But then, maybe he was there for a purpose, to save Mona and to shut down the whole dreadful operation.

Curtis began to run, like he was running for Mona's life. His legs moved beneath him without intent at first, just in a flight of fear and desperation. He ran through the vegetation and then out on the walkway. Not remembering the wheel barrel until the last second, he leaped over it to avoid yet another clumsy fall. He hated to leave the woman alone, but he knew that the only chance he had of saving her was to get off this damn island and get the authorities. It was time for a swim, regardless of the risk. The thought of commandeering a boat crossed his mind, however, he had not seen a harbor or boats tied up anywhere, and he was disoriented as to the location of the dock, where he had arrived a few weeks earlier. He couldn't waste a lot of valuable time trying to find such a resource in the dark. So, it was time to swim.

Curtis ran the entire mile and a half back to his house in a full sprint. This was something he could not have done before his intensive conditioning program. He had another hard fall on the road once when he tripped over an irregularity in the pavement. As he was lying on the ground, he considered darting directly toward the beach. But he wanted his cellphone, just in case he made it to cell coverage. He also needed something for floatation and thought he would have a better chance of finding such a device at his house than in the woods.

He tore through the door of his house like a deranged gazelle grabbing his phone as he went through the kitchen. The night before, he had taken apart his charger. He placed the bare wires into the outlet holes and then hooked up the phone. The phone indicated it was charging, but he had a heck of a time keeping the loose wires in place, and he wasn't sure it had paid off. Fortunately, it was now fully charged.

He threw open the door of the refrigerator and looked in. He grabbed a jar of kosher pickles, dumped out the contents into the sink, turned his phone back off, and placed it inside the jar. He grabbed the electrical cord from the charger, tied it around the mouth of the jar, and hung it from his belt. He needed something to help him float and needed it quickly. He looked around. He darted to the living area and felt the pillows on the couch. He knew that they would eventually become waterlogged and drag him down. He looked back in the refrigerator and saw a liter of milk in a plastic jug. He dumped out the milk, put the cap back on, and tied the empty bottle to his other side. He still needed more, but he was running out of time.

Curtis raced to the sliding door, opened it, and looked to the east. A breeze of salty air greeted him and would have been refreshing in any other context. The red line of dawn was making an appearance through the chalky horizon of haze. At least he could see where the beach started. He ran back inside and grabbed his day pack and emptied out its contents. He took out the couch pillow and stuffed it into a plastic trash bag, tied it up, and then stuffed it inside his day pack. The pickle jar was banging on his knee as he ran for the beach. Just before entering the water, he took the jar with the phone inside and tied it to his pack to keep it out of the way.

While the early morning air was quite cool and damp, the water was thankfully warm, far warmer than Puget Sound where he had last attempted to swim. He found a position where he laid his chest on the daypack, kicked with his feet, and paddled with his arms. The sea was kind to him this morning. The waves had calmed down and were two-footers at best, which was to his advantage. Otherwise, he could have never made it beyond the breakers. Yet, it was a formidable task to survive the churn and mouthfuls of foam until he was past the break zone. Once in smoother water, he was startled when he heard a boat motor start to his far left. Through the thin light of the predawn, he could see a large Zodiac boat leaving the floatplane dock with, what appeared to be, the big metal box on the back. Curtis tried to duck under the water behind his pack. If the sun had been any higher, he would have been spotted for sure. The boat passed by only about seventy-five yards away, but he went unnoticed, or at least he hoped. At that moment, he was filled with regrets. But again, maybe it was his purpose to be there to save Mona and the others who would have come after her. That became his primal focus, and he knew he had to give it his best shot, even though he could die in the process.

Curtis never liked water, at least without a boat. He had this horrible feeling of being on the edge of a panic attack as he watched the shore fading behind him. He was terrified of drowning. He felt a deep sense of betrayal, thinking that Thomas had—most likely—been in on the harvesting, including the harvesting of his own body, if that was their plan. But nothing mattered now except for survival. He would deal with Thomas later… if he made it.

More than once Curtis had a rogue wave break the tranquility and go over his head. Each time he swallowed a mouthful of sea foam. He choked and, despite each episode feeling like it would be the last breath of his life, kept swimming. The next wave poured up through his nostrils and into his sinus cavities, the brine setting his entire face ablaze with a burning pain.

He had heard the familiar stories of how someone's life flashed before their eyes as they encountered a near-death experience. Maybe the thought of those stories stirred up an intentional thought about his life… or maybe it was automatic, an inherent trait within us all. But his mind took him back to his earliest memories of his life. It laid down the years one by one like his 3-D printer. There were glances of his preschool years. Those were quickly layered over with a vivid memory of sitting on his father's lap around age six. The two of them had just returned from church, and his father was reading the Sunday comics section of the *Jonesborough Press* to him. He saw his father's face clearly. He had forgotten that the man had a soft smile and a long, thin mustache.

He remembered looking at the characters on the paper and laughing together. He recalled—richly—as he thrashed in the suffocating waters, his father looking at him and saying, "I love you, boy, more than you will ever know," and kissing him on the top of his head.

Rapidly the years were laid down, through grade school and into high school, while his swimming strokes became automatic. He remembered Sandra. She was standing in her prom dress. It was red with black straps. She was wearing bright red lipstick, carrying a small black purse with rows of diamonds on it. Fake diamonds of course. He saw it clearly. He remembered deciding not to date her anymore after that night, not because he was too shy, but because she was too shallow. It was an intentional parting of ways.

He saw Erika crying as he told her that he was sorry, sorry for giving her hope, when there was none. He, too, was sorry for breaking the promise to save her.

For a moment he envisioned Jennifer, standing below him in the sea with drops of air falling on her, leaving streaks of dryness running down her face, as in a reverse world of our own. She was mouthing something, but with no air in which to form a voice, he couldn't hear her. Then he imagined reaching down and grasping at her hand to pull her up, yet, her hand kept slipping out of his. She was looking up, eyes open, but slowly sinking. The sunlight on her body was retreating upward until only her fearful face was still visible. Her lips continued to move, which he could now read. "You have to love me… you just have to." Then she was swallowed by the murk.

He saw Bryan Rogers standing in the OR, in scrubs with a mask dangling around his neck, and saying, "It's okay, I've got this. They'll ALL walk again." His confidence in the man gave him peace about his dream… even in his absence.

His last thoughts were of Becky, alone in their condo. How would she cope without him? He was worried for her, that her regrets for how she had treated him would haunt her… and he didn't want that. He felt that he must survive… for Becky and Mona.

Before he was out of the lagoon, he felt the first painful sting of a jellyfish on his leg. It stung the same right leg that he had hammered against the wheelbarrow in the dark. The pain was almost paralyzing, and the strength of that leg went down by half. It wasn't long until he had another sting on his back. "Damnit! Why?" shouted Curtis with frustration and pain. He felt that after the surf had been kind to him, now the whole universe was starting to work against him. He had considered a swim to the shipping lane as a difficult feat to start with… but turned out to be worse. While he thought about the many nasty creatures that might encumber him, he had never considered jellyfish as one. With each stroke forward, he was thrown back a half stroke due to the tidal streams. Those he had anticipated.

Somewhere deep in the limbic system of his brain, the layers of memory kept appearing but not in chronological order.

College was where he became consumed with his studies. His destiny was sealed when the University of Michigan was the only medical school that accepted him. Others turned him down, not due to his GPA, but due to his lack of references. He didn't have the social courage to ask professors, practicing physicians, or congressmen or women for support letters like the other applicants.

Then the day he met Erika was another clear layer that hung in his mind for several seconds. What if? What if he had never met her? What if he had never made that promise? What if he had not traded shifts with a fellow medical student that day, who had a bachelor's party to attend?

After a half hour of swimming, with the sun now fully above the horizon, he realized that his daypack flotation device was saturated with water and was no longer helping with buoyancy but was acting only as a drag to his swim. The plastic bag apparently had holes. He slowly released it. He grabbed the pickle jar as it floated away, half submerged. Now, he knew that the only thing that stood between him and drowning was a kosher pickle jar with a phone in it and a sealed liter milk jug. He would pause briefly now and then to rest with the two containers around his head to keep his mouth above the water. Exhaustion poured into him from every direction. The continuous panic attacks and physical exertion had taken the life energy out of him.

The memories continued with the notification of the residency match in neurosurgery with Apple Health. When he opened his certified letter, he had been disappointed. If only he could've been matched with a big university or nonprofit system, how his future might have been different. But the for-profit system set him on an irrevocable course. Yet, at the time, being in New York City seemed like a reasonable trade off.

The lethargy was almost enough to make him give up and succumb to the will of the Andaman Sea. He had lost his resolve to live. Except for the thought of Mona and her parents, he would have drowned then. But Mona had become to him his new Erika. Someone to save. A purpose, somebody else for whom he could dedicate his hope for life. He must make it to a boat, he kept telling himself. He must make it before they came looking for him. He started a side stroke with his face above the water and to the sun. He felt another sting, this time on his face, and he saw the culprit. It was a large, common jellyfish floating on the surface. He feared the infamous, tiny box jellyfish of those waters, whose sting would cause a quick but painful death. These larger, common jellyfish only caused severe pain for no purpose. Meaningless suffering.

He rotated back to a crawl swim stroke. Just four strokes, and he had to rotate to his back and float to rest. He started to swim again, but this time his right hamstring was starting to cramp. With the pain of it, he quickly rotated back to favor the left. In the rapid turn in the water, the milk jug came free and floated away in the current. He held onto the pickle jar like he was a rock climber and it was the one hand hold on a cliff he could use to arrest a fatal fall. But it was not enough. His now lean body, while stronger, was denser and far less buoyant. He felt terror as he started to sink each time he paused from swimming, holding the jar tightly in his hand. The container was not enough to sustain him at the surface.

Curtis tried to look to see where he was. He quickly wiped the water from his face with his hand, but there was nothing to see but more water. He could no longer see the beach. He couldn't see the sun or the direction in which he was to swim. It was a lost cause. He was totally bewildered.

The thought of drowning, while still horrifying for him, was his one respite left. He couldn't save Mona. He couldn't save Becky, Erika, or himself. He was tired. He was tired of it all. He let loose of the jar from his right hand, and it floated upward as he sank. Letting it go was his last act of free will. The last choice of his forty-five years.

Downward he slipped through the planes of the warm brine. His reptilian brain began to take control with more primal memories. The last one was being inside his mother's womb. It seemed real. He felt safe there, being embraced and bathed by the warm brine. Curtis smiled as, in the memory, he felt he could swim freely without the need for air… or lungs. He felt like a fish.

Apart from the vision, in the real world, he gulped a full breath of sea water. It filled his lungs with fire, and he began to cough in silence, coughing out water and inhaling the same. The poison of suffocation began to fill his lungs, his blood, and finally his brain. It was an overwhelming sense of asphyxia. As a scientist, he never imagined that drowning would be so laboring, and the mind would remain so lucid through it all. Death sat, deferred just beyond him. He reached for it with open hands, to embrace the exit from the horror.

The coughing continued in the complete silence of the liquid medium. The jerking of the cough caused his body to spin in slow motion. Feeling once again like a suspended fetus, he sought that peace that was transient. Soon he was there. He could hear his mother's heartbeat. Rhythmic and loud in his ears was the pulsing around and above him, towards her heart. Despite the rising poison of suffocation throughout his body, his lucid mind reappeared. It had identified the heartbeat as not that of his mother's heart, but the rhythmic sounds of a boat propeller. He could see the shadow above him, casting downward through the layers of semi-transparent waters of green and blue, blocking tangential rays of downward light. Without strength, without air left anywhere in his blood, he pulled his hands against the water. Reaching upward with cupped hands, he pulled the sea down. His eyes were wide open, and he drew for the surface where the sun was out. He broke through into the world of gases and coughed out water. He inhaled air and coughed out water again.

He stroked with feeble arms toward the humming, as his uncontrollable coughing absorbed his fragile strength. As soon as he would pause his efforts, his feet started to drift downward again, pulling his whole body in tow as the sea fought to reclaim his soul. He wanted to touch something, but his feet would dangle, madly, reaching downward and finding nothing but the Andaman. When he had been at the surface, his coughing had not paused long enough for him to take in all the air for which his body was desperate.

After a few more strokes, which pulled him back to the surface, he momentarily paused again and tried to quickly wipe the water from his eyes. There, partially hidden by the glare of the sun, was the bow of a small fishing boat, heading directly toward him. The sense of relief was overwhelming. He began to cry, but the tears were washed away by seawater as his head went under, yet again. As the boat came closer, he surfaced to only see the black rubber hull and inhale the air, now infused with bitter gasoline fumes. Then a long brown arm of the fisherman was reaching for him, to save him and hopefully Mona… if it wasn't too late. He grabbed the hand and held on with all his might. The Thai man, to whom it was attached, was his savior, his Calypso.

CHAPTER TWENTY-THREE: PERMUTATION

Carolyn Wagers walked down the long, tiled hallway to the lab. She stepped inside the door, unnoticed. She looked at the six technicians working away. Four of them were from the original New York Sharks group. The fan of a fume hood was roaring at the back of the room. She spoke loudly, "Hey, everybody!" No one seemed to notice her. Then she reached over to the light switch and flickered it off and back on. Everyone looked up. The technician turned off the vent, pushed his safety glasses to the top of his head, and spun around on his stool to listen. She continued, "Dr. Eisner's back in town!"

There were broad smiles on everyone's faces. Then a spontaneous applause echoed through the lab. Jennifer, being totally surprised, asked, "Where is he?"

"Oh, he's up in Thomas's office right now and will be down here soon to start packing his office."

"Packing?" asked Joe, one of the Sharks.

"Yeah," answered Carolyn. "I assume he's gotten his patents relinquished, and he's off to Mayo Clinic. Don't be surprised if he asks some of you to come with him."

Bryan's persistence had eventually paid off and he and Jennifer were now a pair. She sent him a text, "Hey Bry, Curtis is back in town and is in the building. I think he's in Thomas's office."

In a minute a text came back from Bryan, "What? Really? That's great! I'll run up there in a jiffy. Lov Bry."

Bryan had worried about Curtis and had almost, at one point, taken a plane to Thailand to check on him. However, Thomas talked him out of it. Thomas reassured him that Curtis was doing great and loving his long-awaited sabbatical. Bryan did get his weekly, secret text messages via satellite assuring him that all was well. Those things were enough to quell many of his concerns.

Becky didn't have a lot of direct contact with Curtis during the absence because he didn't have cellphone coverage. Thomas, however, kept her up to date. He had her come up to his office to use his video conferencing system for face-to-face chats with Curtis twice. Once during the first month and then there was a long gap due to technical difficulties. But she did conference call him just three weeks before his return. She wanted to do more of them but, per the resort protocol, such virtual visits were strongly discouraged.

When Curtis's stay was extended from three to four and a half, then five months, it was very hard for her. Becky made a couple of plans to travel to Thailand herself, but Thomas kept convincing her that the time away was good for Curtis, and as soon as he was home, she would have him all to herself.

Becky seemed to have reached a place of peace and was almost well again. In Curtis's long absence, she took a couple of trips to Rochester to look at houses. She found a lovely old limestone farm house, northwest of town, near Oronoco. It had a barn and a mother-in-law's suite, perfect for his mom. She imagined seeing children running through the fields with their dog. She was waiting for Curtis to get home to see it and to make an offer before it was gone. Life could be more hopeful for her. She felt their long-awaited lives were about to finally start, and her heart was teeming with anticipation.

Bryan raced from the recovery area to the elevator and went up to the 23rd floor. He arrived at Thomas's closed door and knocked. No one answered, however he heard voices coming from inside. In a moment of impulse, he turned the knob and opened it. There, in the casual area of the big office, sat Thomas with his back toward the door. Across the table from him were two men in suits—which Bryan recognized as Neurogenics lawyers—and another man, whom he didn't recognize, was sitting to Thomas's right. A bottle of Jack Daniels stood tall as a centerpiece on the table. All the solemn men had drinks of amber liquid in front of them. Then he looked closer at the stranger. "Could it be?" he asked himself.

The man looked up. It was Curtis but thirty pounds lighter and bulked up like a neophytic weightlifter. Even his hair was fuller, like he had some hair transplantation. In other words, he looked over ten years younger, deeply tanned. "Damn, boss, you look good!" said Bryan as he—impetuously—walked into the room directly toward Curtis.

Thomas turned, looking over his shoulder with a bit of gravity, "Bryan, please! We're in the middle of something important here." Bryan couldn't stop his emotional momentum and continued walking. Curtis stood. Bryan gave him a big hug. "Great to see you, man!"

Curtis smiled and said in a raspy voice, "And to see you."

Thomas looked up at Bryan and spoke again, "Can you please wait outside? Dr. Eisner will be done in a moment."

Bryan walked back out the door, leaving it ajar, and watched as Curtis signed some documents, which were spread out across the coffee table. He was assuming it was an agreement for Neurogenics to relinquish the patents for the Erika Procedure back to him. The men around the table talked for a while and each raised their glass of Jack Daniels for a toast. The lawyers collected their papers, stuffed them into their briefcases, and left, filing out the door and past Bryan one by one, without making eye contact. Curtis and Thomas spoke quietly between themselves, and then the doctor meandered to the door as the conversation with Thomas slowly washed-out and ended. In the hallway, Bryan grabbed Curtis's hand in a shake and would not let go, "How are ya, boss? I know I said it before, but, man, you look great. Do you feel rested?"

A big, bright smile came across Curtis's face, "I am ecstatic… never been happier in my life! I feel that I've been born again."

They walked down the hall together and boarded the elevator. "So, did you get all your patents?" asked Bryan.

Curtis, with a huge smile on his face, looked down at the floor of the elevator and back up to Bryan, "I've been through a lot in the past few months. Had a lot of time to think. You just wouldn't believe it."

Bryan asked again, "The patents?"

"Uh, well, son, there's been a change of plans. I actually just signed over my patents permanently to Thomas, and I can never do the Erika Procedure again."

Bryan literally fell back against the side of the stainless-steel elevator wall. "Whhhhat? Are you serious?"

"Yes, Bryan, I am. You see, Mack Pendleton passed away from liver disease and has willed most of his liquid assets to me—about $2 billion in cash—so I'll never need to work again."

Bryan was stunned into a speechless stupor. Finally, after a moment, he said in almost a whisper, "Need to? Curtis, when did you ever *need* to work?"

Curtis said nothing. Bryan added, "What about your vision? Do you know what you could do with that amount of money? We could bring the Erika Procedure to the whole damn world… and for free!"

Curtis watched the lights above the elevator door as they went down toward the basement and said nothing. Bryan stood looking at him, up and down. Was this really Curtis? He looked and acted so differently. Or was this an imposter?

They were down to the tenth floor and Bryan said, "Hey, boss, let me see your belly wound." Curtis looked at him with a bewildered look.

"You know, since I sewed it up, I want to make sure it turned out okay." Curtis just continued to stare at him.

Bryan added, "You wanted me to check it immediately after you got back. At least that's what you said." Bryan was making that part up, but he felt the need to see the wound for himself.

Curtis continued looking at him, and his bewilderment over the question didn't seem to waver. However, he sensed that Bryan was doubting his identity. So, without protest, he unbuttoned four buttons on his light blue dress shirt. Bryan looked closely at his belly. Up and down. The obvious suture line scar was still there. Curtis spoke in a strange monotone looking at the top of Bryan's head as he was stooped over looking at the scar on his belly, "Dear Thomas, place your hand in my side and then you will believe."

Bryan reached out and ran his finger down the scar and then straightened back up, with his curiosity seemingly satisfied. "It looks good."

Then Curtis buttoned his shirt back up as the door was opening to the basement.

Now Bryan carried a bewildered look and asked, "Why did you call *me* Thomas?"

Curtis stepped out of the elevator beside him and smiled, "Never mind. I wasn't referring to Thomas upstairs, I was talking about the Biblical Thomas and something Jesus had said to him. But that's not important."

Curtis walked briskly down the hall, toward the lab. Bryan took one step off the elevator and paused, staring at his back as he walked away. The man did not carry Curtis's unique saunter. The elevator door softly closed behind him.

He heard the cheering as Curtis walked into the lab, fifty feet down the hall. Someone had rushed out and bought a bottle of champagne when they heard he was back, and they popped the cork as soon as he walked into the room. Bryan walked slowly in the direction of the noise in a robotic, meditative state, almost oblivious to the world around him. He entered the lab as the impromptu festivities continued. He watched as Curtis grabbed Jennifer by the hand and pulled her past him, out the lab door and down to his office. He tried to follow them, but after Curtis and Jennifer had entered the office door, Curtis closed it behind them. Bryan heard the deadbolt click into the locked position. He saw Curtis drop the vertical blinds, covering the door's frosted window. Bryan stood outside the door but couldn't hear anything from inside. He tried to force the door open. It would not budge.

Jennifer was so happy to have Curtis home, yet confused. It was awkward as he was intruding on her personal space. She walked backward across his office as he marched directly toward her, looking intensely into her eyes. Looking down at a thick envelope on his desk—as they passed it—and back at him, she said, as if to break the awkwardness, "Hey, there's a letter from San Francisco with a return address of Wayne Eisner, could that be your father? It came two months ago."

Ignoring her question, Curtis grabbed her shoulders and pulled her toward him. "Jennifer, I'm a changed man. I now realize that I'm deeply in love with you, and you're all I want." He started to kiss her with a passionate kiss. She flinched and pulled away in shock. Then he grabbed her buttocks with both hands, squeezed, and then pulled her body into his. She was totally stunned and speechless. Curtis continued by whispering in her jasmine-scented ear, "Mack has died and left me a chunk of his fortune, and I'm here on his yacht. I have signed over all my work to Thomas. I'm taking you with me, and we'll live like royalty and explore the world for the rest of our lives. It's gonna be magic, like pixie-dusted destinies."

Jennifer was feeling a total whirlwind of emotions. Not only couldn't she talk, but she couldn't move either, and could only barely breathe. Curtis kissed her again, and then she started kissing him back, but with great internal conflict. She finally mumbled, "But, I'm with Bryan now." Curtis ignored her and continued to kiss her neck. "What about Becky? I thought you were getting back together?" She asked.

He pulled back a couple of inches from her face and smiled softly, "Becky? Becky who?" Then he started to kiss her again.

Then Curtis paused, pushing her back against the bookcase and looked at her muddled eyes. "I have one more piece of business to do, and I will be back. Go pack. You're coming with me. I will be back here in one hour. Don't bring much, as we can buy anything you need."

Curtis turned and opened the door. There stood Bryan still looking perplexed. He turned back to look at Jennifer, "Oh, but don't forget your passport." Curtis pushed pass Bryan, aggressively saying, "Get out of my way, son."

Bryan stepped back dazed and watched him go and hit the elevator button. When the door didn't immediately open, Curtis turned into the stairwell and disappeared, holding his cellphone to his ear.

Bryan entered the messy office. Jennifer was stunned, sitting on the couch with tears streaming down her face. Bryan walked over and picked up her limp hand and held it, "Did he say something rude to you?"

She sat in silence.

He wiped a tear off her dusky face, "Did he hurt you?"

She looked up sobbing and shaking her head to the negative and then looked down at the floor to avoid eye contact. "No… he told me… he told me that he loved me and was taking me with him."

Bryan sat down beside her. He looked as if the blood had drained completely out of him. She was lifeless too and continued looking down at the floor. "Nef, something's wrong here! Curtis has been brainwashed or something. Something isn't right."

She continued to sob, now looking down at her hands as she opened and closed them over and over in a rhythmic ritual of silence.

He pulled her chin up, so that she was looking at him, "Nef, you're not really thinking about going with him... are you?"

She remained inert except to quietly sob and wipe her nose with her bare arm.

Jennifer's restraint from commenting gave Bryan a sinking feeling of uncertainty. Tears began to form in his own eyes. He pulled her head against his chest. "Nef, do you understand I love you, too? I want to take care of you."

Before, when Bryan had said things like that, she seemed offended and responded, "I can take care of myself." This time, however, she said nothing.

Bryan added tear-soaked words, "Nef, I bought you a diamond. It's beautiful, cut just for you. I didn't want to tell you under these circumstances, but I was going to ask you to marry me on your birthday."

These intense words drew nothing out of her, not even a glance. Bryan continued, "Curtis is my hero, too... but he's not right. I've got to figure this out. I need some time. Please don't do anything until I get to the bottom of this."

Jennifer could only sob and nod, but it was an unconvincing, barely detectable nod.

Bryan gathered his own composure and walked out into the hall and then down to the elevator. He was carrying within him a hard hurt. But there was also a sense of urgency, a need for immediate action, but he wasn't sure what to do. Curtis had left the building, and he didn't know where he had gone. He punched the button back up to the 23rd floor, thinking that Thomas would have some answers.

Meanwhile, Curtis had jumped into a taxi, which he had called on the way up the stairs. They drove off to the north toward Lake Union, then around the lake and across the Aurora Bridge toward Ballard.

From the elevator, Bryan called Becky and, fortunately, she answered immediately. He asked, "Hey, Becky, did you know that Curtis is back in town?"

"Yes, I just heard from him a few minutes ago. He texted that he is on his way here."

"Really? Do you know why he's coming there?"

"Why he's coming?" Her intonation suggested that the question was out of place. "Well, he's my husband, and I haven't seen him in almost five months. Why *wouldn't* he be heading here?"

Bryan became speechless as the elevator door opened at his destination. He hung up the phone, placed it in his pocket, and walked down toward Thomas's door.

Becky hung up the phone and mumbled to herself, "That was a little weird."

She continued decorating the condo with balloons, a big "Welcome Home" sign, yellow ribbons everywhere, and a bottle of champagne sitting on the coffee table. She had to work in haste because Curtis's impromptu homecoming had caught her off guard. She had the things ready for the eventuality of his return but wasn't prepared for just a twenty-minute notice. She also had special lingerie, which she had bought for the occasion and to show off her own new body after losing a lot of weight. She had a large photo of the stone farmhouse, with its red trim and shutters, taped on the refrigerator. She felt so happy that this was the beginning, the very first day, of their brand-new life. She had never been more in love with Curtis, and the long absence only sealed that adoration.

Momentarily, a taxi pulled up in front of the house. She thought it was odd that no one drove him home and dropped him off, as was customary when he didn't have his car. She watched him get out of the taxi. She couldn't believe the transformation in his physique. She knew he would come back in better shape, but he looked just like the man she had married seven years earlier, except even younger and more fit. He was so handsome to her. She felt intimidated by his appearance. She had put herself on a diet and exercise program, working with a personal trainer, during his absence, yet didn't have

514

near the results that Curtis's program apparently had. She was hoping to surprise him with her new body, but now she had been outdone. To prop up her sudden feelings of insecurity, she reflected on his words in the restaurant in Ballard, that her size didn't matter to him.

She opened the front door and stared at him with a big smile. Her heart felt like it could literally burst with excitement. Curtis hadn't noticed her yet, or at least it didn't appear that way. He spoke to the taxi driver through his window. But the driver didn't leave. Curtis walked up the sidewalk and toward the door. He flashed a brief, superficial smile but then said, almost with a question mark on his face, "Becky?"

She put her arms around his neck and kissed him on the lips, "I'm so glad to have you home!" She noticed the kiss was cold and stiff, and her hug was not reciprocated.

He looked serious and pointed ahead. "Let's go inside."

She walked back inside, and Curtis followed her but seemed to be oblivious to the decorations and her work. She looked at him with a concerned smile. "Curtis are you alright?"

He spoke, "This won't take long. I'm here to serve you divorce papers. They're final, as of today, and all I need is your signature."

As soon as the word "divorce" came out of his mouth, Becky's great joy was instantly transmuted into an abrupt feeling of horror and insatiable bewilderment. Was he joking? What did those words mean? Within a second, the tears started to flow as if her subconscious understood before her conscious mind had finished processing the semantics. She tried to listen. She wanted to say something but found herself totally deprived of the ability to speak—even one word—as if her jaws were made of concrete. She couldn't even find air from which to form a single sigh.

"I should've done this a long time ago." Curtis continued, "You are nothing but a bitch that has been holding me back. You can have this damn stinky dump and my car… just keep your fat face the hell out of my life and my stuff. Sign these papers!"

By the time the last words got out of Curtis's mouth, Becky had fallen backward to sit but missed the overstuffed chair. She slid down the front of it and landed on the floor. Racer jumped off the back of the chair and ran toward the bedroom. The whole world was being pulled away from her, and things were growing dark, silent, and incoherent. She was the epicenter of an expanding universe, that was moving away from her in all directions, leaving her crouching in its vacuum. She could see Curtis's lips moving in slow motion, but her ears had closed out the insufferable utterances. She was sobbing and hyperventilating. Curtis stooped down on one knee beside her, making no attempt to console her or even to help her up. He placed a pen in her limp, right hand and laid a legal form on his thigh, making sure the signature line was on the flattest surface of his leg. She remained limp. "Sign it, bitch!" he yelled.

She could barely lift her arm. He impatiently grabbed her hand—the one holding the pen—forcing it to scribble her name on the blank line. He stood up and looked at the form, mumbling out loud, "I guess this'll have to do."

He pulled a manila envelope out of his jacket pocket and threw it in her direction. She made no attempt to catch it, and it landed on her hyperventilating chest. He walked toward the door... then suddenly stopping and turned. He looked back at her, still on the floor with the envelope laying as it had landed. He pointed at it. "I advise you to read that... it has all the details of our settlement." Her face was bright red, and tears were flowing down her cheeks. He turned to leave but then quickly turned back again and added, "You look pathetic. Cheer up... like I said, this entire dump is yours as are the cars... debt free. You should be happy."

Curtis went out the door, and she heard the taxi start. She tried to get up and stumbled forward and fell face down on the carpet. "Cur... Curt... Curtis!" She said in a whispered scream, the only words that could slip out of her tight throat. She was shaking and sobbing harder than she had ever before in her life. Suddenly realizing this could be the last time she would ever see the man, the only true love of her life, she tried to crawl to the door, where she pulled herself up. He was getting in the taxi.

Her weeping was totally out of control, and she could see nothing through the tears. She ran across the yard, losing her right Birkenstock in the dirt of her rhododendron row, and she fell again. The taxi had pulled away and into the neighbor's driveway, waiting for traffic to clear so it could back out and complete the turnaround. She could see Curtis looking at her with a facial expression of pity as he shook his head. She stood up and stumbled to her VW and got inside, only realizing then that the keys were in the house. The taxi passed by her condo again as she stepped out of the VW. The driver paused at the stop sign at the end of the block, waiting for a row of cars to pass. She stumbled up the driveway to the garage. She was going to take the Jeep, but then realized that she couldn't back around the VW. The taxi pulled away from the stop sign and continued down the street. In the corner of the garage was her blue, balloon-tired Schwinn. She threw the shoeless foot across the bike and turned to go down the driveway. The tears filled her eyes to the point she was blinded. She ran off the concrete onto the dirt and fell over. She got back on the bike again, wiping her tears with her hand, and took off down the driveway and turned into the street, going in the same direction as the taxi. Due to the small, congested street, the taxi was still in view, although fading. Finally, she could speak, "Curtis! Curtis!" she screamed in a strained voice, thinking, as if by magic, he could hear her. "Curtis... I found us a house! Its beautiful!" The tears were a torrent.

Bryan banged and banged on Thomas's door, but there was no answer. He attempted to call Jennifer, but she didn't answer, either. He frantically called Karla, one of the sharks, who was in the lab. "Hey, what's up?" she asked.

"Where's Jennifer?" he demanded.

"Uh, she's not here."

"Where the hell is she?" shouted Bryan.

"Cool down, Bryan. What's the matter? I don't know where she is. I mean, she left right after you and Curtis left."

"She's in danger and if she comes back, don't let her leave, not even with Curtis."

"Okay, but what's going on?"

"I'll explain later, but that man is an imposter."

Bryan stuck the phone in his pocket without hanging it up. He banged on Thomas's door one more time, and there was again no answer. "Damn you, Thomas, if you're in there… I know you're in on this! Coward!" Then he kicked the door with his foot as hard as he could, but it didn't come open.

Bryan marched down the hall toward the elevator. He called Jennifer's phone again. There was still no answer. He left a voicemail. "Jennifer don't go with him! Something's seriously wrong, and I don't know what it is yet, but give me the chance to find out!"

The elevator opened, and he stepped in. He didn't know what to do or where to go. He could get to his car… and then go where? Go to Jennifer's apartment? Go to Curtis's house? While driving, he could miss both. The doors opened on the 20th floor. A man in coveralls, carrying a large chuck of thick wood, was standing there wanting to get on.

Across the hall from the elevator was the conference room with its double doors wide open. Bryan pushed past the man and ran into the room and to the window. He looked down. From that vantage point, he could see the entrance, which led to the basement lab. By observing, he would know if anyone came or left the building. He called Becky again, and she didn't answer. "Damnit!" he screamed. He was startled by the abrupt and loud sound of an electric, circular saw coming from right behind him. Being startled, he turned and looked at another man in coveralls stooping in the floor over the upside-down table. "Do you have to make so much damn noise!" Bryan asked in an annoyed voice.

The man looked at him. "Hey, chief, Mr. Howell wanted this table out of here. We gotta saw it into pieces here to get it out of the door. I don't know how they got it in here."

Bryan looked around the room and there were chunks of wood scattered around the floor. "Why?"

"Why are we taking it out?" the carpenter asked in response.

"Yeah."

"Uh, he has a new table coming in. A real high-end piece." He paused to line up his saw from his next cut. When finished, he looked back up through his safety googles. "It's made from solid, exotic Pahudia wood. A gift from Thailand or something… I think." He made his next cut and another quarter of the table fell off. He dropped his ear protectors, so he could hear Bryan better and dusted sawdust off his pants. He stood up and looked at him and added, "I've heard it's hand-carved and worth about a half a million… and that's just for the table. So, we must get this piece of faux crap out of here, so they can move that one in."

Bryan turned and looked out the window again. Thailand? It seemed like Thailand was connected to everything. He felt like he was standing inside a snow globe filled with an agitated cloud of a thousand dots, dots that he just couldn't connect. But they were slowly starting to settle.

As Bryan continued looking out of the window, raindrops started to fall and glance off the glass. He was trying to decide if he should run to the lab. If he headed down the elevator, he was afraid that he would miss Jennifer. It was about that time he saw a cab pull up. Bryan pressed his face against the glass to see past the distortion made by the water drops. He watched carefully. Curtis, or whoever the hell he was, got out and handed the driver some money. It dawned on Bryan that Curtis was using his left hand to pay the man. That was odd. Then he recalled the contract signing in Thomas's office. He reconstructed the scene in his mind. Something looked strange to him then. He now realized that Curtis was also using his left hand to sign the contracts. Curtis was also drinking Jack Daniels. Curtis hated hard whisky, especially Jack Daniels. "What's going on?" Bryan kept asking himself. The dots were coalescing in some form that he still couldn't completely construe. He dialed Jennifer's number again, leaving yet another voicemail, "Hey, Nef, don't go with that man. It's not Curtis. Has the real Curtis ever called you 'Jennifer' before? He always calls you 'Nef.' I repeat, that man isn't Curtis. He's an imposter! Nef, hon, please listen to me!"

He was a flood of emotions. He felt a betrayal that Jennifer would even consider going with Curtis, or at least a man she thought was Curtis. Was he still her true love? But, most of all, he felt like he needed to protect her from something dreadful.

While holding his phone, he pulled up the conversation via texts that he had with Curtis while he was in Thailand. He looked at his first one, "I'm here and all is well." Then his next one, "Hey, Bryan, the first week has gone very well, and I'm enjoying it here." Then, two weeks later, came the text asking Bryan to check the Sand-dude web site. Then the next week check in, where he said, "Bryan, things are great here, don't worry." But then strangely at his sixth week check in, and each week after that, the texts sometimes addressed him as "Brian." Curtis had never spelled his name with an "i" before. Was it a voice recognition that spelled it that way? Did the satellite device even have voice recognition? Curt always texted with his thumbs.

"If he's an imposter, how did he have the identical abdominal wall scar as Curtis? The exact same scar that had a J-shape at the bottom?

Bryan put his face against the glass again as the rain came down harder. The dots inside his mental snow globe were now forming a picture right before his eyes. He began to weep and mumble out loud, "Oh, God no! God, please don't let it be." Chills ran down his body. With his face still pressed against the window, there were soon tears running down the inside of the glass, acting as comrades to the rain on the outside. He slid down and sat on the floor.

Momentarily, Jennifer's green Prius pulled up in front of the building. Bryan jumped back up in a jolt to a standing position. The Curtis imposter came running out of the building and jumped into her car.

Bryan lifted his head to watch. They pulled away from the building and turned down E. Madison Street, heading toward the waterfront. Bryan dropped to the floor again and turned away, resting his back to the glass, looking back at the carpenters still working. Through his tears, he picked up his phone and called Jennifer one more time, but in a subdued voice, "Jen, hon, listen to me! It wasn't Mack who died... it was Curtis. He was murdered. Nef, please, for God's sake, pick up. Nef, call me back!"

He thought of calling the police... and telling them what? If he tried to tell them the real story, they would think he was a lunatic. Plus, there were a lot of details he didn't know yet. Any investigation would be drawn out for weeks or months and the Curtis impostor would be long gone, sailing off the map.

Breaking into a full sob, Bryan lay face-down on the floor and began speaking to the blue, Berber carpet. "You were the greatest man I've ever known, and you didn't even see it. What the hell have they done to you?" He couldn't do anything but cry. He felt himself giving up on a hopeless cause.

Bryan didn't notice, but the carpenter walked over and stood directly over him. He reached down and put a hand on his shoulder, "Hey, pal. Are you okay?"

"No," he said as the man in white coveralls helped him back to his feet. Bryan looked out the window again. He could now see the harbor better as the rain had washed out some of the fog that had been hanging over the city the entire morning. What looked like Mack's yacht was moored off the docks. Only the dock used for cruise ships was large enough to accommodate the huge boat. Bryan staggered toward the door and tripped over a piece of thick pressboard from the old table. He looked at the wood for a moment, then kicked it aside. He went into the hall and ran up three flights of stairs back to Thomas's office. He kicked as hard as he could to knock the door down, with no effect. He ran back down to the conference room and back to the window. He looked out, and the big yacht was just leaving its berth. Bryan banged on the glass wall with both fists and screamed at the top of his lungs, "Bastards! Sons of bitches! You don't know what you've done!" Bryan watched for thirty minutes as the big boat disappeared into the impenetrable fog of Puget Sound.

Bryan sat in a space of despondency for at least a half an hour. He stood and looked out. With the storm now waning, the big-tinted window was left with thousands of tiny raindrops clinging delicately to the outside. The shy sun was now divulging a taste of glory as bright rays were breaking through, here and there. The refractive nature of the glass, the water drops, and the air seemed to distort, then to clarify, the immediate world outside. For the first time, Bryan clearly saw the parallelograms and rhomboids in the street layout, which only Curtis had seen before. All the street corners were skewed, running parallel with the geographical ridges, which— in turn—were aligned with the mountains and the sea. There was an external reference point, giving meaning to everything. Only Curtis saw the real meaning and everyone else was lost in the illusion of the immediate, the greed, and the ordinary.

The carpenters were finishing setting up the new table. The Pahudia wood had tight grains, mostly golden with a few ebony streaks. It was delicate and beautiful with engravings of vines, frogs, snakes, birds, and turtles all around the sides. But the table was a real rectangle. The carpenters stepped back and were looking at it and muttering between themselves about how it didn't fit the room... despite its glory. Between themselves, they expressed bafflement, not understanding why it seemed so out of place. Bryan knew why. He looked back toward the window and mumbled, "I'll find you, Jen. I'll save you, I promise."

Becky pedaled harder than she ever had before. She was screaming for the sake of her own ears, "Becky, you fool! You fool! You stupid woman... you lost him!" Due to the series of red lights at cross streets, she was gaining on the taxi at times, only to see it pull away when it had an unhindered route. When the taxi turned right, onto Aurora Avenue, it became a hopeless chase. Yet she continued along the busy highway toward Seattle.

Becky was never seen again. Her bike was found leaning against the rusty-white rail of the pedestrian lane, at the middle of the Aurora Bridge. Her left Birkenstock laid on the asphalt; dirty, mashed, and torn, having encountered countless car tires. She had pedaled over six miles from her condo. Evidently, her acrophobia was not enough to thwart her heart's dismay.

They say that when you fall from the 167-foot structure, the impact of the dense, cold water eviscerates the body. It then quickly fills with the brackish mix, causing a loss of buoyancy. At the bottom of the canal, it meets the outflows from the lakes and follows the release of water from the locks. There it is swept out into Puget Sound. The remains are eventually carried away out to the Pacific by the ensuing tides. In the big waters, the remaining pieces become sustenance to the little blue fish… which swim in the sea.

Mount Erie Press would like to thank you for purchasing *Waters of Bimini*. We are a small independent press, striving to showcase new writers who have something important to say and can say it in a fascinating way. If you found this book worth your read, please encourage your friends and associates, either by personal contact or social media, to purchase their own copy.

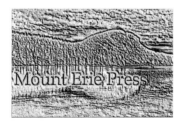

CPSIA information can be obtained
at www.ICGtesting.com
Printed in the USA
LVHW02s0035300818
588620LV00004B/67/P